# Methods in Molecular Biology™



For further volumes:
http://www.springer.com/series/7651

# Antibody Methods and Protocols

Edited by

**Gabriele Proetzel**

*The Jackson Laboratory, Bar Harbor, ME, USA*

**Hilmar Ebersbach**

*NIBR Biologics Center, Novartis Institutes for BioMedical Research, Basel, Switzerland*

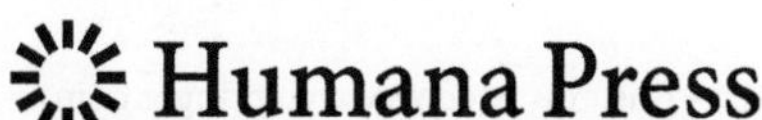

*Editors*
Gabriele Proetzel
The Jackson Laboratory
Bar Harbor, ME, USA

Hilmar Ebersbach
NIBR Biologics Center
Novartis Institutes for BioMedical Research
Basel, Switzerland

ISSN 1064-3745 ISSN 1940-6029 (electronic)
ISBN 978-1-61779-930-3 ISBN 978-1-61779-931-0 (eBook)
DOI 10.1007/978-1-61779-931-0
Springer New York Dordrecht Heidelberg London

Library of Congress Control Number: 2012938221



*Cover illustration*: Artwork provided by Michael V. Wiles, PhD.

Printed on acid-free paper

Humana Press is part of Springer Science+Business Media (www.springer.com)

# Preface

Antibodies play such a central role in research and development due to their high versatility and universal applicability that research without them would be inconceivable. Their use ranges from protein localization, cell separation, and screening to functional assays being applied in many formats including high-throughput assays. With the breakthrough in the generation of monoclonal antibodies, the practical potential of antibodies due to their almost-designer specificities was immediately recognized, especially regarding their applications in diagnostics and therapeutics. However, surprisingly it still took until the 1990s for antibodies to begin to make a substantial impact in drug development and to be applied as effective therapeutics. The industry has since grown into a multibillion-dollar market, and 34 therapeutic antibodies have been FDA approved, most of them still being on the market in 2012. Additionally, literally hundreds of antibodies are now in the development pipeline. These are being generated by a variety of platforms incorporating many technical enhancements, such as improved half-life and effector functions. This rapidly growing field is the result of many advancing technologies allowing current developments to take advantage of molecular engineering to create tailor-made antibodies. New antibody formats and scaffolds are being explored, exemplified by bispecifics and antibody drug conjugates.

This volume, *Antibody Methods and Protocols*, attempts to provide insight into the generation of antibodies using in vitro and in vivo approaches, as well as technical aspects for screening, analysis, and modification of antibodies and antibody fragments. Even though this volume covers subjects as diverse as classical methods, such as hybridoma technology and phage display, to the more recent developments including Fc engineering, it is still beyond the scope of any single volume to present the multitude of techniques now available for antibody isolation, screening, and modification. Instead, we have focused on basic protocols for isolating antibodies and, at the same time, selected a range of specific areas with the aim of providing guides for the overall process of antibody isolation and characterization as well as protocols for enhancing classical antibodies and antibody fragments. The antibody process begins with antigen generation and presentation; this is discussed in the first chapter. An overview of in vitro approaches is presented in the chapters by Ron Geyer, Dev Sidhu, Konstantin Petropoulos, Christoph Rader, Georg Thom, and Elisabetta Traggiai. These cover phage display, ribosome display, as well the use of human B cells for antibody isolation. Chapters by E-Chiang Lee, Michel Cogné, and Chonghui Zhang discuss the usefulness of mice in the development of antibodies, in particular genetically engineered mice to develop human and humanized antibodies directly in the mouse. We touch upon biophysical and biochemical characterization, affinity measurements by surface plasmon resonance, and glycosylation analysis with chapters by Michael Schräml and Christiane Jäger. Further, we have included a description of antibody fragments, cloning approaches, and modification by pegylation presented in chapters by Christoph Rader and Simona Jevševar. More recent developments in the field of antibody engineering addressing half-life extension, effector function modulation, and the rising field of bispecific antibodies, as well as approaches for antibody decoration including antibody drug conjugates, are covered in chapters by Ulrich Brinkmann, Gloria Meng, and Michel Cogné. While we cannot address all the new and exciting developments in this fast-developing field, we believe that this volume provides a broad and useful background to support ongoing efforts and encourages the development of new imaginative approaches.

The assembly of this volume would not have happened without the commitment of all contributors, their discussions and rapid responses, making this a valuable and relevant contribution to antibody methods and protocols. We are also grateful to Dr. Michael V. Wiles for his help in editing of this volume and providing many dinners.

We like to thank Dr. John Walker for the opportunity to assemble this work and his encouragement and help throughout the process. We wish to thank also the team from Humana Press, especially David Casey, for continuous support.

We hope that this volume will provide useful insights for both experts and novices and that it will stimulate further development of antibody approaches and encourage the community to continuously share ideas and protocols.

***Bar Harbor, ME, USA*** — ***Gabriele Proetzel***
***Basel, Switzerland*** — ***Hilmar Ebersbach***

# Contents

## Contributors

MATTHIAS BIEHL • *Roche Diagnostics GmbH, Penzberg, Germany*
ANDREW R.M. BRADBURY • *Los Alamos National Laboratory, Los Alamos, NM, USA*
ULRICH BRINKMANN • *Large Molecule Research, Roche Pharma Research and Early Development, Penzberg, Germany*
MICHEL COGNÉ • *CNRS UMR6101, Contrôle des Réponses Immunes B et Lymphoproliférations, Université de Limoges, Limoges, France*
STEFAN DÜBEL • *Technische Universität Braunschweig, Braunschweig, Germany*
HILMAR EBERSBACH • *NIBR Biologics Center, Novartis Institutes for BioMedical Research, Basel, Switzerland*
CLAUDIA FERRARA • *pRED, Pharma Research and Early Development, Roche Glycart AG, Schlieren, Switzerland*
C. RONALD GEYER • *University of Saskatchewan, Saskatoon, SK, Canada*
MICHAEL GROTE • *Large Molecule Research, Roche Pharma Research and Early Development, Penzberg, Germany*
MARIA GROVES • *MedImmune Ltd, Cambridge, UK*
ALEXANDER K. HAAS • *Large Molecule Research, Roche Pharma Research and Early Development, Penzberg, Germany*
CHRISTIANE JÄGER • *pRED, Pharma Research and Early Development, Roche Glycart AG, Schlieren, Switzerland*
SIMONA JEVŠEVAR • *Sandoz Biopharmaceuticals, Mengeš, Lek Pharmaceuticals d.d, Mengeš, Slovenia*
ROBERT F. KELLEY • *Antibody Engineering, Genentech Inc, South San Francisco, CA, USA*
MAJA KENIG • *Sandoz Biopharmaceuticals, Mengeš, Lek Pharmaceuticals d.d, Mengeš, Slovenia*
CHRISTIAN KLEIN • *Large Molecule Research, Roche Pharma Research and Early Development, Schlieren, Switzerland*
HANS KOLL • *pRED, Pharma Research and Early Development, Roche Diagnostics GmbH, Penzberg, Germany*
MATEJA KUSTERLE • *Sandoz Biopharmaceuticals, Mengeš, Lek Pharmaceuticals d.d, Mengeš, Slovenia*
BRICE LAFFLEUR • *CNRS UMR6101, Contrôle des Réponses Immunes B et Lymphoproliférations, Université de Limoges, Limoges, France*
E-CHIANG LEE • *Kymab Ltd, Meditrina, Cambridge, UK*
KLAUS MAYER • *Large Molecule Research, Roche Pharma Research and Early Development, Penzberg, Germany*
JOHN MCCAFFERTY • *University of Cambridge, Cambridge, UK*

Y. GLORIA MENG • *Biochemical and Cellular Pharmacology, Genentech Inc, South San Francisco, CA, USA*
MICHAEL OWEN • *Kymab Ltd, Meditrina, Cambridge, UK*
VIRGINIE PASCAL • *CNRS UMR6101, Contrôle des Réponses Immunes B et Lymphoproliférations, Université de Limoges, Limoges, France*
KONSTANTIN PETROPOULOS • *MorphoSys AG, Martinsried/Planegg, Germany*
GABRIELE PROETZEL • *The Jackson Laboratory, Bar Harbor, ME, USA*
LEOPOLD VON PROFF • *Roche Diagnostics GmbH, Penzberg, Germany*
CHRISTOPH RADER • *Experimental Transplantation and Immunology Branch, Center for Cancer Research, National Cancer Institute, National Institutes of Health, Bethesda, MD, USA; Department of Cancer Biology and Department of Molecular Therapeutics, The Scripps Research Institute, Scripps Florida Jupiter, FL, USA*
JÖRG THOMAS REGULA • *pRED, Pharma Research and Early Development, Roche Diagnostics GmbH, Penzberg, Germany*
WOLFGANG SCHAEFER • *Large Molecule Research, Roche Pharma Research and Early Development, Penzberg, Germany*
MICHAEL SCHRÄML • *Roche Diagnostics GmbH, Penzberg, Germany*
SACHDEV S. SIDHU • *University of Toronto, Toronto, ON, Canada*
CHRISTOPHE SIRAC • *CNRS UMR6101, Contrôle des Réponses Immunes B et Lymphoproliférations, Université de Limoges, Limoges, France*
GEORGE THOM • *MedImmune Ltd, Cambridge, UK*
ELISABETTA TRAGGIAI • *Translational Science, Novartis Institute for Biomedical Research, Basel, Switzerland*
PABLO UMAÑA • *pRED, Pharma Research and Early Development, Roche Glycart AG, Schlieren, Switzerland*
JIAHUI YANG • *Experimental Transplantation and Immunology Branch, Center for Cancer Research, National Cancer Institute, National Institutes of Health, Bethesda, MD, USA*
ANNE ZECK • *NMI, Naturwissenschaftliches und Medizinisches Institut, Universität Tübingen, Reutlingen, Germany*
CHONGHUI ZHANG • *NIBR Biologics Center, Novartis Institutes for BioMedical Research, Cambridge, MA, Switzerland*

# Chapter 1

# Antigen Presentation for the Generation of Binding Molecules


## Hilmar Ebersbach, Gabriele Proetzel, and Chonghui Zhang



## Abstract

In the last few decades, several new methods have been established to isolate full antibodies and fragments thereof, some even using alternative scaffolds from in vivo and in vitro sources. These methods encompass robust techniques including immunization and hybridoma technology or phage display and also more laborious and novel approaches including ribosome display or B-cell immortalization. All methodologies are dependent upon proper antigen presentation for isolation, screening, and further characterization of the selected binding molecules. Here, antigens are classes of molecules including soluble or membrane proteins, part or domains thereof (extracellular domains of GPCRs), peptides, carbohydrates, and small-molecular-weight moieties. Presentation of the antigen in a functional state or perhaps even mimicking the intended application is crucial for successful isolation of useful binding molecules. Moreover, it is also necessary to consider the expression host and any posttranslational modifications of target proteins. The increasing demand to target more complex antigens, for instance, receptors and ion channels, is leading to the development of alternative procedures to present these proteins appropriately, for example by the use of virus-like particles and DNA immunization. This chapter describes in general approaches for the preparation of different forms of immunogens including synthetic peptides, proteins, cell-based antigens for immunization and in vitro display systems and in detail the preparation of a soluble protein as antigen.



**Key words:** Adjuvant, Antigen presentation, DNA, Hybridoma, Immunogen, Immunization, In vitro display, Monoclonal antibody, Peptide, Protein, Protein expression, Transformation


## 1. Introduction

Fundamental to antibody or binding molecule isolation is the antigen preparation and presentation. A main principle of immunization is the presentation of the antigen to the immune host in a format that elicits the strongest and at the same time, the most specific immune response. Therefore, the quality, integrity, and folding state of an antigen are crucial parameters for successful antibody generation. The antigen characteristics need to mimic as closely as possible its


Gabriele Proetzel and Hilmar Ebersbach (eds.), *Antibody Methods and Protocols*, Methods in Molecular Biology, vol. 901, DOI 10.1007/978-1-61779-931-0_1, © Springer Science+Business Media, LLC 2012

condition in the later application. If this is done correctly, this will dramatically increase the value and applicability of the isolated antibodies. This chapter describes approaches for the preparation of different forms of immunogens, including synthetic peptides, proteins, and cell-based antigens for immunization and in vitro display systems.

The use of peptides as immunogens for hybridoma generation is fast and straightforward. Peptides can be used as surrogates for protein domains or even complete proteins. This is especially useful when the required amount of functional antigen is difficult to produce by protein expression or other means. Cell surface receptors are of high interest currently representing a class of immunogens for which peptide antigens have been successfully used in immunization or phage display (1, 2). However, immunization with peptide antigens derived of cell surface targets may pose special challenges. This type of immunization depends not only on how well an appropriate immunogenic peptide sequence is selected from the target protein, but also on whether the anti-peptide mAbs generated by this approach subsequently recognize the native antigen on the cell surface. The successful generation of mAbs to peptide antigens usually requires coupling of the peptide to a carrier protein, for example, keyhole limpet hemocyanin (KLH) or bovine serum albumin (BSA) (see Note 1).

In vitro display systems require also the use of carrier proteins due to the small size of peptide antigens. The coating of the plastic surface of microtiter plates with unconjugated peptides will render them masked and inaccessible, during the blocking of free binding sites of the plastic surface with BSA or milk.

Peptide antigens can also be biotinylated either at the C or N terminus or via endogenous lysines. This allows for the addition of antigen to displayed binding molecules and facilitates capture of the full binding complex via streptavidin or NeutrAvidin, following a standard panning cycle (3, 4).

Soluble proteins can be either complete proteins, for example, cytokines, or protein domains thereof, or soluble expressible extracellular domains of receptors, for example, GPCRs. Overall, the methodologies applied are similar to those used for peptide antigens. It is however, important that proteins used are homogenous, properly folded and presented such that the critical epitopes are accessible. Protein oxidation, aggregation, and degradation are known issues which can affect the outcome of antibody generation severely. Therefore, there is a need to carefully monitor, for example, by mass spectroscopy or functional assays the quality of the antigen. In case of recombinant protein preparation, posttranslational modification such as deamidation may be critical to the successful isolation of antibodies and needs to be appreciated (5, 6). For example, abnormal glycosylation could lead to the obscuring of an epitope as known for hyperglycosylation in yeast (7). In the case of *E. coli* derived antigens which lack glycosylation, antibodies may be generated against epitopes that are not accessible in the mammalian system and hence of little value (8). For antigen presentation by means of in vitro display applications, proteins can be directly coated on to plastic surfaces, or immobilized to the plastic via biotin and streptavidin or NeutrAvidin. In case of immunization, peptide or protein antigens are usually formulated with an adjuvant. The use of an adjuvant, such as Freund's adjuvant, not only lowers the amount of antigen required but also prolongs the antigen stimulation of the immune host. Even though in recent years there is a growing number of new adjuvant reagents available, Freund's adjuvant has remained the first choice for working with antigens that have poor immunogenicity in the immune host (9–11). Freund's adjuvant contains heat-inactivated bacterial elements, which enhances the immune response by directly stimulating the activity of antigen-presenting cells; however, it also elicits a local inflammatory reaction that may cause a necrotic appearance at the site of injection in the animal. To minimize or eliminate this side effect of Freund's adjuvant, it is necessary to utilize a minimal dose of the antigen and complete Freund's adjuvant mixture in the first injection and subsequent injections (see Notes 2, 3 and 4).

Instead of defined polypeptides, whole cells can be used for immunization and in vitro display. This is of special use for the identification and characterization of novel cell surface biomarkers, where normal or cancerous human cells are potent immunogens for the generation of mAbs (12–14). In contrast to soluble antigens such as proteins and peptides, whole cells are a particular type of antigen presenting vehicle. They are also considerably more immunogenic and result in the production of a stronger immune response in animals. For cell-based immunization, cells can be collected from tissue culture or isolated from tissue samples. For tissue culture derived material, it is necessary that they are washed thoroughly to eliminate any unwanted antigenic proteins from the culture medium (see Note 5).

In vitro display systems often use human cells or peripheral blood mononuclear cells (PBMC) as antigen source. Besides a high level of endogenous expressed target all other surface expressed proteins are potential antigens as well. Here, one needs to choose a cell type that overexpresses a large amount of the antigen in question and in addition it is necessary to have low endogenous level or no antigen expressing cell line for counter selection. Overall extensive screening is required to be successful in isolating highly specific binding molecules (15, 16). But often endogenous expressed antigens are the only valuable source due to their presence and functionality in complexes with other proteins.

Another strategy makes use of transfected cells or cell lines, which helps to overcome the difficulty of purifying cell membrane-bound proteins for use as immunogens and the inefficiency of screening for mAbs that recognize the native antigens. In contrast to human cells or PBMC these are recombinantly expressed target

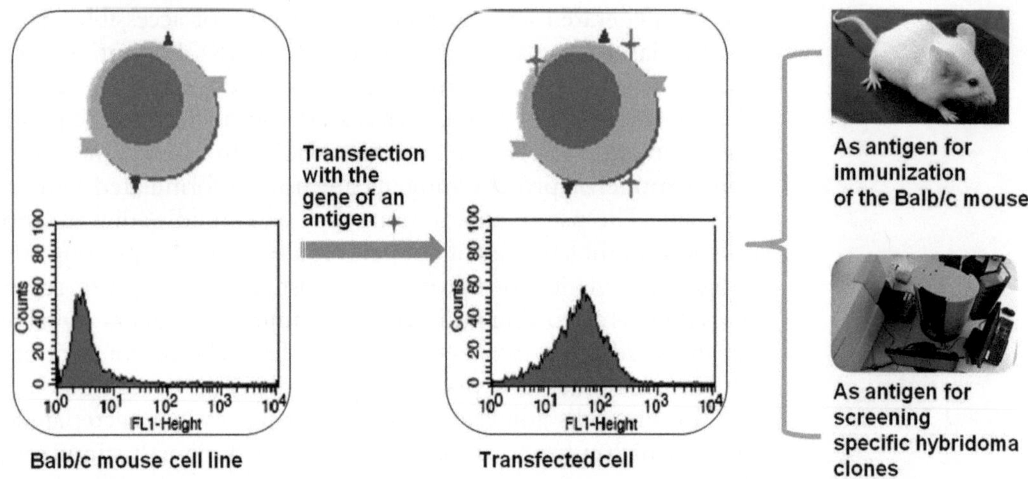


Fig. 1. Transfected cells as antigen for immunization and for the subsequent mAb screening. A human target antigen is overexpressed on the surface of a mouse cell line derived from the BALB/c strain. The stably transfected cells are used as an antigen for immunizing BALB/c mice and for the differential screening of hybridoma supernatants of the transfected versus nontransfected cells by flow cytometry. Example expression profiles of antigen on transfected and nontransfected cells are shown.

proteins which have to be proven for their functionality in chosen cell line. To maximize the specific antibody response in the mouse, human target antigens are cloned into and overexpressed on the surface of mouse cell lines derived from a strain syngeneic to the immunization host strain, e.g., BALB/c mice. The stably transfected cells are used for immunizing the syngeneic mouse strain and for the subsequent screening of hybridoma clones derived from cell fusions while the non transfected cell serves as the negative control (Fig. 1). In comparison to using human cells, transfected murine cells will typically have a significantly reduced background response when using the syngeneic inbred mouse strain, as the cells are genetically identical to the mouse strain apart for the transfected and expressed target molecule. The key benefits of the transfected cell-based immunization strategy are (1) dramatic improvement in the immune response of animals to cell surface antigens, (2) significant increase in the yield of mAbs that identify the native form of antigens expressed by the cells, and (3) obviation of lengthy protocols for the purification of membrane-bound proteins. In addition, it is also possible to use cell-based immunization to generate mAbs against the secreted forms of antigens by tethering the secreted proteins, such as serum proteins and cytokines, to the cell surface as antigens for immunization.

The technical platform which has been established for cell-based immunization enables effective generation of high-quality mAbs to cell surface targets. The procedure for immunizing mice with stably transfected cells is similar to that used for human and other cell lines. Another advantage of this approach, which is also reflected by increasing use of such cell lines in phage display, is the ease of generation of a counter selection cell line in exactly identical genetic background. Parental cell lines without any expression of desired antigen are used for isolation of highly specific antibodies, as described above.

Another option for antigen immunogen presentation is the use of virus-like particles (VLPs). This has been shown to be especially effective for cell receptor or ion channel antigens. A number of different approaches exist; however, they all follow the same principle of co-overexpressing the antigen with a virus coat protein for encapsulation of the antigen into a so-called VLP. The main benefit of this approach over transfected cells is a higher expression or concentration of the antigen combined with a better defined surface, i.e., less presentation of irrelevant proteins from the parental cell line. It is also very easy to produce "null" particles in an identical parental cell line which do not express the target antigen allowing for counter selection (17, 18).

A strategy for dealing with difficult to express antigens is to use a DNA immunization approach. This method exploits the flexibility and ease of working with DNA, allowing the generation of many different DNA constructs encoding peptides, protein domains or full proteins. DNA can also be delivered by many different means, including injection (hypodermic needle), gene gun using DNA-coated gold beads, pneumatic injection, and lipid formulations (19) become routine when immunizing rodents in the laboratory.

A further specialized technique uses in vivo phage display, where antibody libraries are injected into animals. The phage enriched to bind to the target is then recovered by isolation of cells or even tissues of interest, for example, to specific cancer cell targets (20).

Other more specialized techniques to address identification of novel biomarkers or to adapt the screening to optimize the intended purpose of the binding protein are not addressed here as they are beyond the scope of this chapter. All the above-described techniques should be properly considered in advance of any antibody generation campaign to aim for a highly valuable binding molecule.

## 2. Materials

### *2.1. Transformation of DNA*

1. Vector for periplasmatic expression in *E. coli*: pet20b(+) (Novagen, Merck KGaA, Darmstadt, Germany) (Fig. 2) (see Note 6).
2. Competent Cells: BL21 (DE3) chemical competent cells (Invitrogen, Life Technologies).
3. Purified DNA (DNA plasmid purification kit; Qiagen, Hilden, Germany) of the construct that includes a $His_6$-Tag (see Note 7).

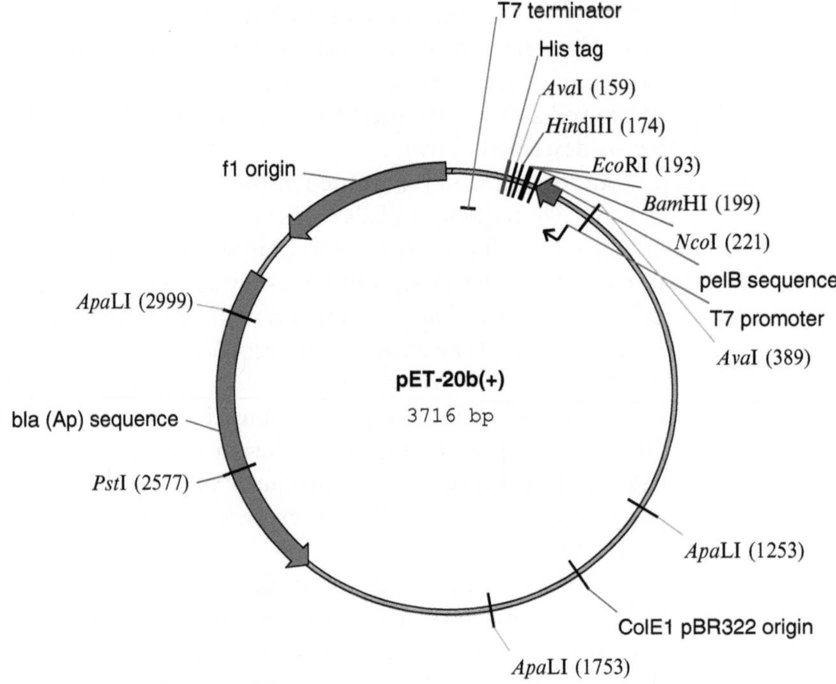


Fig. 2. Plasmid DNA map of expression vector pET20-20b(+). The pET-20b(+) vector includes an N-terminal pelB signal sequence for potential periplasmic localization and an optional C-terminal His·Tag sequence. Image generated by use of Vector NTI Advance 11 (Invitrogen, Life Technologies, Carlsbad, USA).

4. 2× YT or SOC medium.
5. 2× YT/ampicillin (100 μg/mL)/0.1% glucose, 1.5% agar as selection plates.

### 2.2. Protein Expression

1. 2× YT/Amp/Glu medium: 2× YT, 100 μg/mL ampicillin, 0.1% glucose.
2. 1 M IPTG in double distilled (dd) water (BioSolve, Lexington, MA, USA).

### 2.3. Whole Bacteria Cell Lysis

1. 0.1% Lysozyme (Roche, Indianapolis, IN, USA).
2. Benzonase (Merck KGaA, Darmstadt, Germany).
3. Complete EDTA-free protease inhibitor cocktail tablets (cat. no. 11873580001, Roche).
4. Lysis Buffer: 25 mM Tris pH 8.0, 0.5 M NaCl, 0.1% lysozyme, 2 mM $MgCl_2$, 10 U/mL benzonase, one tablet complete EDTA-free protease inhibitor cocktail in a total volume of 50 mL.
5. Syringe filter (low protein binding): 0.2 μm, inherently hydrophilic polyethersulfone membrane, Serum Acrodisc (Pall Corporation, Port Washington, NY, USA).

#### 2.4. Protein Purification

1. Aekta Express (GE Healthcare, UK).
2. IMAC column: HiTrap 1 mL chelating HP (GE Healthcare).
3. IMAC-A buffer: 20 mM Na-Phosphate buffer pH 7.4, 500 mM NaCl, 20 mM imidazole.
4. IMAC-B buffer: 20 mM Na-Phosphate buffer pH 7.4, 500 mM NaCl, and 300 mM imidazole.
5. Gel filtration column (SEC): HiLoad 16/60 Superdex 75 (GE Healthcare).
6. SEC buffer: 1× PBS, pH 7.2.
7. 96-Well, 1.2 ml deep well plate, polypropylene (Greiner, Frickenhausen, Germany).

## 3. Methods

#### 3.1. Transformation of DNA

1. Use 20 μL BL21 (DE3) chemical competent cells per transformation.
2. Add 1.5 μL of a 10 ng/μL dilution of vector DNA, purified via DNA plasmid purification kit.
3. Incubate for 30 min on ice.
4. Incubate for 45 s at 42°C.
5. Incubate for 2 min on ice.
6. Add 100 μL 2× YT or SOC medium.
7. Incubate for 1.5 h at 37°C by 220 rpm shaking.
8. Plate each sample on a small agar selection plates.
9. Incubate at 37°C overnight (O/N).

#### 3.2. Protein Expression (500 mL)

1. Inoculate a preculture of 10 mL 2× YT/Amp/Glu, using a single colony from the transformation plate and incubate for 3 h at 30°C.
2. Transfer the preculture to 500 mL culture in 2× YT/Amp/Glu in a 5-L flask (ratio volume 1:10), nonbaffled, cotton stopper.
3. Incubate until $OD_{600nm}$ reaches 0.5 at 30°C. (This takes about 3–4 h.)
4. For induction of expression add IPTG to a final concentration of 0.75 mM (375 μL of 1 M solution).
5. Express protein at 30°C O/N shaking at 220 rpm shaking.
6. Pellet bacteria at 5,000 × *g* for 30 min at 4°C.
7. Freeze pellet at –20°C.

### 3.3. Whole Bacteria Cell Lysis

1. Resuspend bacterial pellet in 25 mL lysis buffer by pipetting up and down.
2. Transfer suspension to centrifuge tubes and incubate for 45 min at RT on a shaker.
3. Centrifuge to remove bacterial debris for 30 min at 16,000 × *g* at 4°C.
4. Filter supernatant through a 0.2-μm filter.

### 3.4. Protein Purification

This is a two-step purification using AektaExpress with an IMAC column and gel filtration.

1. The IMAC purification of protein antigen with His6-Tag is most easily done with Aekta Express, which allows fully automated purification at room temperature (20°C).
2. Equilibrate IMAC column with ten column volumes (CV) IMAC-A buffer.
3. Load filtered samples on the IMAC column at 1 mL/min flow rate.
4. Wash the IMAC-bound sample with 20 CV IMAC-A buffer to remove unbound material at 1 mL/min flow rate.
5. Elute samples with five CV IMAC-B buffer at 1 mL/min in Aekta Express sample collection loop.
6. Directly apply eluted fraction on gel filtration column (equilibrated in SEC buffer).
7. Run gel filtration column with SEC buffer at 0.8 mL/min.
8. Elute purified protein into a 96-well deep well plate.
9. Pool elution fractions at expected size (in comparison to protein standard run under identical conditions).
10. Determine the protein concentration by OD measurement at 280 nm.
11. Check integrity and quality of protein preparation by mass spectroscopy.

## 4. Notes

1. The choice of animal species for the immune host in hybridoma generation depends largely on the origin of the immunogen available and on the downstream application of mAbs to be generated. Several animal species can be immunized for hybridoma generation. Most commonly used are mice, rats, rabbits, and sheep. For practical reasons rodents represent a good choice for routine mAb generation due to the ease of

rodent handling, the smaller amount of antigen required, and the wide availability of good fusion partners.

2. The choice of an efficient adjuvant for antigen preparation can be difficult, but the decision can be made by evaluating its potency and the side-effects it may mediate in animals. Despite a number of new synthetic adjuvants available for human vaccinations, Freund's adjuvant has remained the most commonly used adjuvant for immunization of laboratory animals due to its effectiveness and low cost.

3. In the routine immunization protocol, a mouse is injected subcutaneously or intraperitoneally with 50 μL of protein or peptide antigen mixed with an equal volume of Freund's adjuvant every other week. After 3–4 boosts with the antigen–adjuvant mixture, the immunized mice are euthanized and the spleen is collected for cell fusion.

4. The standard immunization protocol in which animals are boosted with an antigen at regular intervals often yields higher titers and a better quality of antibodies; however, the development of a repetitive multiple site immunization strategy (RIMMS) enables us to expedite the generation of mAbs (21). In addition, genetic immunization, by which the gene encoding a protein antigen is directly introduced into the immune host, has offered a unique method for hybridoma generation with no requirements for antigen purification and adjuvant administration (22, 23).

5. Mice are immunized subcutaneously or intraperitoneally with approximately $5 \times 10^6$ cells in 100–200 μL of PBS per mouse. The multiple injections are performed every 2 weeks for standard immunizations or twice a week in a quick immunization protocol. After 8–10 weeks for the standard immunization or 2–3 weeks for the quick immunization protocol, mice are sacrificed and spleens are prepared for cell fusion.

6. Proteins can be recombinantly expressed in *E. coli* in cytosolic or via a specific transport mechanism in periplasmatic space. For soluble and functional expression of disulfide bridged proteins an export in periplasm via specific signal sequences (e.g., pelB) is preferred. Prokaryotic organisms keep their cytoplasm reduced and, consequently, disulfide bond formation is impaired in this subcellular compartment. In contrast, bacteria periplasm is oxidizing and contains certain enzymatic activities to produce properly folded disulfide-bonded proteins (24).

7. Polyhistidine-tags are a very common and easy to use system for affinity purification of recombinant proteins expressed in *E. coli* and usually results in relatively pure protein sample (25). Affinity media contain bound metal ions, either nickel or cobalt to which the polyhistidine-tag binds with micromolar affinity.

High concentrations of imidazole or EDTA in elution fraction of samples can be removed by subsequent application of a size-exclusion chromatography.

## References


1. Axelsen TV, Holm A, Christiansen G et al (2011) Identification of the shortest Abeta-peptide generating highly specific antibodies against the C-terminal end of amyloid-beta42. Vaccine 29:3260–3269
2. Huang L, Sato AK, Sachdeva M et al (2005) Discovery of human antibodies against the C5aR target using phage display technology. J Mol Recognit 18:327–333
3. Zahnd C, Sarkar CA, Pluckthun A (2010) Computational analysis of off-rate selection experiments to optimize affinity maturation by directed evolution. Protein Eng Des Sel 23:175–184
4. Derda R, Tang SK, Li SC et al (2011) Diversity of phage-displayed libraries of peptides during panning and amplification. Molecules 16: 1776–1803
5. Srebalus Barnes CA, Lim A (2007) Applications of mass spectrometry for the structural characterization of recombinant protein pharmaceuticals. Mass Spectrom Rev 26:370–388
6. Jenkins N, Murphy L, Tyther R (2008) Post-translational modifications of recombinant proteins: significance for biopharmaceuticals. Mol Biotechnol 39:113–118
7. Singh MB, Bhalla PL (2006) Recombinant expression systems for allergen vaccines. Inflamm Allergy Drug Targets 5:53–59
8. Konthur Z, Hust M, Dubel S (2005) Perspectives for systematic in vitro antibody generation. Gene 364:19–29
9. Sanchez Y, Ionescu-Matiu I, Dreesman GR et al (1980) Humoral and cellular immunity to hepatitis B virus-derived antigens: comparative activity of Freund complete adjuvant alum, and liposomes. Infect Immun 30:728–733
10. Billiau A, Matthys P (2001) Modes of action of Freund's adjuvants in experimental models of autoimmune diseases. J Leukoc Biol 70:849–860
11. Odunsi K, Qian F, Matsuzaki J et al (2007) Vaccination with an NY-ESO-1 peptide of HLA class I/II specificities induces integrated humoral and T cell responses in ovarian cancer. Proc Natl Acad Sci USA 104:12837–12842
12. Kung P, Goldstein G, Reinherz EL et al (1979) Monoclonal antibodies defining distinctive human T cell surface antigens. Science 206:347–349
13. Zhang C, Xu Y, Gu J et al (1998) A cell surface receptor defined by a mAb mediates a unique type of cell death similar to oncosis. Proc Natl Acad Sci USA 95:6290–6295
14. Zhang CH, Davis WC, Grunig G et al (1998) The equine homologue of LFA-1 (CD11a/CD18): cellular distribution and differential determinants. Vet Immunol Immunopathol 62:167–183
15. Jahnichen S, Blanchetot C, Maussang D et al (2010) CXCR4 nanobodies (VHH-based single variable domains) potently inhibit chemotaxis and HIV-1 replication and mobilize stem cells. Proc Natl Acad Sci USA 107:20565–20570
16. Popkov M, Rader C, Barbas CF (2004) Isolation of human prostate cancer cell reactive antibodies using phage display technology. J Immunol Methods 291:137–151
17. Willis S, Davidoff C, Schilling J et al (2008) Virus-like particles as quantitative probes of membrane protein interactions. Biochemistry 47:6988–6990
18. Yao Q, Bu Z, Vzorov A et al (2003) Virus-like particle and DNA-based candidate AIDS vaccines. Vaccine 21:638–643
19. Robinson HL, Pertmer TM (2001) Nucleic acid immunizations. Curr Protoc Immunol Chapter 2:Unit 2.14
20. Rivinoja A, Laakkonen P (2011) Identification of homing peptides using the in vivo phage display technology. Methods Mol Biol 683:401–415
21. Kilpatrick KE, Wring SA, Walker DH et al (1997) Rapid development of affinity matured monoclonal antibodies using RIMMS. Hybridoma 16:381–389
22. Bates MK, Zhang G, Sebestyen MG et al (2006) Genetic immunization for antibody generation in research animals by intravenous delivery of plasmid DNA. Biotechniques 40:199–208
23. Tang DC, DeVit M, Johnston SA (1992) Genetic immunization is a simple method for eliciting an immune response. Nature 356: 152–154
24. de Marco A (2009) Strategies for successful recombinant expression of disulfide bond-dependent proteins in *Escherichia coli*. Microb Cell Fact 8:26
25. Hengen P (1995) Purification of His-Tag fusion proteins from *Escherichia coli*. Trends Biochem Sci 20:285–286

# Chapter 2

# Recombinant Antibodies and In Vitro Selection Technologies

**C. Ronald Geyer, John McCafferty, Stefan Dübel, Andrew R.M. Bradbury, and Sachdev S. Sidhu**

## Abstract

Over the past decade, the accumulation of detailed knowledge of antibody structure and function has enabled antibody phage display to emerge as a powerful in vitro alternative to hybridoma methods for creating antibodies. Many antibodies produced using phage display technology have unique properties that are not obtainable using traditional hybridoma technologies. In phage display, selections are performed under controlled, in vitro conditions that are tailored to suit demands of the antigen and the sequence encoding the antibody is immediately available. These features obviate many of the limitations of hybridoma methodology, and because the entire process relies on scalable molecular biology techniques, phage display is also suitable for high-throughput applications. Thus, antibody phage display technology is well suited for genome-scale biotechnology and therapeutic applications. This review describes the antibody phage display technology and highlights examples of antibodies with unique properties that cannot easily be obtained by other technologies.

**Key words:** In vitro selection, Phage display, Antibodies

## 1. Introduction

Methods for generating antibodies were initially developed more than a century ago with the production of polyclonal antibody preparations from animal immunizations (1). The advent of hybridoma technology in 1975 enabled the production of monoclonal antibodies through the fusion of myeloma cells with antibody producing B-cells (2). Hybridoma technology advanced our capacity for research and diagnostics by providing homogenous, purified antibody preparations that improved tracking, detection, and quantitation of target molecules in cells and serum. The hybridoma technology, however, is not without its limitations. With regard to generating human therapeutics, hybridoma antibodies are typically from murine sources, which limits their therapeutic

Gabriele Proetzel and Hilmar Ebersbach (eds.), *Antibody Methods and Protocols*, Methods in Molecular Biology, vol. 901, DOI 10.1007/978-1-61779-931-0_2, © Springer Science+Business Media, LLC 2012

applications due to human anti-mouse antibody reaction (3, 4). A variety of strategies have been developed to address this problem, including chimerization and humanization strategies (5–9), and transgenic animals with human immunoglobulin loci (10–14). Despite these efforts, the generation of antibodies by hybridoma technology is still costly and time-consuming. Further, since these antibodies are produced in animals, it is difficult to generate them against toxic and highly conserved antigens (15) as well as antigens that are not stable in animal systems.

Alongside the hybridoma technology, methods have been established to generate antibodies using in vitro display technologies. The first such method was antibody phage display, introduced 20 years ago (16–18), followed by yeast, ribosome, puromycin-based plasmid, and bacterial display systems (19–22). Selection platforms (23–25) and the design of antibody fragments (26, 27) for making libraries have been widely dealt with in previous reviews. The purpose of this review is to illustrate how in vitro selection, especially phage display, has yielded antibodies with remarkable properties that are difficult to obtain using traditional immunization methods.

Principles behind methods used in all in vitro display systems are similar whatever the display platform, and center on the coupling of genotype (gene) to phenotype (binding protein). In practice, this comprises the creation of DNA libraries encoding binding molecules such as antibodies, the display of the encoded proteins, the application of selective pressure based on the binding properties of the encoded proteins, followed by growth and screening of individual clones. Since in vitro display methods are performed in bacterial or yeast systems, the turnaround time for antibody generation is less, and the potential for high-throughput generation of binders is greater (28). The power of in vitro antibody selection is further enhanced by the ability to precisely control selection conditions. In contrast to animal immunization, where there is little control over the nature of antibodies produced, manipulation of selection conditions can be carried out in vitro, for example, by presentation of specific conformations of the target antigen or by including competitors to direct selection towards targets or epitopes of interest. In vitro selection methods also overcome the problem of tolerance, which limits the potential for making anti-self antibodies. As tolerance is applied to specific variable heavy (VH) and light (VL) domain combinations that recognize self-antigens, when in vitro libraries are created from natural sources new combinations with the capacity to recognize self-antigens can be created. This has been proven for example by the selection of hundreds of human antibodies from naive libraries to human targets (29–32). For libraries that are constructed using synthetic diversity, the concept of tolerance does not apply. This enables the selection of antibodies against highly conserved targets such as ubiquitin (33, 34), histones (35), hemoglobins (36), and posttranslational modifications (37–39).

Another advantage of in vitro selected antibodies is that the gene encoding the antibody is cloned simultaneously with selection. This is perhaps the most crucial difference between hybridoma and in vitro selection technologies and provides many advantages for engineering selected antibodies. For example, affinity maturation of selected antibodies can be easily performed using in vitro selection technologies. Maturation of antibody affinity to the picomolar range (40–44) has become relatively routine and, at least in one case, femtomolar affinity has been achieved (45). These affinities are far higher than those that can be obtained by immunization, which are limited to ~100 pM by the physiological mechanisms of B-cell activation (46–48). In addition, antibody specificities can be broadened or narrowed by appropriate selection conditions. As a result, in vitro selection has yielded antibodies with remarkable properties that are either a direct result of the flexibility and control that can be applied to all aspects of the selection processes, or novel properties developed as a direct result of the recombinant nature of selected proteins. Finally, the availability of the antibody gene allows the creation of a large variety of antibody derivatives with added functions by simple subcloning.

## 2. Phage-Displayed Antibody Libraries

Antibody libraries for in vitro selections can be generated from immunized repertoires, natural naïve repertoires, or designed "synthetic" repertoires. Strategies to generate antibody libraries have been described extensively (49, 50) and are discussed briefly here. Immune antibody libraries are generated by cloning antibody fragments, either single-chain variable fragments (scFvs) or antigen binding fragments (Fabs), from IgG mRNAs obtained from activated B-cells (49, 50). These libraries are biased for members that bind a specific antigen and require that a new library be generated for each antigen of interest. Immune antibody libraries have been generated against a number of different species (51, 52). Human immune libraries have been constructed from virus-infected patients to generate neutralizing antibodies and from cancer patients to isolate tumor specific antibodies (53–57).

Although natural naïve antibody libraries have been generated using IgM or IgG mRNAs from resting B-cells, initial results indicated that libraries based on IgM mRNA yield more binders (17), probably because the IgG fraction is biased towards recent immune responses. Naturally rearranged variable region genes have been used to construct large antibody fragment libraries (32, 58–61). In contrast to immune libraries, naïve libraries can be used to generate antibodies against a variety of antigens; however; they generally bind with lower affinity and may need to be affinity matured.

In synthetic antibody libraries, antibody diversity is designed and synthesized in a controlled manner. In these libraries, the composition of complementarity determining regions (CDRs) can be precisely defined. A number of approaches have been used to design synthetic libraries and they vary in the number of variable framework regions used, the design of CDR diversity, and the library construction method. Synthetic libraries have been constructed using a variety of different variable framework genes (62–65), with diversity introduced into the CDRs, primarily in CDRH3 and CDRL3. Results from selections with these libraries have shown that larger libraries yield antibodies with higher affinity and greater specificity (50), and that specific variable framework regions are over represented in the selected antibody fragments. This observation led to the development of libraries using a single VH and VL combination (66–68). A number of different libraries have been devised that differ in the variable gene and the diversification strategy. Most libraries use a common VH domain (VH3–23) as it is stable, expressed well in bacteria and on phage, and pairs with most VL domains. Synthetic libraries are constructed by cloning oligonucleotides into the CDRs of defined antibody fragments, and thus, these libraries are not limited to the diversity present in natural repertoires. However, libraries have been created by grafting natural CDRs into single frameworks (69), as well as by using designed oligonucleotides that mimic the CDR diversity observed in natural repertoires (68, 70). Libraries have also been designed with restricted diversity in the CDRs, based on the observation that tyrosine and serine are enriched in the antigen-binding sites of antibodies (71–73).

In addition to variable domain and CDR design, antibody fragments must be fused to the phage coat protein in order to establish the genotype/phenotype connection. Phage display requires that antibody fragments be displayed rather than IgGs. The two most popular antibody fragments used to display the variable antigen binding domains are the Fab and the scFv. The Fab is a heterodimer consisting of the variable and first constant domains of heavy and light chains. The scFv consists of the variable domains from the light and heavy chains joined by a peptide linker. These antibody fragments are most commonly displayed on phage by fusing them to pIII or pVIII coat proteins. The pVIII coat protein can potentially enable the display of multiple polypeptides on the phage surface, as approximately 2,500 copies of pVIII are present on each phage particle (74). However, large proteins are not well tolerated as pVIII fusions, which limits their use for displaying antibody fragments (75), and in direct comparisons, pIII display appears to be more efficient than pVIII (76). Thus, antibody fragments are more commonly fused to the pIII coat protein. There are approximately five pIII coat proteins on one tip of the phage particle. Fusion to the pIII coat protein results in low-level display of antibody fragments using phagemid systems (49), and display levels can easily be switched between monovalent and oligovalent display (77), which allows selections from large libraries to be optimized for obtaining higher affinity antibody fragments by avoiding avidity effects.

### *2.1. Diverse Applications of Antibody Phage Display*

Since the invention of antibody phage display, intellectual property issues have delayed its broad use and have limited the number of synthetic antibodies in the clinic during the 1990s. Nonetheless, as of 2010, phage display technology has been used to generate at least 35 human antibodies that are in clinical development (78). The FDA has approved two of these antibodies (adalimumab and belimumab) and one is under review (raxibacumab). The success of phage-derived antibodies in clinical trials is similar to monoclonal antibodies derived from other technologies (78). The number of antibodies generated using phage display is rapidly expanding and a comprehensive catalog is beyond the scope of this review. Below, we highlight some examples of phage-derived antibodies generated against extracellular targets as well as some of the unique features of antibodies that can be generated using phage display technologies.

### *2.2. Antibodies Against Extracellular Targets*

Phage display technologies are extremely powerful for generating functional antibodies that disrupt normal or pathological extracellular signaling. Phage display selects for antibodies that bind their target with high affinity, however this does not guarantee that they will have the desired function. Phage display, however, can produce many antibodies that bind a given target, increasing the chance that some of the antibodies will possess the desired properties. One such example was the use of phage display to generate more than 1,200 antibodies against the B-lymphocyte stimulator (Blys) (79), a potent cytokine for B-cell proliferation and differentiation. Biochemical and cellular assays were used to subsequently identify antibodies, many with subnanomolar affinities, which blocked B-cell activation by inhibiting the interaction between Blys and its receptor. One of these antibodies, which showed specificity for secreted Blys, was affinity matured and shown to be a potent inhibitor of Blys signaling (80). This antibody, belimumab, has been approved by the FDA in March 2011 for use in treatment of systemic lupus erythematosus.

A second example of an antibody isolated by phage display against a cytokine target is the tumor necrosis factor alpha (TNFα) blocking antibody, adalimumab. TNFα is a proinflammatory mediator implicated in autoimmune conditions. Adalimumab has been approved for the treatment of several conditions including rheumatoid arthritis, ankylosing spondylitis, chronic plaque psoriasis, and Crohn's disease, which was the first fully human antibody approved by the FDA in 2002. A number of other antibodies against soluble ligands have been generated by phage display and are in advanced clinical trials (81).

Another strategy to block receptor signaling is to target receptor sites that prevent ligand binding. A recent series of studies highlights the use of phage-derived antibodies to block Insulin-like Growth Factor 1 Receptor (IGF-1R) signaling (82–84). Phage display was used to generate antibodies against two unique epitopes of IGF-1R. Both antibodies blocked binding of Insulin-like Growth Factor 1 (IGF-1) and Insulin-like Growth Factor 2 (IGF-2), but they did so by either directly competing for ligand binding or by an allosteric mechanism, which decreased the affinity of ligand binding (84). Interestingly, cotreatment with both antibodies improved both the potency and extent of IGF-1 and IGF-2 blockade compared to treatment with either antibody alone. Similar results have been observed with Her2 (Human Epidermal growth factor Receptor 2), where combinations of antibodies that bind unique epitopes have greater activity than either antibody alone (85).

Antibodies have also been generated to block ligand-induced conformational changes in Notch receptors (86). The ectodomain of the Notch receptor contains multiple epidermal growth factor (EGF) repeats and ligand binding induces a conformational change at the juxtamembrane negative regulatory region, which causes a protease cleavage site to be exposed. Subsequent proteolysis causes the intracellular domain to be translocated to the nucleus. Phage display was used to generate antibodies that target the juxtamembrane negative regulatory regions of Notch-1 and Notch-2 (86). These antibodies bind and stabilize the "closed" conformation of the Notch receptor, preventing proteolytic cleavage.

Ligands often act either by causing dimerization of their target receptors or by inducing conformational changes in preexisting dimers. Antibodies targeting the ligand-binding domain can, in some instances, mimic the effect of the natural ligand and cause receptor activation rather than inhibition. For example, phage display was used to generate antibodies that bind to Muscle Specific Kinase (MuSK) (87) or CD40 (88) and function as agonists for receptor activation (87). In another recent study, over 500 distinct antibodies were generated against TRAIL receptor-1 (TRAIL-R1) and TRAIL receptor-2 (TRAIL-R2) (89). TRAIL is a homotrimeric ligand that causes multimerization of TRAIL receptors, which in turn leads to apoptosis, particularly in tumor cells overexpressing the receptors. Ten agonistic antibodies specific for TRAIL-R1 and six antibodies acting only on TRAIL-R2 were identified. As expected, these antibodies competed for binding with TRAIL, but surprisingly, they were active agonists as monovalent antibodies in either scFv or Fab formats, and activity was not enhanced upon conversion to IgG. The mechanism of action for this unusual agonistic activity is still unclear.

In addition to selecting antibodies that bind to purified proteins, phage display can be used to select antibodies that recognize targets expressed on the surfaces of cells. A number of selection protocols have been developed to select antibodies that bind cell surface proteins. These include strategies that incorporate negative selections or preabsorption steps (90–94), strategies to remove unbound phage (95, 96), and the pathfinder approach (97, 98). In vitro selection schemes have also been devised to select for antibodies that mediate receptor internalization (99–101). In these selections, phage libraries are incubated with target cells and then phage that bind the cell surface are removed and phage antibodies inside the cell are isolated. This strategy is useful for generating antibodies to deliver drugs to specific cells (102, 103). The ability to perform selections directly on cells with negative selections has proven to be a powerful trait of phage display technology.

### 2.3. Antibodies Against Infectious Disease Targets

Phage display has been used to select antibodies against a variety of infectious agents. For example, antibodies have been isolated that discriminate between strains of Hanta (104), Dengue (105, 106), Influenza (107, 108), Ebola (109), and Venezuelan equine encephalitis virus (110). Further, phage display selections do not require purified virus. For the Venezuelan equine encephalitis virus selection, the use of competitive binding conditions allowed antibodies to be generated against impure virus preparations (110). In these selections, cell extracts from uninfected cells were added to the binding buffer, which eliminated the isolation of antibodies against components of the host cell and allowed antibodies to be generated against the viral envelope. Human antibodies have also been selected against a number of bacterial bio-threat targets, including *Brucella melitensis* (111), *Burkholderia mallei*, *Burkholderia pseudomallei* (112), and anthrax toxins (113–117) and spores (118).

In one study, antibodies were used to block protein interactions associated with influenza entry into target cells. Phage display was used to generate antibodies that recognize the H5 hemagglutinin influenza ectodomain (119, 120). Structural characterization of one of these antibodies bound to H5 showed that it binds to hemagglutinin by inserting its heavy chain into a highly conserved pocket in the stem region, which prevents structural reorganizations required for membrane fusion. This conserved epitope is found in many different influenza viruses and this antibody was shown to neutralize H5N1, H1N1, H2N2, H6N1, H6N2, H8N4, and H9N2 viruses. Although antibodies have not been generated against this epitope by traditional immunization, and antibodies with this specificity do not normally arise during infection, antibodies with similar VH gene usage and neutralizing activity have been selected from phage antibody libraries created from human IgM + memory B-cells from recently infected individuals (121).

### 2.4. Antibodies with Ultra-High Specificity

With protein targets, antibodies have been selected that display high specificity for a chosen target. For example, antibodies have been generated that differentiate between chicken and quail lysozyme, which differ by only four amino acids (122). Another example is the isolation of antibodies that distinguish between the SH2 domains of ABL1 and ABL2 tyrosine kinase (29, 123), which differ by only 11%, and for which it has not been possible to obtain specific antibodies by immunization. In such studies, negative selection steps have been incorporated into phage display selections to generate antibodies with desired specificity. For example, antibodies were generated that recognize only fetal and not adult hemoglobin (124). In this study, antibodies that recognize adult hemoglobin were depleted by preincubating the antibody phage library with adult hemoglobin prior to each round of selection against fetal hemoglobin. Phage display has also been used to generate antibodies that recognize specific protein complexes, for example the generation of antibodies that recognize unique peptides in the context of specific MHC molecules (125–128).

The technology has also been applied to selectively target alternatively spliced fibronectin variants associated with tumor neovasculature. Extra-domain A (EDA) and B (EDB) are fibronectin variants each of which contain an additional domain, both being highly conserved between human and mouse. Using a synthetic antibody library, it was possible to select human/mouse cross-reactive scFvs against each of the recombinantly purified extra domains (129, 130), and these antibodies were effective for immunohistochemical analysis in vitro and for biodistribution studies in vivo. In the case of the anti-EDB antibody (130), the modular nature of the scFv was exploited to engineer numerous fusion proteins with potential for cancer therapy (131), and three of these derivatives are now in clinical trials.

### *2.5. Antibodies Against Specific Protein Conformations*

Phage display has been used to generate antibodies that recognize specific protein conformations. Many signaling proteins exist in specific conformational states that mediate distinct cellular responses. Antibodies that recognize specific protein conformations provide a unique resource for characterizing signaling pathways. These types of antibodies are difficult to generate via immunization strategies, as protein conformations are often unstable in an immunized animal. In contrast, in vitro selection technologies are ideally suited for these applications because selection conditions can be precisely controlled to favor particular conformations. Negative selections can be used to deplete nonspecific binders and affinity maturation strategies can be employed to fine-tune specificity.

Phage display has been used to generate antibody fragments that specifically recognize the GTP-bound form of Rab6 (132) and active and inactive forms of Caspase-1 (133). scFvs specific to the GTP-bound form of the small guanosine triphosphatase (GTPase) Rab6 were generated by performing selections against a

GTP-locked mutant (132). Fabs specific to on and off states of caspase-1 were generated by selecting libraries against capase-1 complexed to small molecules that lock it in the on or off state (133). Fabs were converted into full-length IgGs to produce highly sensitive affinity reagents that could be used to probe the localization of active caspase-1 in cells (133). Conformation-specific antibodies have also been generated against active cell membrane receptors by performing phage selections on whole cells (134).

### 2.6. Antibodies Against Integral Membrane Proteins

Integral membrane proteins absolutely require a membrane or detergent environment to maintain their native conformation. Consequently, the generation of conformation-specific antibodies against membrane proteins by animal immunization is severely limited by the denaturing effects of the serum environment. In contrast, the ability to control selection conditions makes in vitro techniques much more amenable to this task. By performing selections in the presence of detergent, high affinity Fabs were isolated against the citrate transporter CitS from *Klebsiella pneumoniae* (135), as well as against the potassium channel KcsA from *Streptomyces lividans* (136). In the latter case, the Fabs were used as crystallization chaperones that enabled the elucidation of the crystal structure of the full-length potassium channel.

### 2.7. Antibodies Against RNA

Phage display has been used to generate antibodies that recognize structured RNA molecules (137), which have proven to be essentially nonimmunogenic for hybridoma methods. Using a nuclease free selection buffer, high affinity Fabs were isolated against a structured domain from the *Tetrahymena* group I intron. The structure of the Fab/RNA complex was solved to high resolution, highlighting the use of antibody fragments as chaperones for RNA crystallization. Fabs were also obtained against a class I ligase ribozyme and were used as chaperones to obtain the crystal structure (138). One Fab recognized a small, discrete sequence in the ribozyme and retained binding capacity when this sequence was transferred to other RNA structures, providing a novel RNA crystallization chaperone system.

### 2.8. Antibodies Against Posttranslational Modifications

Phage display has been useful for detecting posttranslational modifications that have proven intractable to immunization. For example, sulfotyrosine is a posttranslational modification predicted to occur in 30% of all secretory and membrane proteins (139). Perhaps because of its ubiquitous nature, traditional immunizations have consistently failed to produce anti-sulfotyrosine antibodies. However, using phage display, antibodies were readily generated to recognize proteins containing sulfotyrosine (but not tyrosine or tyrosine phosphate) independently of protein context or sequence (39, 140).

## 3. Exploiting the Recombinant Nature of In Vitro Antibodies

Since phage display is an in vitro selection method, it offers many advantages for engineering antibodies. The phage display system provides the antibody gene and sequence following selection against a particular target. This allows antibodies to be easily further evolved and engineered to improve binding, to narrow or broaden specificity, or to improve expression as IgGs or as fusions to functional moieties.

Antibody fragments isolated from an initial phage display selection can be used directly as an affinity reagent, or they can be used as leads for further improving binding. Since the sequence of isolated antibody fragments are rapidly determined by sequencing, it is straightforward to make second-generation libraries by introducing mutations into antibody fragments. Affinity maturation strategies have been used to generate antibodies with affinities that exceed those of natural antibodies, which are limited to a ceiling of $K_d > 0.1$ nM by the nature of the B cell response (46–48). There are many different approaches for introducing diversity into antibody fragments to improve the affinities obtained from combinatorial libraries. With in vitro affinity maturation selections, randomized antibody fragments undergo selection with increased pressure to identify variants with enhanced affinity (141). In general, there are two approaches for generating diversification: targeted and nontargeted. There are many examples of in vitro affinity maturation, and here we highlight some key studies that demonstrate the power of the process.

Error prone PCR is the most common method for introducing nontargeted mutations (142). In this method, sequence diversity is randomly introduced into the antibody fragment gene by mutagenic PCR strategies (50). The down side of this approach is that deleterious mutations can be introduced into the conserved framework region, which reduces the number of functional antibody fragments in the library. DNA shuffling is another method for introducing nontargeted mutations (143). In this method, a group of closely related sequence are randomly fragmented and then reassembled by PCR, which leads to a shuffling of DNA fragments. The approach can be combined with PCR mutagenesis to further enhance diversity. This method was used to increase the affinity of an scFv for fluorescein by 1,000-fold, resulting in subpicomolar affinity (45).

As an alternative to random PCR mutagenesis, knowledge of the antibody sequence enables precise targeting of mutations for affinity maturation. Targeted mutation strategies have the advantage of focusing mutations to CDR loops, which are most likely to enhance affinity without introducing deleterious mutations in regions that may affect protein folding and stability. Targeted mutagenesis can be performed using degenerate oligonucleotides, which allows for precise control over the locations where diversity is introduced. Further, CDRs can be targeted in either a parallel or sequential fashion. By targeting CDR loops in phage-displayed antibody libraries, an anti-HIV-1 antibody (44) and an anti-c-erbB-2 (43) antibody were affinity matured to the low picomolar range.

In addition to affinity, the specificity of antibodies can be altered by phage display. While absolute specificity for a single antigen is generally the goal of antibody design, cross-reactivity is desirable for certain applications. For example, in the case of antibody therapeutics, species cross-reactivity enables assessment of therapeutic efficacy and toxicity in animal models. Cross-reactive antibodies are often difficult to obtain by hybridoma methods because of the conservation of functional sites on proteins across species. In contrast, in vitro phage antibody libraries are not affected by immune tolerance, and generation of antibodies that target conserved sites across species orthologues has proven to be the rule rather than the exception. For example, antibodies that cross-react with human and mouse VEGF were obtained directly from phage libraries without further selections to broaden specificity (144, 145). For BAFF/BLys receptor 3 (BR3), antibodies generated against human BR3 showed weak cross-reactivity with mouse BR3. In this case, phage display was used to select cross-reactive antibodies from secondary libraries (146). This strategy has also been used to generate antibodies with cross-reactivity towards CXCL10 and CXCL9 homologues (147). In an extreme example, this approach has been used to broaden the specificity of trastuzumab so that it cross-reacts with Erb-B2 and VEGF, two proteins that share no sequence or structural homology (148). In this case, secondary libraries were created by diversifying the light chain, which plays a minor role in Erb-B2 recognition. Extensive affinity maturation produced antibodies with low nanomolar affinity for both ErbB2 and VEGF (148).

The ability to improve affinity and broaden specificity also has major implications for the development of antibodies against infectious disease agents. For the effective inhibition of viral infection and bacterial toxins, antibodies must be of very high affinity, and at the same time, they should be cross-reactive with a variety of antigen subtypes to afford broad protection against pathogen variants. A powerful example of using affinity and specificity selection cycles was demonstrated for an antibody with broad specificity for different subtypes of Botulinum toxins. Remarkably, this antibody is able to recognize Botulinum toxins A, B, E, and F, all the serotypes that afflict humans (149, 150).

The ability to rapidly obtain the gene for a selected antibody fragment allows the antibody to be easily engineered by simple subcloning strategies. Antibody fragments produced from phage display selections can be subcloned into IgG expression systems to produce antibodies in mammalian tissue culture systems (151). Antibody fragments have also been engineered with other functions by fusing them to peptides and proteins that induce dimerization (152) and multimerization (153–155) to facilitate detection and purification, or that provide them with fluorescent (156–158) or enzymatic (159) properties. In vivo peptide biotinylation tags have been fused to the C-termini of antibody fragments to enable antibodies to be immobilized or multimerized (153, 160–163). Antibody fragments have been fused to the dimeric enzyme alkaline phosphatase, which provides both dimerization and alkaline phosphatase activity that greatly enhances functionality and simplifies screening (30, 159). scFvs have also been fused to Fc domains, converting them into antibody-like molecules with properties similar to IgGs (164–167).

Recombinant technologies have enabled the generation of a large variety of bispecific antibodies that recognize two different targets (ref. 168 and see also Chapter 16). This can be accomplished by engineering two different Fc domains to allow heterologous pairing (169, 170). Alternatively, scFvs can be fused recombinantly to IgGs to impart bifunctionality (171). This strategy has recently been used to generate bispecific antibodies against IGF-1R, which blocked ligand binding better that either monospecific IgG (172). The bispecific antibodies also showed an improved ability to reduce the growth of multiple tumor cell lines, to inhibit ligand-induced IGF-1R signaling in tumor cells, and to block in vivo tumor growth (172). Bispecific antibody fragments have also been generated by varying the peptide linker length that connects VH and VL domains in scFvs. This strategy has been used to generate dimers (173–175), trimers (174, 176, 177), and tetramers (178). Various other bispecific antibody designs have also been created (see ref. 179 for a review).

Within the context of improved antibody therapeutics, fusion proteins that can extend the capabilities of natural IgGs have been constructed. By exchanging or engineering the Fc region, antibodies with designed pharmacokinetics and improved effector functions have been obtained (for reviews see refs. 180, 181).

## 4. High-Throughput Antibody Selections and Next-Generation Sequencing

The ease and speed with which antibody fragments can be selected using phage display, usually between 1 and 2 weeks, allows the technology to be implemented in a high-throughput manner (29, 30, 123, 182, 183) and see also Chapters 3–6. Initial experiments using a limited number of targets showed that antibodies could be generated from semiautomated selections using phage antibody libraries (182–184). More recent studies have shown that phage display selections can be scaled up to target a larger number of antigens (29, 30, 123, 182, 183). For example, phage antibody selections were carried out on over 400 different antigens representing 292 proteins. In total, 25% of antibodies screened were positive, and 80% of these were specific when screened against irrelevant antigens (30). The practicality of generating antibodies against a broad array of different targets was further demonstrated in a recent multinational study in which antibodies against 20 different SH2 domains were generated via immunization and hybridoma technology or by phage display technology (31). The phage display selections were successful against all 20 targets and yielded at least ten unique binders for each target. Both phage display and hybridoma technologies produced many binders with low-nanomolar affinities. Antibodies were validated using a number of different assays, including microarrays, immunoblots, immunofluorescence, and immunoprecipitation. Overall, this study shows that antibodies with high affinity and specificity can be efficiently generated using high-throughput phage technologies.

Next-generation sequencing (NGS) technologies have been used to improve the characterization of mouse immunizations and phage display selections and to speed up the identification of antibodies. Several studies have utilized NGS for high-resolution analysis of natural (185) and synthetic (186) antibody repertoires. The 454 sequencing platform, which provides sequencing reads between 250 and 400 bases, was used to provide information on the diversity of CDRs and on VH and VL pairings (185, 187). The Illumina sequencing platform, which provides a higher number of shorter reads (~100 bases), was used to analyze the CDRH3 region of an scFv library (186). NGS platforms provide information on V-gene family frequency, CDR length and diversity, and a comparison of the theoretical and actual properties of the library (188). NGS has also been used to characterize how the immunoglobulin repertoire changes after immunization, where NGS was used to monitor enrichment in antigen specific V-genes (189).

For phage display selections, NGS was used to monitor enrichment of antibody sequences during successive rounds of selection (186). The information generated by NGS can be used to bypass antibody screening, which is time-consuming and expensive. For antibodies generated by mouse immunization, NGS was used to indentify heavy and light chains and pairings between them were inferred based on their frequencies in the repertoire (189). A similar strategy was used to identify antibodies from phage display selections (186). High frequency antibody fragments were identified following rounds of selection and desired antibody fragments were recovered by PCR (186). Identification of antibody sequences following selection eliminates the characterization of redundant clones. Further, it reduces the amount of target protein required to perform and characterize antibodies from immunizations or phage selections. Lastly, NGS was used to characterize an antibody phage display selection against a protein target IL-6, expressed on the surface of *E. coli* (190). This study highlighted the potential for using NGS to characterize phage display selections against complex targets.

## 5. Conclusions and Future Perspectives

It is now well accepted in the scientific community that there is an urgent need to improve antibody quality in general, as an alarmingly high proportion of commercial antibodies either show poor specificity, or fail to even recognize their targets (191–194). At the same time, high-throughput genomics and proteomics technologies have vastly expanded the scope of proteins and pathways that now await detailed analysis at the cell biology level. To deal with the thousands of new proteins revealed by genomics and proteomics projects, there is an urgent need for high quality antibodies, and it is clear that the current hybridoma methods are not suitable for this task.

In this landscape, the emergence of high quality in vitro antibody libraries is both timely and opportune. Numerous studies have reported in vitro repertoires that routinely yield antibodies that rival or surpass hybridoma antibodies in terms of functionality. Moreover, while further improvements in hybridoma technology are likely to be slight, in vitro repertoires and selection methods continue to improve. Universal in vitro libraries that can provide antibodies against virtually any antigen are now a reality, and it is hoped that the technology can be broadly disseminated in the near future.

The recombinant nature of in vitro repertoires is a fundamental advantage that extends the technology beyond the scope of hybridoma technology. With synthetic antibodies in particular, frameworks can be chosen for favorable traits such as low immunogenicity or high stability, initial clones can be rapidly affinity matured and reformatted, and antibodies can be shared and distributed in the form of synthetic DNA. Furthermore, precise control over selection conditions allows for high precision engineering of specificity and affinity. Further standardization of libraries and selection methods will enable the adaptation of the technology to high-throughput pipelines to enable antibody generation on a proteome scale, and the ability to select directly against cells and tissues will further expand the scope of the technology. Clearly, in vitro antibody libraries are ideally suited for addressing the challenges of cell biology in the genomics era, and the technology is poised to play an ever-expanding role in the future of biological research.

## References


1. von Behring E, Kitasato S (1890) Über das zustandekommen der diphtherie-immunität und der tetanus-immunität bei thieren. Deut Med Wochenzeitschr 16:1113–1114
2. Köhler G, Milstein C (1975) Continuous cultures of fused cells secreting antibody of predefined specificity. Nature 256:495–497
3. Courtenay-Luck NS, Epenetos AA, Moore R et al (1986) Development of primary and secondary immune responses to mouse monoclonal antibodies used in the diagnosis and therapy of malignant neoplasms. Cancer Res 46:6489–6493
4. Tjandra JJ, Ramadi L, McKenzie IF (1990) Development of human anti-murine antibody (HAMA) response in patients. Immunol Cell Biol 68:367–376
5. Almagro JC, Fransson J (2008) Humanization of antibodies. Front Biosci 13:1619–1633
6. Hwang WYK, Foote J (2005) Immunogenicity of engineered antibodies. Methods 36:3–10
7. Kashmiri SVS, De Pascalis R, Gonzales NR, Schlom J (2005) SDR grafting—a new approach to antibody humanization. Methods 36:25–34
8. Studnicka GM, Soares S, Better M et al (1994) Human engineered monoclonal antibodies retain full specific binding activity by preserving non-CDR complementarity-modulating residues. Protein Eng 7:805–814
9. Osbourn J, Groves M, Vaughan T (2005) From rodent reagents to human therapeutics using antibody guided selection. Methods 36: 61–68
10. Fishwild DM, O'Donnell SL, Bengoechea T et al (1996) High-avidity human IgG kappa monoclonal antibodies from a novel strain of minilocus transgenic mice. Nat Biotechnol 14:845–851
11. Jakobovits A (1995) Production of fully human antibodies by transgenic mice. Curr Opin Biotechnol 6:561–566
12. Kuroiwa Y, Kasinathan P, Sathiyaseelan T et al (2009) Antigen specific human polyclonal antibodies from hyperimmunized cattle. Nat Biotechnol 27:173–181
13. Lonberg N, Huszar D (1995) Human antibodies from transgenic mice. Int Rev Immunol 13:65–93
14. Weiner LM (2006) Fully human therapeutic monoclonal antibodies. J Immunother 29:1–9
15. Winter G, Milstein C (1991) Man-made antibodies. Nature 349:293–299
16. McCafferty J, Griffiths AD, Winter G et al (1990) Phage antibodies: filamentous phage displaying antibody variable domains. Nature 348:552–554
17. Marks JD, Hoogenboom HR, Bonnert TP et al (1991) By-passing immunization. Human antibodies from V-gene libraries displayed on phage. J Mol Bio 222:581–597
18. Breitling F, Dübel S, Seehaus T (1991) A surface expression vector for antibody screening. Gene 104:147–153
19. Boder ET, Wittrup KD (1997) Yeast surface display for screening combinatorial polypeptide libraries. Nat Biotechnol 15:553–557
20. Feldhaus MJ, Siegel RW, Opresko LK et al (2003) Flow-cytometric isolation of human antibodies from a nonimmune *Saccharomyces cerevisiae* surface display library. Nat Biotechnol 21:163–170
21. He M, Taussig MJ (2007) Rapid discovery of protein interactions by cell-free protein technologies. Biochem Soc Trans 35:962–965
22. Jostock T, Dübel S (2005) Screening of molecular repertoires by microbial surface display. Comb Chem High Throughput Screen 8:127–133
23. Paschke M (2006) Phage display systems and their applications. Appl Microbiol Biotechnol 70:2–11
24. Zahnd C, Amstutz P, Pluckthun A (2007) Ribosome display: selecting and evolving proteins in vitro that specifically bind to a target. Nat Methods 4:269–279
25. Chao G, Lau WL, Hackel BJ et al (2006) Isolating and engineering human antibodies using yeast surface display. Nat Protoc 1: 755–768
26. Benhar I (2007) Design of synthetic antibody libraries. Expert Opin Biol Ther 7:763–779
27. Bradbury AR, Marks JD (2004) Antibodies from phage antibody libraries. J Immunol Methods 290:29–49
28. Dübel S, Stoevesandt O, Taussig MJ et al (2010) Generating recombinant antibodies to the complete human proteome. Trends Biotechnol 28:333–339
29. Mersmann M, Meier D, Mersmann J et al (2010) Towards proteome scale antibody selections using phage display. New Biotechnol 27:118–128
30. Schofield DJ et al (2007) Application of phage display to high throughput antibody generation and characterization. Genome Biol 8:R254
31. Colwill K, Gräslund S, Persson MA et al (2011) A roadmap to generate renewable protein binders to the human proteome. Nat Methods 8:551–561

32. Hust M, Meyer T, Voedisch B et al (2011) A human scFv antibody generation pipeline for proteome research. J Biotechnol 152: 159–170
33. Koide A, Bailey CW, Huang X et al (1998) The fibronectin type III domain as a scaffold for novel binding proteins. J Mol Biol 284: 1141–1151
34. Angenendt P, Wilde J, Kijanka G et al (2004) Seeing better through a MIST: evaluation of monoclonal recombinant antibody fragments on microarrays. Anal Chem 76:2916–2921
35. Philibert P, Stoessel A, Wang W (2007) A focused antibody library for selecting scFvs expressed at high levels in the cytoplasm. BMC Biotechnol 7:1472–6750
36. Parsons HL, Earnshaw JC, Wilton J et al (1996) Directing phage selections towards specific epitopes. Protein Eng 9:1043–1049
37. Lassen KS, Bradbury AR, Rehfeld JF et al (2008) Microscale characterization of the binding specificity and affinity of a monoclonal antisulfotyrosyl IgG antibody. Electrophoresis 29:2557–2564
38. Kehoe JW, Velappan N, Walbol M et al (2006) Using phage display to select antibodies recognizing post-translational modifications independently of sequence context. Mol Cell Proteomics 5:2350–2363
39. Hoffhines AJ, Damoc E, Bridges KG et al (2006) Detection and purification of tyrosine-sulfated proteins using a novel anti-sulfotyrosine monoclonal antibody. J Biol Chem 281:37877–37887
40. Raza A, Garcia-Rodriguez C, Lou J et al (2005) Molecular evolution of antibody affinity for sensitive detection of botulinum neurotoxin type A. J Mol Biol 351:158–169
41. Lee CV, Liang WC, Dennis MS et al (2004) High-affinity human antibodies from phage-displayed synthetic Fab libraries with a single framework scaffold. J Mol Biol 340: 1073–1093
42. Hanes J, Schaffitzel C, Knappik A et al (2000) Picomolar affinity antibodies from a fully synthetic naive library selected and evolved by ribosome display. Nat Biotechnol 18: 1287–1292
43. Schier R, McCall A, Adams GP et al (1996) Isolation of picomolar affinity anti-c-erbB-2 single-chain Fv by molecular evolution of the complementarity determining regions in the center of the antibody binding site. J Mol Biol 263:551–567
44. Yang WP, Green K, Pinz-Sweeney S et al (1995) CDR walking mutagenesis for the affinity maturation of a potent human anti-HIV-1 antibody into the picomolar range. J Mol Biol 254:392–403
45. Boder ET, Midelfort KS, Wittrup KD (2000) Directed evolution of antibody fragments with monovalent femtomolar antigen-binding affinity. Proc Natl Acad Sci USA 97: 10701–10705
46. Foote J, Eisen HN (1995) Kinetic and affinity limits on antibodies produced during immune responses. Proc Natl Acad Sci USA 92: 1254–1256
47. Foote J, Eisen HN (2000) Breaking the affinity ceiling for antibodies and T cell receptors. Proc Natl Acad Sci USA 97:10679–10681
48. Batista FD, Neuberger MS (1998) Affinity dependence of the B cell response to antigen: a threshold, a ceiling, and the importance of off-rate. Immunity 8:751–759
49. Sidhu SS (2005) Phage display in biotechnology and drug discovery. CRC Press, Baco Raton, FL
50. Ponsel D, Neugebauer J, Ladetzki-Baehs K et al (2011) High affinity, developability and functional size: the holy grail of combinatorial antibody library generation. Molecules 16:3675–3700
51. Azzazy HM, Highsmith WE Jr (2002) Phage display technology: clinical applications and recent innovations. Clin Biochem 35: 425–445
52. Benhar I (2007) Design of synthetic antibody libraries. Expert Opin Biol Ther 7:763–779
53. Burton DR, Barbas CF III, Persson MA et al (1991) A large array of human monoclonal antibodies to type 1 human immunodeficiency virus from combinatorial libraries of asymptomatic seropositive individuals. Proc Natl Acad Sci USA 88:10134–10137
54. Kramer RA, Marissen WE, Goudsmit J et al (2005) The human antibody repertoire specific for rabies virus glycoprotein as selected from immune libraries. Eur J Immunol 35:2131–2145
55. de Carvalho NC, Williamson RA, Parren PW et al (2002) Neutralizing human Fab fragments against measles virus recovered by phage display. J Virol 76:251–258
56. Zebedee SL, Barbas CF III, Hom YL et al (1992) Human combinatorial antibody libraries to hepatitis B surface antigen. Proc Natl Acad Sci USA 89:3175–3179
57. Cai X, Garen A (1995) Anti-melanoma antibodies from melanoma patients immunized with genetically modified autologous tumor cells: selection of specific antibodies from single-chain Fv fusion phage libraries. Proc Natl Acad Sci USA 92:6537–6541

58. Vaughan TJ, Williams AJ, Pritchard K et al (1996) Human antibodies with sub-nanomolar affinities isolated from a large non-immunized phage display library. Nat Biotechnol 14:309–314
59. Lloyd C, Lowe D, Edwards B et al (2009) Modelling the human immune response: performance of a 1011 human antibody repertoire against a broad panel of therapeutically relevant antigens. Protein Eng Des Sel 22: 159–168
60. Sheets MD, Amersdorfer P, Finnern R et al (1998) Efficient construction of a large nonimmune phage antibody library: the production of high-affinity human single-chain antibodies to protein antigens. Proc Natl Acad Sci USA 95:6157–6162
61. De Haard HJ (2002) Construction of large naive Fab libraries. Methods Mol Biol 178: 87–100
62. Nissim A, Hoogenboom HR, Tomlinson IM et al (1994) Antibody fragments from a 'single pot' phage display library as immunochemical reagents. EMBO J 13:692–698
63. de Kruif J, Boel E, Logtenberg T (1995) Selection and application of human single chain Fv antibody fragments from a semi-synthetic phage antibody display library with designed CDR3 regions. J Mol Biol 248: 97–105
64. Griffiths AD, Williams SC, Hartley O et al (1994) Isolation of high affinity human antibodies directly from large synthetic repertoires. EMBO J 13:3245–3260
65. Hoogenboom HR, Winter G (1992) By-passing immunisation. Human antibodies from synthetic repertoires of germline VH gene segments rearranged in vitro. J Mol Biol 227:381–388
66. Pini A, Viti F, Santucci A et al (1998) Design and use of a phage display library. Human antibodies with subnanomolar affinity against a marker of angiogenesis eluted from a two-dimensional gel. J Biol Chem 273: 21769–21776
67. Hoet RM, Cohen EH, Kent RB et al (2005) Generation of high-affinity human antibodies by combining donor-derived and synthetic complementarity-determining-region diversity. Nat Biotechnol 23:344–348
68. Lee CV, Liang WC, Dennis MS et al (2004) High-affinity human antibodies from phage-displayed synthetic Fab libraries with a single framework scaffold. J Mol Biol 340: 1073–1093
69. Söderlind E, Strandberg L, Jirholt P et al (2000) Recombining germline-derived CDR sequences for creating diverse single-framework antibody libraries. Nat Biotechnol 18:852–856
70. Rothe C, Urlinger S, Lohning C et al (2008) The human combinatorial antibody library HuCAL GOLD combines diversification of all six CDRs according to the natural immune system with a novel display method for efficient selection of high-affinity antibodies. J Mol Biol 376:1182–1200
71. Sidhu SS, Li B, Chen Y, Fellouse FA et al (2004) Phage-displayed antibody libraries of synthetic heavy chain complementarity determining regions. J Mol Biol 338:299–310
72. Fellouse FA, Wiesmann C, Sidhu SS (2004) Synthetic antibodies from a four-amino-acid code: a dominant role for tyrosine in antigen recognition. Proc Natl Acad Sci USA 101:12467–12472
73. Fellouse FA, Li B, Compaan DM, Peden AA et al (2005) Molecular recognition by a binary code. J Mol Biol 348:1153–1162
74. Russel M, Linderoth NA, Sali A (1997) Filamentous phage assembly: variation on a protein export theme. Gene 192:23–32
75. Iannolo G, Minenkova O, Petruzzelli R et al (1995) Modifying filamentous phage capsid: limits in the size of the major capsid protein. J Mol Biol 248:835–844
76. Kretzschmarm T, Geiser M (1995) Evaluation of antibodies fused to minor coat protein III and major coat protein VIII of bacteriophage M13. Gene 155:61–65
77. Rondot S, Koch J, Breitling F et al (2001) A helper phage to improve single chain antibody presentation in phage display. Nat Biotechnol 19:75–78
78. Nelson AL, Dhimolea E, Reichert JM (2010) Development trends for human monoclonal antibody therapeutics. Nat Rev Drug Discov 9:767–774
79. Edwards BM, Barash SC, Main SH et al (2003) The remarkable flexibility of the human antibody repertoire; isolation of over one thousand different antibodies to a single protein, BLyS. J Mol Biol 334:103–118
80. Baker KP, Edwards BM, Main SH et al (2003) Generation and characterization of LymphoStat-B, a human monoclonal antibody that antagonizes the bioactivities of B lymphocyte stimulator. Arthritis Rheum 48:3253–3265
81. Lloyd C, Lowe D, Edwards B et al (2009) Modelling the human immune response: performance of a 1011 human antibody repertoire against a broad panel of therapeutically relevant antigens. Protein Eng Des Sel 22:159–168

82. Dong J, Demarest SJ, Sereno A et al (2010) Combination of two insulin-like growth factor-I receptor inhibitory antibodies targeting distinct epitopes leads to an enhanced antitumor response. Mol Cancer Ther 9: 2593–2604
83. Doern A, Cao X, Sereno A et al (2009) Characterization of inhibitory anti-insulin-like growth factor receptor antibodies with different epitope specificity and ligand-blocking properties: implications for mechanism of action in vivo. J Biol Chem 284:10254–10267
84. Dong J, Sereno A, Snyder WB et al (2011) Stable IgG-like bispecific antibodies directed toward the type I insulin-like growth factor receptor demonstrate enhanced ligand blockade and anti-tumor activity. J Biol Chem 286: 4703–4717
85. Baselga J, Gelmon KA, Verma S et al (2010) Phase II trial of pertuzumab and trastuzumab in patients with human epidermal growth factor receptor 2-positive metastatic breast cancer that progressed during prior trastuzumab therapy. J Clin Oncol 28:1138–1144
86. Wu Y, Cain-Hom C, Choy L et al (2010) Therapeutic antibody targeting of individual Notch receptors. Nature 464:1052–1057
87. Xie MH, Yuan J, Adams C et al (1997) Direct demonstration of MuSK involvement in acetylcholine receptor clustering through identification of agonist ScFv. Nat Biotechnol 15:768–771
88. Ellmark P, Andersson H, Abayneh S et al (2008) Identification of a strongly activating human anti-CD40 antibody that suppresses HIV type 1 infection. AIDS Res Hum Retroviruses 24:367–373
89. Dobson CL, Main S, Newton P et al (2009) Human monomeric antibody fragments to TRAIL-R1 and TRAIL-R2 that display potent in vitro agonism. MAbs 1:552–562
90. Eisenhardt SU, Schwarz M, Bassler N et al (2007) Subtractive single-chain antibody (scFv) phage-display: tailoring phage-display for high specificity against function-specific conformations of cell membrane molecules. Nat Protoc 2:3063–3073
91. Huie MA, Cheung MC, Muench MO et al (2001) Antibodies to human fetal erythroid cells from a nonimmune phage antibody library. Proc Natl Acad Sci USA 98:2682–2687
92. Noronha EJ, Wang X, Desai SA et al (1998) Limited diversity of human scFv fragments isolated by panning a synthetic phage-display scFv library with cultured human melanoma cells. J Immunol 161:2968–2976
93. Ridgway JB, Ng E, Kern JA et al (1999) Identification of a human anti-CD55 single-chain Fv by subtractive panning of a phage library using tumor and nontumor cell lines. Cancer Res 59:2718–2723
94. Van Ewijk W, de Kruif J, Germeraad WT et al (1997) Subtractive isolation of phage-displayed single-chain antibodies to thymic stromal cells by using intact thymic fragments. Proc Natl Acad Sci USA 94:3903–3908
95. Giordano RJ, Cardo-Vila M, Lahdenranta J et al (2001) Biopanning and rapid analysis of selective interactive ligands. Nat Med 7: 1249–1253
96. Williams BR, Sharon J (2002) Polyclonal anti-colorectal cancer Fab phage display library selected in one round using density gradient centrifugation to separate antigen-bound and free phage. Immunol Lett 81:141–148
97. Osbourn JK, Derbyshire EJ, Vaughan TJ et al (1998) Pathfinder selection: in situ isolation of novel antibodies. Immunotechnology 3:293–302
98. Osbourn JK, Earnshaw JC, Johnson KS et al (1998) Directed selection of MIP-1 alpha neutralizing CCR5 antibodies from a phage display human antibody library. Nat Biotechnol 16:778–781
99. Poul MA, Becerril B, Nielsen UB et al (2000) Selection of tumor-specific internalizing human antibodies from phage libraries. J Mol Biol 301:1149–1161
100. Zhou Y, Marks JD (2009) Identification of target and function specific antibodies for effective drug delivery. Methods Mol Biol 525:145–160
101. Crépin R, Goenaga AL, Jullienne B et al (2010) Development of human single-chain antibodies to the transferrin receptor t, hat effectively antagonize the growth of leukemias and lymphomas. Cancer Res 70: 5497–5506
102. Park JW, Kirpotin DB, Hong K et al (2001) Tumor targeting using anti-her2 immunoliposomes. J Control Release 74:95–113
103. Nielsen UB, Kirpotin DB, Pickering EM et al (2002) Therapeutic efficacy of anti-ErbB2 immunoliposomes targeted by a phage antibody selected for cellular endocytosis. Biochim Biophys Acta 1591:109–118
104. Velappan N, Martinez JS, Valero R et al (2007) Selection and characterization of scFv antibodies against the Sin Nombre hantavirus nucleocapsid protein. J Immunol Methods 321:60–69

105. Cabezas S, Rojas G, Pavon A et al (2009) Phage-displayed antibody fragments recognizing dengue 3 and dengue 4 viruses as tools for viral serotyping in sera from infected individuals. Arch Virol 154:1035–1045

106. Cabezas S, Rojas G, Pavon A et al (2008) Selection of phage-displayed human antibody fragments on Dengue virus particles captured by a monoclonal antibody: application to the four serotypes. J Virol Methods 147: 235–243

107. Lim AP, Chan CE, Wong SK et al (2008) Neutralizing human monoclonal antibody against H5N1 influenza HA selected from a Fab-phage display library. Virol J 5:130

108. Okada J, Ohshima N, Kubota-Koketsu R et al (2010) Monoclonal antibodies in man that neutralized H3N2 influenza viruses were classified into three groups with distinct strain specificity: 1968–1973, 1977–1993 and 1997–2003. Virology 397:322–330

109. Meissner F, Maruyama T, Frentsch M et al (2002) Detection of antibodies against the four subtypes of ebola virus in sera from any species using a novel antibody-phage indicator assay. Virology 300:236–243

110. Kirsch MI, Hülseweh B, Nacke C et al (2008) Development of human antibody fragments using antibody phage display for the detection and diagnosis of Venezuelan equine encephalitis virus (VEEV). BMC Biotechnol 8:66

111. Hayhurst A, Happe S, Mabry R et al (2003) Isolation and expression of recombinant antibody fragments to the biological warfare pathogen Brucella melitensis. J Immunol Methods 276:185–196

112. Zou N, Newsome T, Li B et al (2007) Human single-chain Fv antibodies against *Burkholderia mallei* and *Burkholderia pseudomallei*. Exp Biol Med (Maywood) 232:550–556

113. Maynard JA, Maassen CB, Leppla SH et al (2002) Protection against anthrax toxin by recombinant antibody fragments correlates with antigen affinity. Nat Biotechnol 20:597–601

114. Wild MA, Xin H, Maruyama T et al (2003) Human antibodies from immunized donors are protective against anthrax toxin in vivo. Nat Biotechnol 21:1305–1306

115. Steiniger SC, Altobell LJ 3rd, Zhou B, Janda KD (2007) Selection of human antibodies against cell surface-associated oligomeric anthrax protective antigen. Mol Immunol 44:2749–2755

116. Pelat T, Hust M, Laffly E et al (2007) High-affinity, human antibody-like antibody fragment (single-chain variable fragment) neutralizing the lethal factor (LF) of Bacillus anthracis by inhibiting protective antigen-LF complex formation. Antimicrob Agents Chemother 51:2758–2764

117. Cirino NM, Sblattero D, Allen D et al (1999) Disruption of anthrax toxin binding with the use of human antibodies and competitive inhibitors. Infect Immun 67:2957–2963

118. Zhou B, Wirsching P, Janda KD (2002) Human antibodies against spores of the genus *Bacillus*: a model study for detection of and protection against anthrax and the bioterrorist threat. Proc Natl Acad Sci USA 99:5241–5246

119. Sui J, Hwang WC, Perez S et al (2009) Structural and functional bases for broad-spectrum neutralization of avian and human influenza A viruses. Nat Struct Mol Biol 16:265–273

120. Sun L, Lu X, Li C et al (2009) Generation, characterization and epitope mapping of two neutralizing and protective human recombinant antibodies against influenza A H5N1 viruses. PLoS One 4:e5476

121. Throsby M, van den Brink E, Jongeneelen M et al (2008) Heterosubtypic neutralizing monoclonal antibodies cross-protective against H5N1 and H1N1 recovered from human IgM+memory B cells. PLoS One 3:e3942

122. Ayriss J, Woods T, Bradbury A, Pavlik P (2007) High-throughput screening of single-chain antibodies using multiplexed flow cytometry. J Proteome Res 6:1072–1082

123. Pershad K, Pavlovic JD, Gräslund S et al (2010) Generating a panel of highly specific antibodies to 20 human SH2 domains by phage display. Protein Eng Des Sel 23:279–288

124. Parsons HL, Earnshaw JC, Wilton J et al (1996) Directing phage selections towards specific epitopes. Protein Eng 9:1043–1049

125. Mutuberria R, Satijn S, Huijbers A et al (2004) Isolation of human antibodies to tumor-associated endothelial cell markers by in vitro human endothelial cell selection with phage display libraries. J Immunol Methods 287:31–47

126. Cohen CJ, Denkberg G, Lev A et al (2003) Recombinant antibodies with MHC-restricted, peptide-specific, T-cell receptor-like specificity: new tools to study antigen presentation and TCR-peptide-MHC interactions. J Mol Recognit 16:324–332

127. Engberg J, Krogsgaard M, Fugger L (1999) Recombinant antibodies with the

antigen-specific, MHC restricted specificity of T cells: novel reagents for basic and clinical investigations and immunotherapy. Immunotechnology 4:273–278

128. Stryhn A, Andersen PS, Pedersen LO et al (1996) Shared fine specificity between T-cell receptors and an antibody recognizing a peptide/major histocompatibility class I complex. Proc Natl Acad Sci USA 93:10338–10342
129. Villa A, Trachsel E, Kaspar M et al (2008) A high-affinity human monoclonal antibody specific to the alternatively spliced EDA domain of fibronectin efficiently targets tumor neo-vasculature in vivo. Int J Cancer 122:2405–2413
130. Pini A, Viti F, Santucci A et al (1998) Design and use of a phage display library. Human antibodies with subnanomolar affinity against a marker of angiogenesis eluted from a two-dimensional gel. J Biol Chem 273: 21769–21776
131. Schliemann C, Neri D (2010) Antibody-based vascular tumor targeting. Recent Results Cancer Res 180:201–216
132. Nizak C, Monier S, del Nery E et al (2003) Recombinant antibodies to the small GTPase Rab6 as conformation sensors. Science 300:984–987
133. Gao J, Sidhu SS, Wells JA (2009) Two-state selection of conformation-specific antibodies. Proc Natl Acad Sci USA 106:3071–3076
134. Eisenhardt SU, Schwarz M, Bassler N, Peter K (2007) Subtractive single-chain antibody (scFv) phage-display: tailoring phage-display for high specificity against function-specific conformations of cell membrane molecules. Nat Protoc 2:3063–3073
135. Rothlisberger D, Pos KM, Pluckthun A (2004) An antibody library for stabilizing and crystallizing membrane proteins - selecting binders to the citrate carrier CitS. FEBS Lett 564:340–348
136. Uysal S, Vásquez V, Tereshko V et al (2009) Crystal structure of full-length KcsA in its closed conformation. Proc Natl Acad Sci USA 106:6644–6649
137. Ye JD, Tereshko V, Frederiksen JK et al (2008) Synthetic antibodies for specific recognition and crystallization of structured RNA. Proc Natl Acad Sci USA 105:82–87
138. Koldobskaya Y, Duguid EM, Shechner DM et al (2010) A portable RNA sequence whose recognition by a synthetic antibody facilitates structural determination. Nat Struct Mol Biol 18:100–106
139. Monigatti F, Gasteiger E, Bairoch A, Jung E (2002) The Sulfinator: predicting tyrosine sulfation sites in protein sequences. Bioinformatics 18:769–770
140. Kehoe JW, Velappan N, Walbolt M et al (2006) Using phage display to select antibodies recognizing post-translational modifications independently of sequence context. Mol Cell Proteomics 5:2350–2363
141. Thie H, Voedisch B, Dübel S et al (2009) Affinity maturation by phage display. Methods Mol Biol 525:309–322
142. Cadwell RC, Joyce GF (1994) Mutagenic PCR. PCR Methods Appl 3:S136–S140
143. Stemmer WP (1994) DNA shuffling by random fragmentation and reassembly: *in vitro* recombination for molecular evolution. Proc Natl Acad Sci USA 91:10747–10751
144. Fellouse FA, Wiesmann C, Sidhu SS (2004) Synthetic antibodies from a four-amino-acid code: a dominant role for tyrosine in antigen recognition. Proc Natl Acad Sci USA 101:12467–12472
145. Liang WC, Wu X, Peale FV et al (2006) Cross-species vascular endothelial growth factor (VEGF)-blocking antibodies completely inhibit the growth of human tumor xenografts and measure the contribution of stromal VEGF. J Biol Chem 281:951–961
146. Lee CV, Hymowitz SG, Wallweber HJ et al (2006) Synthetic anti-BR3 antibodies that mimic BAFF binding and target both human and murine B cells. Blood 108:3103–3111
147. Fagète S, Ravn U, Gueneau F et al (2009) Specificity tuning of antibody fragments to neutralize two human chemokines with a single agent. MAbs 1:288–296
148. Bostrom J, Yu SF, Kan D et al (2009) Variants of the antibody herceptin that interact with HER2 and VEGF at the antigen binding site. Science 323:1610–1614
149. Volk WA, Bizzini B, Snyder RM et al (1984) Neutralization of tetanus toxin by distinct monoclonal antibodies binding to multiple epitopes on the toxin molecule. Infect Immun 45:604–609
150. Zwick MB, Labrijn AF, Wang M et al (2001) Broadly neutralizing antibodies targeted to the membrane-proximal external region of human immunodeficiency virus type 1 glycoprotein gp41. J Virol 75:10892–10905
151. Cheson BD, Leonard JP (2008) Monoclonal antibody therapy for B-cell non-Hodgkin's lymphoma. N Eng J Med 359:613–626
152. de Kruif J, Logtenberg T (1996) Leucine zipper dimerized bivalent and bispecific scFv antibodies from a semi-synthetic antibody phage display library. J Biol Chem 271: 7630–7634

153. Thie H, Binius S, Schirrmann T et al (2009) Multimerization domains for antibody phage display and antibody production. New Biotechnol 26:314–321
154. Hudson PJ, Kortt AA (1999) High avidity scFv multimers; diabodies and triabodies. J Immunol Methods 231:177–189
155. Dübel S, Breitling F, Kontermann R et al (1995) Bifunctional and multimeric complexes of streptavidin fused to single chain antibodies (scFv). J Immunol Methods 178:201–209
156. Huang D, Shusta EV (2006) A yeast platform for the production of single-chain antibody-green fluorescent protein fusions. Appl Environ Microbiol 72:7748–7759
157. Hink MA, Griep RA, Borst JW et al (2000) Structural dynamics of green fluorescent protein alone and fused with a single chain Fv protein. J Biol Chem 275:17556–17560
158. Casey JL, Coley AM, Tilley LM et al (2000) Green fluorescent antibodies: novel in vitro tools. Protein Eng 13:445–452
159. Griep RA, van Twisk C, Kerschbaumer RJ et al (1999) pSKAP/S: an expression vector for the production of single-chain Fv alkaline phosphatase fusion proteins. Protein Expr Purif 16:63–69
160. Al-Mrabeh A, Ziegler A, Cowan G et al (2009) A fully recombinant ELISA using in vivo biotinyla.ted antibody fragments for the detection of potato leafroll virus. J Virol Methods 159:200–205
161. Predonzani A, Arnoldi F, Lopez-Requena A et al (2008) In vivo site-specific biotinylation of proteins within the secretory pathway using a single vector system. BMC Biotechnol 8:41
162. Warren DJ, Bjerner J, Paus E et al (2005) Use of an in vivo biotinylated single-chain antibody as capture reagent in an immunometric assay to decrease the incidence of interference from heterophilic antibodies. Clin Chem 51: 830–838
163. Cloutier SM, Couty S, Terskikh A et al (2000) Streptabody, a high avidity molecule made by tetramerization of in vivo biotinylated, phage display-selected scFv fragments on streptavidin. Mol Immunol 37:1067–1077
164. Moutel S et al (2009) A multi-Fc-species system for recombinant antibody production. BMC Biotechnol 9:14
165. Hu S, Shively L, Raubitschek A et al (1996) Minibody: a novel engineered anti-carcinoembryonic antigen antibody fragment (single-chain Fv-CH3) which exhibits rapid, high-level targeting of xenografts. Cancer Res 56:3055–3061
166. Gilliland LK, Norris NA, Marquardt H et al (1996) Rapid and reliable cloning of antibody variable regions and generation of recombinant single chain antibody fragments. Tissue Antigens 47:1–20
167. Shan D, Press OW, Tsu TT et al (1999) Characterization of scFv-Ig constructs generated from the anti-CD20 mAb 1F5 using linker peptides of varying lengths. J Immunol 162:6589–6595
168. Kontermann RE (2010) Alternative antibody formats. Curr Opin Mol Ther 12:176–183
169. Merchant AM, Zhu Z, Yuan JQ et al (1998) An efficient route to human bispecific IgG. Nat Biotechnol 16:677–681
170. Ridgway JB, Presta LG et al (1996) 'Knobs-into-holes' engineering of antibody CH3 domains for heavy chain heterodimerization. Protein Eng 9:617–621
171. Coloma MJ, Morrison SL (1997) Design and production of novel tetravalent bispecific antibodies. Nat Biotechnol 15:159–163
172. Dong J, Sereno A, Snyder WB et al (2011) Stable IgG-like bispecific antibodies directed toward the type I insulin-like growth factor receptor demonstrate enhanced ligand blockade and anti-tumor activity. J Biol Chem 286:4703–4717
173. Kortt AA, Dolezal O, Power BE et al (2001) Dimeric and trimeric antibodies: high avidity scFvs for cancer targeting. Biomol Eng 18: 95–108
174. Lawrence LJ, Kortt AA, Iliades P et al (1998) Orientation of antigen binding sites in dimeric and trimeric single chain Fv antibody fragments. FEBS Lett 425:479–484
175. Perisic O, Webb PA, Holliger P et al (1994) Crystal structure of a diabody, a bivalent antibody fragment. Structure 2:1217–1226
176. Atwell JL, Breheney KA, Lawrence LJ et al (1999) scFv multimers of the anti-neuraminidase antibody NC10: length of the linker between VH and VL domains dictates precisely the transition between diabodies and triabodies. Protein Eng 12: 597–604
177. Pei XY, Holliger P, Murzin AG et al (1997) The 2.0-A resolution crystal structure of a trimeric antibody fragment with noncognate VH-VL domain pairs shows a rearrangement of VH CDR3. Proc Natl Acad Sci USA 94:9637–9642
178. Le Gall F, Kipriyanov SM, Moldenhauer G et al (1999) Di-, tri- and tetrameric single chain Fv antibody fragments against human CD19: effect of valency on cell binding. FEBS Lett 453:164–168

179. Muller D, Kontermann RE (2010) Bispecific antibodies for cancer immunotherapy: current perspectives. BioDrugs 24:89–98
180. Beck A, Wagner-Rousset E, Bussat MC et al (2008) Trends in glycosylation, glycoanalysis and glycoengineering of therapeutic antibodies and Fc-fusion proteins. Curr Pharm Biotechnol 9:482–501
181. Presta LG (2008) Molecular engineering and design of therapeutic antibodies. Curr Opin Immunol 20:460–470
182. Hallborn J, Carlsson R (2002) Automated screening procedure for high-throughput generation of antibody fragments. Biotechniques Suppl, 30–37
183. Lou J, Marzari R, Verzillo V et al (2001) Antibodies in haystacks: how selection strategy influences the outcome of selection from molecular diversity libraries. J Immunol Methods 253:233–242
184. Kawe M, Forrer P, Amstutz P et al (2006) Isolation of intracellular proteinase inhibitors derived from designed ankyrin repeat proteins by genetic screening. J Biol Chem 281: 40252–40263
185. Glanville J, Zhai W, Berka J et al (2009) Precise determination of the diversity of a combinatorial antibody library gives insight into the human immunoglobulin repertoire. Proc Natl Acad Sci USA 106:20216–20221
186. Ravn U, Gueneau F, Baerlocher L et al (2010) By-passing in vitro screening-next generation sequencing technologies applied to antibody display and in silico candidate selection. Nucleic Acids Res 38:e193
187. Ge X, Mazor Y, Hunicke-Smith SP et al (2010) Rapid construction and characterization of synthetic antibody libraries without DNA amplification. Biotechnol Bioeng 106: 347–357
188. Fischer N (2011) Sequencing antibody repertoires: the next generation. MAbs 3: 17–20
189. Reddy ST, Ge X, Miklos AE et al (2010) Monoclonal antibodies isolated without screening by analyzing the variable-gene repertoire of plasma cells. Nat Biotechnol 28: 965–969
190. Zhang H, Torkamani A, Jones TM et al (2011) Phenotype-information-phenotype cycle for deconvolution of combinatorial antibody libraries selected against complex systems. Proc Natl Acad Sci USA 108: 13456–13461
191. Bordeaux J, Welsh A, Agarwal S et al (2010) Antibody validation. Biotechniques 48: 197–209
192. Pozner-Moulis S, Cregger M, Camp RL et al (2007) Antibody validation by quantitative analysis of protein expression using expression of Met in breast cancer as a model. Lab Invest 87:251–260
193. Grimsey NL, Goodfellow CE, Scotter EL et al (2008) Specific detection of CB1 receptors; cannabinoid CB1 receptor antibodies are not all created equal! J Neurosci Methods 171:78–86
194. Saper CB (2005) An open letter to our readers on the use of antibodies. J Comp Neurol 493:477–478

# Chapter 3

# Phage Display


## Konstantin Petropoulos



### Abstract

Phage display has emerged as one of the leading technologies for the selection and generation of highly specific antibodies, offering a number of advantages over traditional ways of antibody generation such as mouse hybridoma techniques. While there are various possibilities to conduct phage display, selection of antibodies via solution panning is an elegant way to circumvent conformation changes of antigen, which may arise when performing panning with antigen immobilized on a solid surface. Here, a standard solution panning procedure using a Fab based antibody library including primary screening for selectivity is described.



**Key words:** Antibody fragment, Phage display, Antibody library, Fab, Solution panning


## 1. Introduction

The healing potential of antibodies has first been described in the 1890s, when Emil von Behring and colleagues—despite the fact that the exact source of cure was still undiscovered then—were able to demonstrate the ability of immune serum to eliminate the effects of diphtheria toxin (1, 2). However, the real quest for monoclonal antibodies as potential therapeutics started to emerge more than 80 years later when Köhler and Milstein published their hallmark paper on the generation of hybridoma cells for the generation and secretion of specific antibodies in 1975 (3). Since then, a plethora of researchers has spent decades to invent, develop, and improve alternatives for the discovery and development of target specific antibodies by new techniques circumventing both animal hosts and hybridoma technology. Phage display as today's probably most abundantly applied new concept has first showed up in 1985 and was initially implemented in 1989/1990 (4, 5). Being the first molecular diversity selection platform, phage display has emerged to become one of the leading technologies for the discovery and identification of (fully human) antibodies out of


Gabriele Proetzel and Hilmar Ebersbach (eds.), *Antibody Methods and Protocols*, Methods in Molecular Biology, vol. 901, DOI 10.1007/978-1-61779-931-0_3, © Springer Science+Business Media, LLC 2012

libraries with several billion different clones, applicable for both academic research and drug discovery. Of note, this technology not only is limited to the screening of antibody libraries, but naturally can be extended to screening peptide, antibody fragment or other scaffold libraries as well. Besides phages, a variety of other display techniques have arisen in recent years such as ribosomal-, mRNA- or cell based display technologies with yeast as probably the most commonly applied one within cell based display systems. Still, most if not all display techniques harbor the same common features: genotypic diversity, genotype–phenotype coupling, selection pressure, and amplification (6). Within phage display technology for the selection of antibodies, applied libraries generally are differentiated between naïve and immune libraries. While naïve libraries are generated from healthy donors, the latter is derived from immunized donors. In addition, a variety of synthetic libraries has been generated, and the topic of library generation is extensively discussed in a number of excellent reviews in recent years, e.g., refs. 4, 6, 7. Nowadays, there is an additional range of synthetic libraries such as the human combinatorial antibody library (HuCAL), which are generated by several different techniques such as TRIM (trinucleotide-directed mutagenesis) or ligation-based strategy for chemical gene synthesis (8, 9), yet only few "ready to use" libraries are purchasable for academic research (e.g., libraries generated at UK based Medical Research Center, distribution via www.lifesciences.sourcebioscience.com). Centerpiece of phage display, however, is its ability to selectively enrich for target specific antibodies through several rounds of selection. There is an broad collection of methodologies available for the separation of binding from nonbinding clones with different variants of phage display which are described in detail elsewhere (e.g., refs. 4, 7, 10–12) and also see Chapters 4 and 5. Here, phage display using a Fab based antibody library applying the option of solution panning is presented. For additional information on library and vectors used in this chapter, please refer to ref. 13.

## 2. Materials

All solutions prepared should use ultrapure or double-distilled (deionized) water. Solutions and media should be autoclaved before use if not otherwise indicated. For this protocol, we used a phagemid vector based library harboring a chloramphenicol-resistance gene. Gene pIII and Fab heavy and light gene expression is inducible and regulated by an IPTG-inducible lac promoter region. All reagents should be stored as indicated; otherwise, storage at room temperature is recommended. Waste disposal regulations should be considered when disposing of waste materials.

### 2.1. Isolation of Antibody Fragments by Solution Panning with Biotinylated Antigen

#### 2.1.1. Blocking of Phage and Beads Prior to Selection

1. Antigen of interest, biotinylated.
2. 2× ChemiBLOCKER™ (e.g., Millipore, Billerica, MA, USA).
3. Tween20 (e.g., Merck KGaA, Darmstadt, Germany).
4. Streptavidin-coupled magnetic beads (e.g., Dynabeads® M-280 Streptavidin, Invitrogen, Paisley, UK).
5. Magnetic separator (e.g., Dynal®, Invitrogen, San Diego, CA, USA).
6. TG1 *E. coli* competent cells.
7. Phosphate buffered saline (1× PBS): 136 mM NaCl, 2.68 mM KCl, 8.1 mM $Na_2HPO_4$, 1.46 mM $KH_2PO_4$ in $H_2O$. This solution is also needed in subsequent chapters.
8. 2-YT medium: for 1 L of medium, add 31 g 2-YT dehydrated culture media (e.g., BD, Franklin Lakes, NJ, USA). This medium is needed in subsequent chapters.

#### 2.1.2. Selection Process: Binding of Phage to Specific Biotinylated Antigen and Bead Capture

1. Wash buffer: 1× PBS, 0.05% Tween20.
2. LB/Cam agar plates (small: 10 cm diameter/big: 15 cm diameter): 40 g of ready-to-use LB (Luria–Bertani), 24.4 mL of 40% glucose solution, and 1 mL of a chloramphenicol (Cam) stock solution (34 mg/mL) are added to a final volume of 1 L $H_2O$. The mixture is stirred by a magnetic rotator and heated to 70°C. After that, 25 and 50 mL are poured into small and big dishes, respectively, with subsequent drying at sterile conditions.
3. LB/Kan agar plates (small: 10 cm diameter): 40 g of ready-to-use LB (Luria Bertani), 24.4 mL of 40% glucose solution, and 1 mL of a kanamycin (Kan) stock solution (50 mg/mL) are added to a final volume of 1 L $H_2O$. Mixture is stirred by a magnetic rotator and heated to 70°C. After that, 25 mL is poured into small dishes with subsequent drying at sterile conditions.

#### 2.1.3. Elution of Selected Phage and Bacteria Infection

1. 100 mM Glycine–HCl, pH 2.2: 100 mM glycine, 0.5 M NaCl, in $H_2O$. After dissolving, adjust pH with 37% HCl from initial pH (~6.2) to 2.2. Do not autoclave, but include a sterile filtration step instead.
2. 2 M Tris base: add 2.42 g of Tris powder to $H_2O$ up to a final volume of 10 mL.
3. Sterile glass beads (e.g., Roth, Karlsruhe, Germany).
4. 70% Ethanol and 3% RBS 35 detergent for workbench cleaning.

#### 2.1.4. Recovery of Panning Output

1. Pasteur pipette (e.g., VWR, Radnor, PA, USA).
2. Freezing medium: 2-YT liquid medium containing final conc. 34 μg/mL chloramphenicol, 1% glucose, and 15% glycerol for

freezing of stock cultures. This medium will be needed in subsequent chapters.

3. 2-mL Microtubes (Sarstedt, Nuembrecht, Germany).
4. Growth medium: 2-YT liquid medium containing final conc. 34 μg/mL chloramphenicol and 1% glucose.

*2.1.5. Phage Production and Precipitation*

1. VCSM13 helper phage (e.g., Agilent Technologies, Santa Clara, CA, USA).
2. Induction medium #1: 2-YT liquid medium supplemented with 34 μg/mL chloramphenicol, 50 μg/mL kanamycin, and 0.25 mM IPTG final conc.
3. PEG/NaCl solution: 20% PEG 6000, 2.5 M NaCl in $H_2O$.

### 2.2. Subcloning of Selected Phages into Expression Vector

1. Mini DNA preparation kit (e.g., Qiagen, Hilden, Germany).
2. *Xba*I, *Eco*RI-HF, NEBuffer 4, BSA (New England BioLabs, Ipswich, MA, USA).
3. 10× Gel loading buffer (e.g., Invitrogen, San Diego, CA, USA).
4. DNA ladder (e.g., Thermo Scientific, Rockford, IL, USA).
5. Agarose (e.g., Invitrogen, San Diego, CA, USA).
6. T4 DNA ligase and ligase buffer (e.g., Invitrogen, San Diego, CA, USA).
7. 2-Butanol (e.g., Sigma-Aldrich, St. Louis, MO, USA).
8. 70% Ethanol.
9. Glycogen (Roche, Indianapolis, IN, USA).
10. *E. coli* competent cells (e.g., DH5α, Invitrogen, San Diego, CA, USA).
11. Electroporation system (e.g., Gene Pulser II, Bio-Rad, Hercules, CA, USA).
12. Electroporation cuvette (e.g., VWR, Radnor, PA, USA).
13. SOB medium: 2% (w/v) tryptone, 0.5% yeast extract, 10 mM NaCl, 2.5 mM KCl, 10 mM $MgCl_2$, 10 mM $MgSO_4$, in $H_2O$.

### 2.3. Preparation of Selection Plates for Subsequent Primary ELISA Screening

1. Toothpicks (autoclaved).
2. 96-Well microtiter plates, round bottom (e.g., Sigma-Aldrich, St. Louis, MO, USA).
3. Low glucose medium: 2-YT medium supplemented with 34 μg/mL chloramphenicol and 0.1% glucose.
4. Aluminum foil seal/gas-permeable foil seal (e.g., Thermo Scientific, Rockford, IL, USA).
5. Induction medium #2: 2-YT liquid medium supplemented with 34 μg/mL chloramphenicol, 50 μg/mL kanamycin, and 3 mM IPTG final conc.

6. BEL buffer: 24.7 g/L boric acid, 18.7 g/L NaCl, 1.4 g/L EDTA, pH 8.0, 2.5 mg/mL lysozyme (e.g., Roche, Indianapolis, IN, USA, add freshly before use), 12.5 U/mL Benzonase® (Merck KGaA, Darmstadt, Germany, add freshly before use).
7. Blocking buffer #1: 1× PBS, 12.5% (w/v) skim milk powder, 0.05% Tween20.

#### *2.4. Primary ELISA Screening*

1. NeutrAvidin 96-well coated plate (Thermo Scientific, Rockford, IL, USA).
2. Blocking buffer #2: 1× PBS, 5% (w/v) skim milk powder.
3. Incubation buffer #1: 1× PBS, 5% (w/v) skim milk powder, 0.05% Tween20.
4. Tris-buffered saline (1× TBS): 50 mM Tris, 150 mM NaCl in $H_2O$. Adjust pH to 7.4 with 37% HCl acidic solution (pH is temperature dependent).
5. Dilution buffer: 1× PBS, 0.5% skim milk powder, 0.05% Tween20.
6. AP labeled α-human Fab detection antibody (e.g., AbD Serotec, Oxford, UK).
7. AttoPhos® (Roche, Indianapolis, IN, USA).

## 3. Methods

#### *3.1. Isolation of Antibody Fragments by Solution Panning with Biotinylated Antigen*

##### *3.1.1. Blocking of Phage and Beads Prior to Selection*

A prerequisite for solution pannings is the biotinylation of respective antigen of choice as well as confirmation of retained activity of the biotinylated antigen. In general, biotinylation of an antigen can be achieved via a specific tag (e.g., Avitag™ (14, 15)) or by chemical or enzymatic biotinylation of reactive groups within the protein such as primary amines, sulfhydryls, carboxyls as well as carbonyls in case of glycosylated proteins. Apart from specific tags, the latter may even be best suited for phage display, as biotinylation of glycoepitopes will not interfere with functionality of nonglycosylated epitopes of the antigen, which in general are preferred for antibody selection. For a brief introduction on biotinylation, Thermo Scientific's educational webpage is recommended (16), for an excellent and in-depth overview of biotinylation techniques please refer to ref. 17 (see Note 1). The overall process is shown in Fig. 1.

1. Preblocking of library phage and beads (see Note 2).
   (a) Mix the required amount of phage of the respective library (recommended: covering 1,000-fold the diversity) with the same volume of 2× ChemiBLOCKER™ containing 0.1% Tween20 in a low binding 2 mL tube (the working

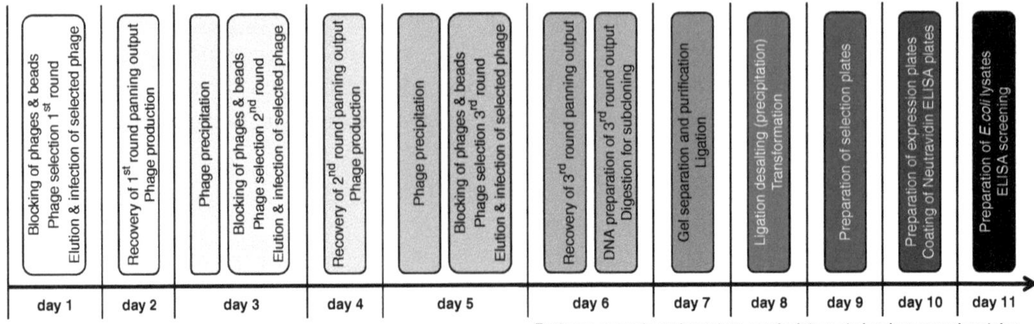


Fig. 1. Solution panning process overview: after three rounds of solution panning, DNA of third round panning output is extracted and subcloned into a respective expression vector. After transformation, selection plates, expression plates, and *E. coli* lysates are prepared for subsequent ELISA screening.

volume should not exceed 1.5 mL). Incubate for 2 h at room temperature on a rotator (see Note 3).

(b) Parallel to step a, prepare two tubes with 1 mg Streptavidin-coupled magnetic beads and one tube with 2 mg Streptavidin-coupled magnetic beads for each selection. Capture the beads for 5 min on a magnetic separator and remove the supernatant. Wash the beads three times with 1× PBS and resuspend the bead pellet of each tube in 200 μL 1× ChemiBLOCKER™. Incubate for 1 h at room temperature on a rotator to block the beads (see Note 4).

2. For each library panning, 15 mL 2-YT medium is inoculated with *E. coli* (e.g., TG1) in a phage-free working space. This *E. coli* culture later will be used for infection with the selected phage (step 2 in Subheading 3.1.3). Shake the culture at 250 rpm and 37°C until an $OD_{600nm}$ of 0.6–0.8 is reached. Keep *E. coli* on ice until required for infection with the eluted phage. Use a phage-free or disposable flask for *E. coli* incubation to avoid any contamination with library phage or helper phage (see Note 5).

3. Capture beads from step 1b for at least 3 min on a magnetic separator. Remove and discard the supernatant.

4. For a first preadsorption step, resuspend a pellet of 1 mg beads in the preblocked phage and incubate for 30 min at room temperature on a rotator (here, unspecific phage binding to the beads are removed).

5. Capture the beads with a magnetic separator as done before and transfer the phage containing supernatant into a new tube containing a pellet of 1 mg beads. Incubate for 30 min at room temperature on a rotator (= second preadsorption step). The phage samples are now preadsorbed and ready for selection.

*3.1.2. Selection Process: Binding of Phage to Specific Biotinylated Antigen and Bead Capture*

1. Mix the supernatant containing the preadsorbed phage samples with the biotinylated antigen in a new low binding 2-mL tube and incubate for 2 h at room temperature on a rotator (see Note 6).
2. Transfer the phage antigen mix to a new tube containing a pellet of 2 mg blocked beads and incubate for 10 min at room temperature on a rotator. Capture the beads with a magnetic separator for at least 3 min. Remove the supernatant carefully and discard it.
3. Wash the magnetic beads repeatedly with 1 mL wash buffer. In order to achieve considerable selectivity, at least five quick washes with subsequent discarding of the supernatant should be applied, followed by two steps of 5 min incubation with washing buffer. Make sure that for the 5 min washing steps phages are incubated on a rotator. End the washing procedure with three quick washing steps in 1 mL of 1× PBS in order to get rid of residual Tween20. In between the washing steps, capture the beads as described before, and remove and discard the supernatant carefully (see Note 7).
4. With the last washing step, transfer the suspension of magnetic beads with the captured antigen–phage complex into a fresh tube. Capture the beads as described before, and remove the supernatant carefully and discard it.

*3.1.3. Elution of Selected Phage and Bacteria Infection*

1. Elute selected phage by adding 300 μL of 100 mM glycine-HCl, pH 2.2 and incubate for 10 min at room temperature without shaking. Avoid prolonged incubation time in order to prevent reduced infection efficiency.
2. Collect the beads with a magnetic separator and transfer the eluate to a sterile 2-mL low binding tube. Add ~18 μL of a 2 M Tris base for neutralization and add the neutralized eluate to ~14 mL *E. coli* culture. If *E. coli* was stored on ice, it should be prewarmed to 37°C just prior to eluate addition. The phage tube used is flushed once with 300 μL 1× PBS and added to the *E. coli* culture. Incubate the *E. coli* culture for 45 min in a water bath at 37°C without shaking (see Note 8).
3. Determine the phage selection titer of each selection via spot titration (refer to Subheading 3.1.6). For spot-titration, remove 200 μL of infected cells into a separate tube prior to centrifugation. For a better workflow, spot titration should be performed later (after step 5). Centrifuge the remaining infected *E. coli* TG1 for 5 min at 4,000 ×*g* and 4°C.
4. Check the remaining uninfected *E. coli* TG1 culture for phage contamination by plating 50 μL on a small LB/Cam agar plate and 50 μL on a small LB/Kan agar plate. Incubate the agar plates overnight at 37°C (see Note 9).

5. Discard the supernatant (step 3) and resuspend each pellet in ~600 μL 2-YT medium. Plate the cell suspension evenly on 2–3 large LB/Cam agar plates using sterile glass beads or other devices applicable for bacteria plating (see Note 10). Incubate the large LB/Cam plates overnight at 30°C. If the colonies are still very small on the following morning, continue incubation at 37°C for 1–2 h.
6. Perform spot titration for the determination of the output titers (see Subheading 3.1.6). Clean working bench with 3% RBS solution and 70% EtOH.
7. (Next day) The output titer of each selection round is calculated from the colony forming units (cfu) on the spot titration agar plate prepared in step 3 the day before (see Note 7).

*3.1.4. Recovery of Panning Output*

1. (Next day) Scrape off the bacteria (which contain the selected phagemids) from each large selection agar plate with 3 mL freezing medium using a new, sterile Drygalski spatula (e.g., prepared from a Pasteur pipette). Collect the bacterial suspensions belonging to the same selection in a 15-mL disposable tube. Take care to prepare homogeneous bacteria suspensions.
2. Prepare 2–3 aliquots of each selection pool in 2-mL microtubes and keep on ice. For each antigen selection, inoculate 10 mL growth medium in a 50-mL disposable tube with 10–50 μL bacterial suspension from the bacterial suspension resulting in an $OD_{600nm} < 0.3$. Store the microtubes with the remaining bacteria suspension labeled correctly at −80°C (e.g., "yyyymmdd_panning output_antigen'x'_1st round output").
3. For the procedure after the last round of panning, refer to Subheading 3.2 step 1.
4. Incubate the cultures for 30–90 min at 37°C in a shaker at 250 rpm until an $OD_{600nm}$ of 0.5–0.6 is reached.

*3.1.5. Phage Production and Precipitation*

1. Transfer ~5 mL of the *E. coli* culture containing the selected phagemids (see Subheading 3.1.4) to a 13-mL disposable snap cap tube and add a proper amount of VCSM13 helper phage, equivalent to at least 4× 10E10 total units phage per 5 mL bacterial culture. Incubate for 30 min in a water bath at 37°C without shaking and then for 30 min at 37°C shaking at 250 rpm (see Note 11).
2. To check for helper phage infection, prepare 1:1,000 dilutions of the selection cultures before and after infection. Plate 30 μL of the dilutions each on a LB/Kan agar plate and incubate overnight at 37°C. It is not necessary to count the colonies, but a significant increase in the number of colonies after helper phage infection should be visible. In general, it takes ~48 h for the infected bacteria to grow on LB/Kan agar plates.
3. Spin down the bacteria at 4,000 × *g* for 5 min at 4°C and discard the helper phage containing supernatant. Add 1 mL

induction medium #1 to the pellet containing the infected bacteria in the snap cap tube and carefully resuspend the bacteria (see Note 12).

4. Transfer the culture to 19 mL induction medium #1 in a shake flask or 50-mL Falcon tube (= final volume of 20 mL). Ensure proper circulation of oxygen (e.g., by not closing but only loosely attaching the lid of the Falcon tube with tape) and incubate overnight at 22°C, shaking at 250 rpm (for 18–20 h).
5. (Next day) Spin down the bacteria from the overnight culture for 10 min at 4,000 × *g* at 4°C using a 50-mL disposable tube. Transfer the supernatant containing the Fab-presenting phage to a new 50-mL disposable tube and discard the bacterial pellet.
6. The cleared phage-containing supernatant should be purified and concentrated by a precipitation step as described next:
   (a) Add 5 mL chilled PEG/NaCl solution (precooled to −10°C) to the phage-containing supernatant, mix and incubate for at least 30 min on ice (see Note 13).
   (b) Spin down the precipitated phage for a minimum of 30 min at 12,000 × *g* and 4°C. Discard the supernatant and tap the tube on a stack of paper towels to remove residual PEG/NaCl. Allow to stand upside down on the paper towels for about 5 min.
   (c) Resuspend the phage pellet in 500–100 μL sterile 1× PBS and transfer the phage suspension to a sterile 1.5-mL reaction tube. Pellet residual bacterial debris at max. speed in a tabletop microcentrifuge for 2 min at room temperature and transfer the supernatant again into a new sterile 1.5-mL reaction tube.
   (d) Rotate the phage suspension for more than 30 min at 4°C to completely resolve the phage.
7. Determine the input phage titer for the next round of panning by spot titration (Subheading 3.1.6). Use a total phage input of at least 10E10 phages for the next panning round (see Note 14).
8. The number of total panning rounds may be chosen individually dependent on the size and quality of the applied library. We suggest three rounds of panning in order to ensure sufficient selectivity. More rounds are possible, yet at the caveat of increased amplification of a reduced number of selective clones (see Note 15).

#### 3.1.6. Spot Titration (for Determination of Input and Output Titer)

1. Dry a large LB/Cam agar plate (15 cm diameter) by preincubation of plate with open lid for ~2 h at 37°C in an incubator. The use of dry plates is essential. Perform all determinations in duplicates.
2. Add 40 μL 2-YT medium to wells A2–B8 of a 96-well round-bottom microtiter plate using a multichannel pipette

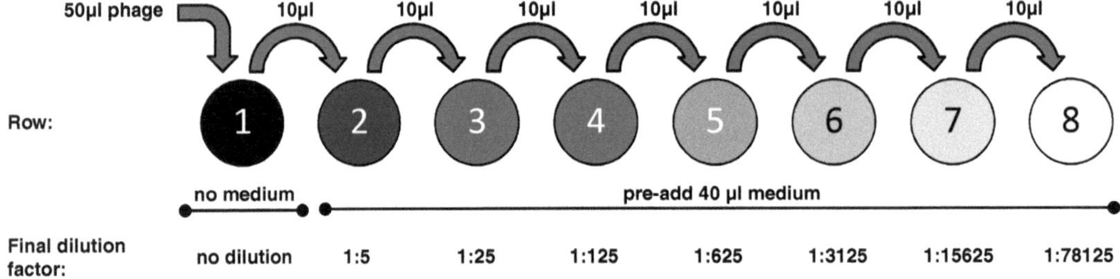


Fig. 2. Determination of panning output titer via spot titration: *rows 2–8* of a 96-well microtiter plate are prefilled with 40 μL medium. Fifty microliter bacterial suspension of panning output is added to *row 1* and 10 μL each is then transferred to the next row to generate a serial dilution covering a range from undiluted to roughly 1:80,000. For the determination of phage input titers, 1:10 dilutions from *row 2* to *12* are recommended.

(see Fig. 2). Add 50 μL of each bacterial suspension to wells A1 and B1, respectively, and perform a serial dilution by transferring 10 μL to the next row (A2–A8 and B2–B8) using a multichannel pipette (Fig. 2). Proceed until dilution number seven (wells A8–B8). Mix each well by pipetting the liquid up and down and change tips before each transfer.

3. Spot 5 μL from each well onto a dry large LB/Cam agar plate using a multichannel pipette. Incubate all plates overnight at 37°C.
4. (Next day) Count the colonies from those spots in which single colonies can clearly be identified (= less than 30 colonies per spot). Determine bacterial titer (bacteria/mL) according to the following equation:

$$\text{Panning input/output} = \text{counted colonies} \times 200 \times \text{dilution factor} \times \text{volume of bacterial suspension}$$

5. This protocol can also be used to determine the phage titer after phage precipitation: for this, make 1/10 dilution steps instead of 1/5 dilutions and include rows 9–12 in order to increase titration range.

### 3.2. Subcloning of Selected Phages into Expression Vector

While an initial ELISA screening is feasible with pIII fusion protein (10), we would highly recommend subcloning of the panning output into an expression vector system in which Fab is produced as soluble protein without being fused to pIII. Pool subcloning into an expression system prior to specific binding analysis offers the advantage that after specific binding analysis single positive hits are already in an appropriate format for further in-depth characterization or purification. In contrast, analysis within a display vector system would trigger subsequent cloning of a multitude of positive hits compared to a single pool subcloning step, thus significantly increasing work load. Within the vector system used herein the Fab encoding region is flanked by unique restriction sites and enables subcloning into an expression vector using *Xba*I and *Eco*RI restriction enzymes, but other digestion strategies may be needed when working with different phagemid vector systems.

1. After the last selection round of the panning procedure, scrape off the bacteria from each large selection agar plate with 3 mL freezing medium using a new, sterile Drygalski spatula. Collect the bacterial suspensions belonging to the same selection in a 15-mL disposable tube and prepare 1–2 mL aliquots of each selection pool in 2-mL microtubes. Keep aliquots on ice.
2. Determine the $OD_{600nm}$ of a 1:200 diluted bacterial suspension of each panning strategy. Calculate which volume equals the amount of bacteria contained in 1 mL of an $OD_{600nm}$ 12 suspension according to the equation below and use this volume for a DNA preparation. Store rest of the aliquots at –80°C (see Note 16).

$$V\,(\text{bacterial suspension})\,[\mu\text{L}] = \frac{\text{OD}_{600\text{nm}}\text{desired} \times 1{,}000\mu\text{L}}{\text{OD}_{600\text{nm}}(\text{bacterial suspension}) \times \text{dilution factor}}.$$

3. Wash the bacteria twice to remove the glycerol: add 2-YT medium for a final volume of ~1–2 mL, pellet the bacteria by centrifugation for 8 min at 4°C and 4,000 × *g* and discard the glycerol containing supernatant. Repeat washing with 2-YT a second time. Glycerol has to be removed as it may impair DNA preparation efficiency.
4. Perform two plasmid DNA preparations using a suitable DNA preparation kit according to instructor's manual. Determine the plasmid DNA concentration, e.g., by absorbance at 260 nm (see Note 17).
5. Digest 5 μg of the polyclonal DNA in a final volume of 200 μL with appropriate amounts of restriction enzymes *Eco*RI and *Xba*I according to Table 1a. Also digest 5 μg of the expression vector in a similar manner. It is advisable to use restriction enzymes from a supplier allowing a double digest. Digest for 2–3 h at 37°C. After the digestion incubation time, inactivate the restriction enzymes in the sample for 20 min at 65°C.
6. (Next day) Mix the digested samples with 20 μL 10× gel loading buffer and run with an appropriate DNA ladder on a preparative 1% agarose gel at about 10 V/cm gel distance (~2–3 h).
7. Cut out the bands of the digested Fab-encoding DNA and the expression vector. Extract DNAs from the agarose gel slice using an appropriate gel extraction kit and elute with 50 μL nuclease-free $H_2O$.
8. Quantify the eluted DNA samples on a 1% analytical agarose gel by loading a mix of 5 μL DNA, 4 μL $H_2O$, and 1 μL 10× gel

**Table 1**
**(a) Digestion setup. (b) Ligation setup. (c) Controls for ELISA screening**

| (a) Digestion | (b) Ligation | | |
|---|---|---|---|
| **5 mg DNA** | **Ligation** | **Vector BG ctrl.** | **Insert BG ctrl.** |
| 20 μL of 10× buffer 4 | 4 μL of 5× ligase buffer | 20 μL of 5× ligase buffer | 4 μL of 5× ligase buffer |
| 2 μL of 100× BSA | 1 μL of vector DNA (50 ng) | 1 μL of vector DNA (50 ng) | |
| 40 U *XbaI* | Insert DNA (5× molar excess to vector) | | Insert DNA (5× molar excess to vector) |
| 20 U *EcoRI-HF* | 1 μL T4 DNA ligase | 1 μL T4 DNA ligase | 1 μL T4 DNA ligase |
| $H_2O$ ad 200 μL | $H_2O$ ad 20 μL | $H_2O$ ad 200 μL | $H_2O$ ad 20 μL |

*BG: background*

**(c) Controls for ELISA screening**

| Well | Purpose | Coating | Primary antibody | Secondary antibody | Detection reagent |
|---|---|---|---|---|---|
| E12 | pos. ctrl | Control antigen | BEL of control antibody | α-Human Fab AP | AttoPhos® |
| F12 | Neg. ctrl | Antigen of interest | BEL of control antibody/ 1× PBS | α-Human Fab AP | |
| G12 | Neg. ctrl | Antigen of interest | BEL of control antibody/ 1× PBS | Dilution buffer | |
| H12 | Background | 1× PBS | BEL of control antibody | α-Human Fab AP | |

loading buffer. Also load 2 and 4 μL of an appropriate DNA ladder on the gel to estimate the amount of insert DNA. Separate the DNA by electrophoresis at 10 V/cm gel distance.

9. For ligation of the digested Fab-encoding fragment with the prepared expression vector fragment calculate ~5× molar excess of insert compared to vector and set up 20 μL ligations according to Table 1b. Include a negative control ligation without insert DNA to check the vector background, as high numbers of resulting clones might indicate only partially digested vector DNA or truncated plasmids. Ligate also insert without vector DNA to check for the presence of truncated plasmids.
10. Mix the calculated volume of sterile distilled water, vector, and DNA insert in a sterile 1.5-mL tube, heat to 56°C in a water bath for 10 min and cool to room temperature. Add temperature sensitive ligase buffer and ligase to the samples and incubate the ligation mix for at least 2 h at room temperature (or overnight at 16°C). Heat the reaction to 65°C for 10 min to inactivate ligase to improve the transformation efficiency.
11. (Next day) For preparation of the transformation, desalt the sample by precipitation:
    (a) Fill the ligation samples to 50 μL with sterile $H_2O$, add 500 μL 2-butanol and 1 μL glycogen, and incubate for at least 5 min at room temperature on a rotator. Spin down the precipitated DNA for 30 min at max. speed and 4°C in a tabletop centrifuge (at least 20,000 × *g*).
    (b) Carefully remove the supernatant (the pellet of precipitated DNA might be hardly visible). Add 500 μL 70% ethanol precooled to −20°C and spin for 15 min at max. speed and 4°C.
    (c) Carefully remove the ethanol and air-dry the DNA for about 15 min. Resuspend the precipitated DNA samples in 10 μL sterile $H_2O$ and incubate on a shaker for about 30 min at 37°C to ensure that the DNA got dissolved completely.
12. Transform competent *E. coli* cells (e.g., XL1-Blue or DH5α) with 5 μL desalted ligation sample. Perform transformation as follows (see Note 18):
    (a) Thaw competent cells on ice and precool electroporation cuvettes at −20°C. For each transformation sample, prewarm 950 μL SOB medium in a sterile 2 mL tube. Mix 5 μL of the ligated DNA sample with 45 μL competent cells and transfer the mixture into a chilled electroporation cuvette. Store the rest of the ligation at −20°C.
    (b) Dry the cuvette with a paper towel and perform electroporation as suggested by the manufacturer. Immediately after

electroporation, transfer the electroporated cells into prewarmed SOB medium and incubate for 1 h at 37°C shaking at ~750 rpm.

(c) Centrifuge the bacterial suspension for 5 min at 1,500 × *g*. Discard the supernatant and resuspend the pellet in 500–1,000 μL SOB medium.

13. Plate an appropriate volume of the transformation sample onto large LB/Cam agar plates to obtain single colonies. Incubate all plates overnight at 30°C (see Note 19).

### 3.3. Preparation of Selection Plates for Subsequent Primary ELISA Screening

1. (Next day) For each panning, prepare one round-bottom 96-well microtiter plate with 100 μL growth medium per well. Inoculate each well with a single colony picked from the LB/Cam agar plates prepared, e.g., using a sterile toothpick. Seal the inoculated microtiter plates with gas-permeable foil, put the lid on top and shake overnight at 400 rpm and 30°C. These plates will be the master plates (see Note 20).
2. (Next day) Prepare one round-bottom 96-well microtiter plate per master plate with 100 μL low glucose medium per well. These plates will be used for ELISA screening ("expression plates"). Carefully remove the gas-permeable seals from the master plates and inoculate each well of the expression plate with 5 μL from the corresponding well of the master plate (see Note 21). Add 100 μL 2-YT containing 30% glycerol to each well of the master plates, seal plates with aluminum foil and store master plates at –80°C (see Note 22).
3. Place a lid on the inoculated expression plates and shake at 30°C and 400 rpm until the cultures become slightly turbid (~2–4 h) with an $OD_{600nm}$ of ~0.5. Add 20 μL induction medium #2 to each well (final IPTG concentration is 0.5 mM). Seal the expression plates with gas-permeable foil, put a lid on top and shake overnight at 400 rpm and 22°C (see Note 23).
4. (Next day) Add 40 μL BEL buffer to each well of the expression plate and shake for 60 min at 400 rpm and 22°C to lyse the bacteria.
5. For a subsequent ELISA screening block the Fab-containing *E. coli* lysates by adding 40 μL blocking buffer #1 to each well and shake the expression plates for at least 30 min at 400 rpm and 22°C (see Note 24).

### 3.4. Primary ELISA Screening

1. For each panning, coat one NeutrAvidin plate with 100 μL antigen solution (e.g., diluted in 1× PBS) per well at a suited concentration of the biotinylated antigen. Do not coat well H12. Coat well E12 with a control antigen (refer to Table 1c).

Seal the plates with laminated foil and incubate overnight at 4°C (see Notes 25–28).

2. (Next day) Remove the antigen solution from the coated NeutrAvidin plate, wash wells once with 1× PBS containing 0.05% Tween20 and tap the plates on a stack of paper towels to remove residual buffer. Block NeutrAvidin plate with 400 μL blocking buffer #2 for 2 h at room temperature, shaking gently (see Note 29).
3. Rinse the blocked ELISA plates once with 1× PBS and tap them on a stack of paper towels to remove residual buffer. Transfer 100 μL of the blocked *E. coli* lysates (prepared as described in Subheading 3.3) from the expression plate to the corresponding well of the blocked NeutrAvidin plate. Transfer *E. coli* lysates of an irrelevant Fab or 100 μL 1× PBS to the negative control wells F12 and G12 (see Table 1c).
4. Incubate NeutrAvidin plate for 90 min at room temperature, shaking gently. Wash plate 5× quickly with wash buffer and tap it on a stack of paper towels to remove residual buffer.
5. Add 100 μL Fab specific secondary antibody (AP-labeled) diluted as proposed by the manufacturer in dilution buffer. Add 100 μL dilution buffer to well G12 (do not add antibody). Incubate 60 min at room temperature.
6. Wash the plate quickly, 5× with wash buffer and once with 1× TBS. Tap plate on a stack of paper towels to remove residual buffer. Add 100 μL AttoPhos® substrate to each well and measure fluorescence at an excitation of 440 ± 25 nm and an emission of 550 ± 35 nm. Full signal intensity is typically reached after 5–15 min at room temperature (see Note 30).
7. Check signals of controls (see Note 31):
   (a) Well E12: positive control for preparation of *E. coli* lysates and ELISA procedure.
   (b) Well F12: background of Fab detection antibody on screening antigen.
   (c) Well G12: background of AttoPhos® substrate on screening antigen.
   (d) Well H12: background of ELISA plate.
8. Determine the hit rate of the primary screenings. Positive signals should be at least 5× higher than background signal. Positive hits can then be selected from the respective position on the master plate and subjected to sequencing for CDR uniqueness, subsequent large scale expression and in-depth functional characterization.

## 4. Notes

1. Of utmost importance is an appropriate quality check of the biotinylated antigen. First parameter to be checked is the quantification of the extent of protein biotinylation in order to ensure proper selection of phage. If a portion of the antigen is not biotinylated, selection of specific phage on this percentage cannot be recovered and will be lost during this process. Second, activity of the protein should be checked and compared prior and after the biotinylation process, e.g., retained ligand/receptor binding or activation by ELISA or other means.
2. This protocol describes panning with a Fab-fragment based library. However, other library types such as scFv-based, scaffold-based, etc. may be applied as well.
3. In general, solutions of skim milk powder are often used as blocking solution; as skim milk powder may contain biotin contaminations, a biotin-free blocking solution is preferable. Phage might stick to the surface of tubes and may therefore be lost. This effect can be reduced by using either standard reaction tubes preblocked with 1× ChemiBLOCKER™ or siliconized, low binding tubes.
4. To deplete biotin binding clones, the Streptavidin-coupled beads intended for preadsorption may be coated with an irrelevant biotinylated protein.
5. For the selection of the *E. coli* strain, it is important to choose a strain harboring an F-pilus positive phenotype ($F^+$), as the presence of F-pili is required for phage infection.
6. In the first selection round, the final concentration of the biotinylated antigen should be in the range of ~100–500 nM, dependent on the library size and potency. If wanted, several antigen concentrations can be tested. If desired, the panning stringency can be increased by applying lower antigen concentrations.
7. The washing stringency of subsequent panning rounds can be adjusted according to the output titer of the previous selection round: in general, output titers (dependent on the input library) should range within 10E3–7 cfu; For output titers >10E7 cfu, number and duration of individual washing steps can be adjusted in the subsequent selection round for a more stringent selection.
8. Previous to step 2, the pH of a glycine–Tris mixture (300 μL glycine and 18 μL Tris base) should be checked for neutral pH, e.g., by pH indicator strips. Avoid prolonged incubation (60–90 min) of cells on ice to prevent reduced efficiency of *E. coli.*

9. Within this experimental setup described, the used library phages harbor a chloramphenicol resistance, while the helper phage VSCM13 helper phages inherit the kanamycin resistance gen. If other antibiotic resistances are used, caution has to be taken with regard to correct use of antibiotics within the used agar plates.
10. Do not use more than ~20 glass beads, as increased amount of glass beads may decrease panning output.
11. For phage production the *E. coli* TG1 carrying the selected phagemids are infected with helper phage which supply all the proteins required for complete assembly of functional phage.
12. The induction medium must not contain glucose which would inhibit the IPTG-induced Fab expression.
13. Usually clouds of precipitating phage become visible after the incubation step on ice.
14. Alternatively, input phage titers can be determined at the same day via measuring the optical density of phages' ssDNA at 268 nm ($OD_{268nm}$). For that, at least 1:10 dilutions of the phage preparations are measured at a respective spectrophotometer devise (e.g., NanoDrop). An $OD_{268nm}$ of 1 equals approximately 5× 10E12 colony forming units/mL (cfu/mL; (18)).
15. Despite preadsorption steps of phages with preblocked beads (refer to Subheading 3.1.1), it may still occur that Streptavidin specific phages are selected and enriched. Additional efforts to circumvent this can be done by applying panning strategies with alternating panning rounds, e.g., solution panning as described within this article in round one and three, while the second panning round can be performed with biotinylated antigen coated on preblocked NeutrAvidin plates.
16. Example: the 1:200 diluted bacterial suspension has an $OD_{600nm}$ of 0.5.

$$V(\text{bacterial suspension})[\mu\text{L}] = \frac{12 \times 1{,}000\mu\text{L}}{0.5 \times 200} = 120\mu\text{L}.$$

    Use 120 μL of the undiluted bacterial suspension for each DNA preparation.
17. When using a DNA preparation kit, try to use a kit which enables removal of endA nuclease, as this might be contained in plasmid preparations from TG1 cells and thus degradation of the DNA is avoided.
18. DH5α *E. coli* cells do not require IPTG to induce expression from the lac promoter even though the strain expresses the Lac repressor, as the copy number of most plasmids exceeds the repressor number in the cells. If you are concerned about

obtaining maximal levels of expression, add IPTG to a final concentration of 1 mM.

19. It is advisable to plate different volumes between 50 and 500 μL which should provide enough single colonies for picking the next day. In order to avoid mixed clones expressing more than one Fab, a second transformation step with diluted DNA from the subcloned phage pool may be performed (e.g., 1:10,000 of initial expression vector pool DNA preparation; for a 1:10,000 dilution, perform a step-wise dilution, e.g., 1 μL in 99 μL $H_2O$, from this dilution take 10 μL in 990 μL $H_2O$).
20. Covering the plates with a lid during overnight incubation is important to reduce evaporation.
21. For 96-well screening, inoculate wells E12 and H12 with a control clone, which will serve as screening control. For ELISA negative controls, inoculate the medium in wells F12 and G12 with an irrelevant Fab, which does not bind to the screening antigen, or leave these wells empty.
22. Do not store master plates at 4°C. Avoid multiple freezing and thawing of master plates, as this will result in a lower number of growing clones after ~3–4 freezing and thawing cycles.
23. Remember to coat plates for the subsequent ELISA screening as described in the following chapter.
24. Screening in 384-well format is possible; however, in this case automated setup would be preferable.
25. Black NeutrAvidin plates are recommended with fluorogenic substrates to avoid signal cross talk between the wells.
26. Counter screening for biotin-specific hits is advisable, as biotin-specific hits would also display positivity in the primary ELISA screening: for that, irrelevant biotinylated protein should be coated at a suited concentration on a MaxiSorp™ plate to allow biotin-specific hits to bind to biotin molecules of the irrelevant protein. Hits positive in both antigen specific and irrelevant antigen ELISAs should be deselected.
27. Start coating of the ELISA plates 1 day before you are ready with the BEL lysate expression plates, then you can omit freezing expression plates. Refreezing expression plates several times may lead to reduced signal intensities in the ELISA. For antigen concentration and coating buffer selection, a coating check ELISA should be performed before pannings. Usually a concentration of 5 μg/mL antigen and 1× PBS as coating buffer is acceptable.
28. If the conformation of the antigen relies on antigen-stabilizing ions such as $Ca^{2+}$, $Mg^{2+}$, or $Mn^{2+}$ and if these ions were therefore added for the panning, they should also be added to all buffers during the Fab screenings.

29. 1× PBS within the wash buffer might be replaced by 1× TBS if phosphate sensitivity is an issue.
30. Alternatively, Fab detection can be performed using α-human Fab-HRP conjugate with Quantablue (excitation: 320 ± 25 nm, emission: 430 ± 35 nm) or with BM Blue Soluble Peroxidase substrate (absorption: 370 nm).
31. Alternatively, well E12 may also be coated with antigen of interest and detected with a primary specific control antibody. If so, an additional Fab expression check of all picked clones is recommended for verification of Fab expression in *E. coli* lysates using for example an Fd specific anti-human IgG as coating antigen.

## References


1. Lindenmann J (1984) Senior overviews. Scand J Immunol 19:281–285
2. Emil von Behring – Biography. Nobelprize.org. http://www.nobeprize.org/nobel_prizes/medicine/laureates/1901/behring.html. Accessed 16 Feb 2012
3. Kohler G, Milstein C (1975) Continuous cultures of fused cells secreting antibody of predefined specificity. Nature 256:495–497
4. Bradbury AR, Sidhu S, Dubel S, McCafferty J (2011) Beyond natural antibodies: the power of in vitro display technologies. Nat Biotechnol 29:245–254
5. Smith GP (1985) Filamentous fusion phage: novel expression vectors that display cloned antigens on the virion surface. Science 228:1315–1317
6. Bradbury AR, Marks JD (2004) Antibodies from phage antibody libraries. J Immunol Methods 290:29–49
7. Hoogenboom HR (2002) Overview of antibody phage-display technology and its applications. Methods Mol Biol 178:1–37
8. Knappik A, Ge L, Honegger A et al (2000) Fully synthetic human combinatorial antibody libraries (HuCAL) based on modular consensus frameworks and CDRs randomized with trinucleotides. J Mol Biol 296:57–86
9. Van den Brulle J, Fischer M, Langmann T et al (2008) A novel solid phase technology for high-throughput gene synthesis. Biotechniques 45:340–343
10. Burton DR, Scott JK, Silverman GJ (2001) Phage display. Cold Spring Harbor Laboratory Press, Cold Spring Harbor, NY, USA
11. Finlay WJ, Bloom L, Cunningham O (2011) Optimized generation of high-affinity, high-specificity single-chain Fv antibodies from multiantigen immunized chickens. Methods Mol Biol 681:87–101
12. Kotlan B, Glassy MC (2009) Antibody phage display: overview of a powerful technology that has quickly translated to the clinic. Methods Mol Biol 562:1–15
13. Rothe C, Urlinger S, Lohning C et al (2008) The human combinatorial antibody library HuCAL GOLD combines diversification of all six CDRs according to the natural immune system with a novel display method for efficient selection of high-affinity antibodies. J Mol Biol 376:1182–1200
14. Løset GÅ, Bogen B, Sandlie I (2011) Expanding the versatility of phage display I: efficient display of peptide-tags on protein VII of the filamentous phage. PLoS One 6(2):e14702
15. Barat B, Wu AM (2007) Metabolic biotinylation of recombinant antibody by biotin ligase retained in the endoplasmic reticulum. Biomol Eng 24:283–291
16. Thermo Scientific Avidin-Biotin Technical Handbook (2009) http://www.piercenet.com/browse.cfm?fldID=84EBE112-F871-4CA5-807F-47327153CFCB
17. Hermanson GT (2008) Bioconjugate techniques, 2nd edn. Academic, New York, NY
18. Clackson T, Lowman HB (2004) Phage display: a practical approach. Oxford University Press, Oxford

# Chapter 4

# Generation of Human Fab Libraries for Phage Display

Christoph Rader


## Abstract

This protocol describes the generation of human antibody libraries in Fab format from $2.5 \times 10^7$ human peripheral blood or bone marrow mononuclear cells for their subsequent selection by phage display. Although it can be applied to the mining of both human naïve and immune antibody repertoires, the procedure is primarily intended for the generation of fully human monoclonal antibodies from patients with endogenous antibody responses of interest and limited availability of clinical specimens.


**Key words:** Immune antibody repertoires, Antibody fragment, Antibody libraries, Fab, Human monoclonal antibodies, Library, Phage display, Phagemid

## 1. Introduction

Monoclonal antibodies (mAbs) are pharmaceuticals of rising importance for the treatment and prevention of cancer, inflammatory diseases, and infectious diseases. Thus far, 32 mAbs have received regulatory approval by the Food and Drug Administration (FDA) in the United States (for a current list, see www.landesbioscience.com/journals/mabs/about). Of these, nine mAbs have sequences that are direct or indirect products of the human genome. These mAbs, referred to as human mAbs, are ideally undetectable by the patient's immune system as they cannot be distinguished from endogenous human antibodies. Flying under the radar of the immune system, human mAbs can be administered repeatedly which is an important advantage over nonhuman mAbs, in particular in chronic diseases that require continual dosing over extended periods of time.

Employing a variety of strategies, human mAbs have been generated from naïve, immune, and synthetic antibody repertoires. In particular, immune repertoires provide a potentially rich source for human mAbs that has not been fully exploited yet. Mining strategies

Gabriele Proetzel and Hilmar Ebersbach (eds.), *Antibody Methods and Protocols*, Methods in Molecular Biology, vol. 901,
DOI 10.1007/978-1-61779-931-0_4, © Springer Science+Business Media, LLC 2012

can be divided into noncombinatorial methods that preserve endogenous heavy and light chain pairs and combinatorial methods that randomly combine heavy and light chains (1). A key concept of combinatorial methods is the selection of antibody libraries by display technologies that physically link a displayed antibody fragment to its cDNA in a defined particle such as a filamentous phage, a ribosome, or a cell. Particles that display antibody fragments to an antigen or an antigen assembly of interest are selected by various panning procedures. Importantly, the physical linkage of phenotype and genotype links recognition and replication, enabling multiple rounds of selection.

Phage display is the most robust and versatile display technology for mining human antibody repertoires. It can be conducted in laboratories with standard molecular biology equipment and expertise. The particle that facilitates the physical linkage of antibody fragment and its cDNA is a filamentous bacteriophage such as M13. M13 features a single-stranded DNA that is encapsulated by a protein core consisting of major coat protein pVIII and minor coat proteins such as pIII (2). Antibody fragments can be recombinantly fused to these coat proteins without impairing the physical and functional integrity of phage (3). The most common display formats are human scFv or Fab fused to the N terminus of either wild-type pIII or a C-terminal fragment of pIII. A system of choice (4) for the selection of human mAbs with high affinity is monovalent human Fab display through a C-terminal fragment of pIII. This system is based on (1) the cloning of a *phagemid library* that encodes a human Fab repertoire recombinantly fused to a C-terminal fragment of pIII, (2) its transformation into *Escherichia coli* with only one phagemid clone persisting in each cell after proliferation, and (3) the infection of transformed *E. coli* with helper phage leading to the assembly of one phage clone in each cell with matching genotype and phenotype. The resulting *phage library* can now be subjected to panning against immobilized antigens, antigens in solution, or more complex antigen assemblies such as viruses or cells. In the recognition phase, each panning round comprises binding, washing, and elution steps. In the replication phase, *E. coli* is infected with eluted phage followed by helper phage. Phage displaying Fab with high affinity for the antigen or antigen assembly of interest are highly enriched after three to five panning rounds. In addition to Fab, scFv and other antibody fragments have been successfully selected in this system. However, due to the aggregation tendency of other antibody fragments, Fab has remained a format of choice for the selection of monovalent affinity rather than multivalent avidity. In addition, based on its natural assembly of light chain and heavy chain fragment, the Fab format is more reliable than other formats of antibody fragments for subsequent conversion to IgG with preserved antigen binding properties. This protocol is based on phagemid pC3C which we designed to facilitate the generation and selection of Fab libraries with human constant domains (Fig. 1) (5).

Antibody light and heavy chain mRNA in human B cells from bone marrow or peripheral blood is the principle ingredient of human antibody libraries. Whereas B cells in secondary lymphoid tissues such as spleen, lymph nodes, and tonsils, all of which are of limited accessibility and availability in humans, are a confined source of immune antibody repertoires, B cells from bone marrow and peripheral blood represent both naïve and immune antibody repertoires (1). Immune antibody repertoires are largely defined by the pool of postgerminal center B cells, plasma blasts, plasma cells, and memory B cells. The mRNA of these B cells is a preferred template for human antibody libraries because it encodes antibodies that have undergone stringent selection and affinity maturation in vivo, resulting in high specificity and affinity. Another consideration is the abundance of antibody light and heavy chain mRNA in plasma cells which mainly reside in the bone marrow. This abundance can lead to a greater representation in antibody libraries and may or may not be a desired bias depending on the natural history of the antibody response that is subject to human mAb mining. Accordingly, total RNA from bone marrow mononuclear cells (BMMC) is considered a preferred source for mining secondary antibody responses and total RNA from peripheral blood mononuclear cells (PBMC) a preferred source for mining primary antibody responses. This protocol was written for the mining of immune antibody repertoires from individual or small cohorts of human subjects with endogenous antibody responses of interest. In a starting material of $2.5 \times 10^7$ PBMC or BMMC, one can expect at least $1 \times 10^6$ different light and heavy chains which, after random combination, can yield $1 \times 10^{12}$ different antibodies. The protocol aims for an antibody library that consists of $10^8$–$10^9$ independent transformants, thus only representing a fraction of the theoretical complexity and favoring the selection of original light and heavy chain pairs of antibodies that dominate the endogenous antibody response of interest.

The mining of endogenous antibody responses provides a concerted antibody and antigen discovery platform that may lead to new diagnostic, preventative, and therapeutic reagents. For example, we applied this protocol to the generation and selection of an antibody library from peripheral B cells of a chronic lymphocytic leukemia patient who revealed an endogenous antitumor antibody response following allogeneic hematopoietic stem cell transplantation (alloHSCT) (6). Several human mAbs directed to a tumor cell surface antigen were selected from this post-alloHSCT antibody library. The same protocol can be applied to the generation of human mAbs from patients treated with other regimens that trigger endogenous antibody responses such as vaccines or immunomodulatory drugs. The protocol also facilitates the mining of

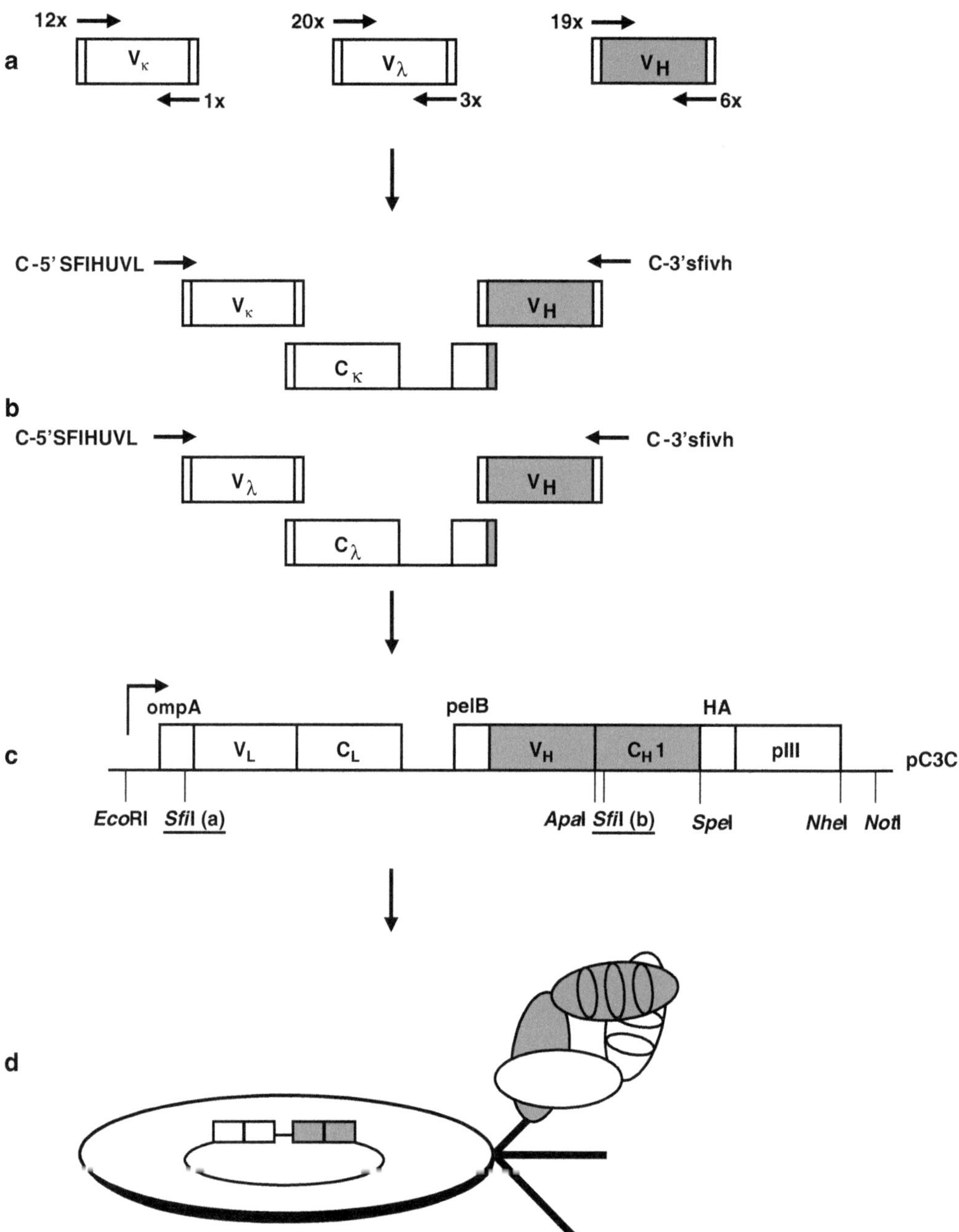


Fig. 1. Generation of a human Fab library in phagemid pC3C. (**a**) Amplification of human variable domains by RT-PCR. The numbers of sense and antisense primers for amplification of Vκ (*white*), Vλ (*white*), and VH (*gray*) encoding sequences are shown. A total of 186 separate amplifications are carried out. (**b**) Assembly of Vκ/Cκ/VH and Vλ/Cλ/VH expression cassettes by overlap extension PCR. (**c**) Asymmetric *Sfi*I sites labeled as "(a)" and "(b)" facilitate the cloning of the VL/CL/VH expression cassette into phagemid pC3C. The design of pC3C (5) is based on phagemids from the pComb3 series (4, 12). A single lacZ promoter drives the synthesis of a dicistronic transcript. Two ribosome binding sites initiate the translation of two separate polypeptide chains, light chain VL-CL (*white*) and heavy chain fragment VH-CH1 (*gray*) fused to a hemagglutinin (HA) decapeptide and the C-terminal pIII protein domain; pIII is the minor coat protein of filamentous phage which is displayed in low copy number at one end of the phage. Through leader peptides ompA and pelB, both polypeptides are transported to the periplasm of *E. coli*, where they associate and form a natural interchain disulfide bridge at their

endogenous antibody responses to autoantigens or infectious agents. The only requirement is access to clinical specimens, commonly blood or bone marrow.

## 2. Materials

All steps in this protocols can be successfully executed in a laboratory with standard molecular and cell biology equipment, including autoclave, Bunsen burner, digital balance with 0.01 g readability, Erlenmeyer flasks (250 mL and 2 L), freezers (–20 and –80°C), freezing container (e.g., Nalgene, www.nalgenelabware.com), glass bottles (500 mL and 1 L), heat blocks (50, 65, and 85°C), hemocytometer (e.g., Hausser Scientific, www.hausserscientific.com), incubator (37°C; e.g., VWR Signature General Purpose Incubator, www.vwr.com), laminar flow hood, light microscope, liquid nitrogen tank with cryoboxes, microfuge (e.g., Eppendorf 5415D, www.eppendorf.com), microwave oven, power supply for agarose gel electrophoresis (e.g., EC 105 Compact Power Supply, Owl Separation Systems, www.owlsci.com), razor blades, refrigerated benchtop centrifuge with swinging bucket rotor and microplate carriers (e.g., Sorvall Legend RT, Thermo Scientific, www.thermoscientific.com), refrigerated microfuge (e.g., Eppendorf 5417R), refrigerated floor centrifuge (e.g., Sorvall Evolution RC, Thermo Scientific) with fixed-angle rotor (e.g., Sorvall SLA-3000 Super-Lite, Thermo Scientific) for 500-mL centrifuge bottles (e.g., Sorvall Dry-Spin Polypropylene Bottles, Fisher Scientific, www.fishersci.com, cat. no. 50-866-922), refrigerator (4°C), Savant SpeedVac concentrator (Thermo Scientific), single-channel and multichannel micropipettes (1–1,000 μL), shaker (e.g., Innova 4000 Benchtop Incubator Shaker, New Brunswick Scientific, www.nbsc.com; two separate shakers, one for phage-free conditions and one for phage are required), UV photometer (e.g., Eppendorf BioPhotometer), vortexer, water bath (70°C), and 96-well thermocyclers (e.g., GeneAmp PCR System 9700; Life Technologies, Applied Biosystems). General disposables such as blood collection tubes (10 mL) and syringes (20 mL) with anticoagulant, centrifuge tubes (15 and 50 mL), cryovials (2 mL), filtered 10 μL,

Fig. 1. (continued) C termini. Addition of helper phage leads to the incorporation of the fusion protein into phage particles (**d**) that display one Fab copy linked to the phage surface by the C-terminal pIII protein domain as their phenotype and, as their genotype, contain the corresponding single-stranded phagemid that encodes the Fab. The six complementarity determining regions (CDRs) of the Fab, three provided by each variable domain, are shown as ovals. Phagemid pC3C was designed to facilitate the cloning of Fab libraries through a VL/CL/VH expression cassette that can be efficiently assembled in one step by overlap extension PCR. *SpeI/NheI* self-ligation of pC3C removes both HA and pIII and results in the expression of soluble Fab which can be enhanced by addition of isopropyl-β-D-thiogalactoside (IPTG).

20 μL, 100 μL, 200 μL, 1 mL pipette tips (e.g., ART, Molecular BioProducts, www.mbpinc.com), 0.22 μm filters (e.g., Millex GP from Millipore, www.millipore.com), microfuge tubes (1.5 and 2 mL), and pipettes (5 mL) are not specially listed. It is recommended to use highly purified water from, e.g., a Picopure 2 UV Plus system (Hydro Service and Supplies, www.hydroservice.com) sterilized by filtration (e.g., Millipore Steriflip Filter Units, cat. no. SCGP00525) and stored at room temperature (RT).

### 2.1. PBMC and BMMC Preparation

1. 50 mL whole blood or 20 mL aspirated bone marrow fluid and cells from human (see Note 1).
2. Phosphate-buffered saline (PBS): 5.6 mM $Na_2HPO_4$, 154 mM NaCl, 1.06 mM $KH_2PO_4$, pH 7.4; diluted in water from 10× PBS (Quality Biological, Gaithersburg, MD, USA, www.quality biological.com, cat. no. 119-069-101); store at RT.
3. Lymphocyte Separation Medium (Lonza, Basel, Switzerland, www.lonza.com, cat. no. 17-829E); store at RT.
4. *(Optional)* ACK Lysing Buffer (Lonza, cat. no. 10-548E); store at RT.
5. Trypan Blue (Lonza, cat. no. 17-942E); store at RT.
6. Recovery Cell Culture Freezing Medium (Life Technologies, Carlsbad, CA, USA, www.invitrogen.com, cat. no. 12648010); store at −20°C.
7. Isopropanol (Sigma-Aldrich, St. Louis, MO, USA, www. sigmaaldrich.com, cat. no. I9516); store at RT.

### 2.2. Total RNA Preparation

1. Fresh or cryopreserved human mononuclear cells (see Subheading 3.1 and Note 1).
2. RNase-free centrifuge tubes (15 and 50 mL).
3. RNase-free 1.5-mL microfuge tubes (e.g., Eppendorf, cat. no. 022600028).
4. PBS (see Subheading 2.1).
5. Trypan Blue (see Subheading 2.1).
6. TRI reagent (Molecular Research Center, Cincinnati, OH, USA, www.mrcgene.com, cat. no. TR 118); store at 4°C.
7. 1-Bromo-3-chloro-propane (BCP; Molecular Research Center, cat. no. BP 151); store at RT.
8. Isopropanol (see Subheading 2.1).
9. For 70% (vol/vol) ethanol, mix 15 mL ethanol (Sigma-Aldrich, cat. no. E7023; store at RT) with 35 mL RNase-free water (Life Technologies, cat. no. AM9906; store at RT) in a 50-mL RNase-free centrifuge tube. Store at RT.
10. RNA Storage Solution [1 mM sodium citrate (pH 6.4), Life Technologies, cat. no. AM7000]; store at−20°C.

11. *(Optional)* Qiagen RNeasy MinElute Cleanup Kit (Qiagen, Hilden, Germany, www.qiagen.com, cat. no. 74204); store at RT.
12. *(Optional)* RNase-free 7.5 M LiCl (Life Technologies, cat. no. AM9480); store at RT.
13. RNase-free 3 M sodium acetate (pH 5.5) (Life Technologies, cat. no. AM9740); store at RT.

### 2.3. RT-PCR Amplification of VH and VL cDNA

1. RNase-free 1.5-mL microfuge tubes (see Subheading 2.2).
2. RNase-free water (see Subheading 2.2).
3. SuperScript III First-Strand Synthesis System for RT-PCR (Life Technologies, cat. no. 18080-051) containing 50 μM oligo(dT), 10 mM dNTP mix, 10× RT buffer [200 mM Tris–HCl (pH 8.4), 500 mM KCl], 25 mM $MgCl_2$, 100 mM DTT, 40 U/μL RNaseOUT, 200 U/μL SuperScript III RT, and 2 U/μL *E. coli* RNase H; store at −20°C.
4. 3 M Sodium acetate (pH 5.2) (Quality Biological, cat. no. 351-035-721); store at RT.
5. Ethanol (see Subheading 2.2).
6. 0.2-mL PCR tubes (e.g., Eppendorf, cat. no. 951010022)
7. Sense and antisense primers diluted to 20 μM in water (Table 1).
8. 5 U/μL Taq DNA polymerase, 10× Taq buffer with $(NH_4)_2SO_4$, and 25 mM $MgCl_2$ (Fermentas, Glen Burnie, Maryland, USA, www.fermentas.com, cat. no. EP0072); store at −20°C.
9. 10 mM dNTP mix: 2.5 mM of each dATP, dCTP, dGTP, and dTTP diluted in water from 100 mM stock concentrations (GE Healthcare, Pittsburgh, PA, USA, www.gelifesciences.com, cat. no. 28-4065-52); store at −20°C.
10. 6× Gel loading dye solution (Fermentas, cat. no. R0611); store at RT.
11. Model D2 Spider Wide Gel Electrophoresis System with two D1-20C combs (Owl Separation Systems).
12. Agarose (Life Technologies, cat. no. 16500500); store at RT.
13. TAE buffer [40 mM Tris-acetate (pH 8.0), 1 mM EDTA; diluted in water from 50× TAE] (Quality Biological, cat. no. 351-008-131); store at RT.
14. SYBR Safe DNA gel stain (Life Technologies, cat. no. S33102); store at RT.
15. 100-bp DNA ladder (Fermentas, cat. no. SM0243); store at RT.
16. Safe Imager blue-light transilluminator (Life Technologies).
17. Model B1A EasyCast Mini Gel Electrophoresis System with preparative combs (Owl Separation Systems).

**Table 1**
**Primer sequences**

| Name | Sequence |
|---|---|
| *VH sense primers (19)* | |
| HUVH1A | GCTGCCCAACCAGCCATGGCCCAGGTGCAGCTGGTGCAGTCTGG |
| HUVH1B | GCTGCCCAACCAGCCATGGCCCAGGTYCAGCTKGTGCAGTCTGG |
| HUVH1C | GCTGCCCAACCAGCCATGGCCCAGGTCCAGCTGGTACAGTCTGG |
| HUVH1D | GCTGCCCAACCAGCCATGGCCCARATGCAGCTGGTGCAGTCTGG |
| HUVH1E | GCTGCCCAACCAGCCATGGCCCAGGTSCAGCTGGTGCARTCTGG |
| HUVH2A | GCTGCCCAACCAGCCATGGCCCAGRTCACCTTGAAGGAGTCTGG |
| HUVH2B | GCTGCCCAACCAGCCATGGCCCAGGTCACCTTGAGGGAGTCTGG |
| HUVH3A | GCTGCCCAACCAGCCATGGCCSAGGTGCAGCTGGTGGAGTCTGG |
| HUVH3B | GCTGCCCAACCAGCCATGGCCGAGGTGCAGCTGTTGGAGTCTGG |
| HUVH3C | GCTGCCCAACCAGCCATGGCCGAGGTGCAGCTGGTGGAGWCYGG |
| HUVH3D | GCTGCCCAACCAGCCATGGCCGAAGTGCAGCTGGTGGAGTCTGG |
| HUVH3E | GCTGCCCAACCAGCCATGGCCCAGGTACAGCTGGTGGAGTCTGG |
| HUVH4A | GCTGCCCAACCAGCCATGGCCCAGSTGCAGCTGCAGGAGTCGGG |
| HUVH4B | GCTGCCCAACCAGCCATGGCCCAGGTGCAGCTACAGCAGTGGGG |
| HUVH4C | GCTGCCCAACCAGCCATGGCCCAGCTGCAGCTGCAGGAGTCCGG |
| HUVH4D | GCTGCCCAACCAGCCATGGCCCAGGTGCAGCTACAACAGTGGGG |
| HUVH5 | GCTGCCCAACCAGCCATGGCCGARGTGCAGCTGGTGCAGTCTGG |
| HUVH6 | GCTGCCCAACCAGCCATGGCCCAGGTACAGCTGCAGCAGTCAGG |
| HUVH7 | GCTGCCCAACCAGCCATGGCCCAGGTGCAGCTGGTGCAATCTGG |
| *VH antisense primers (6)* | |
| hujh1 | CGATGGGCCCTTGGTGGAGGCTGAGGAGACGGTGACCAGGGT GCCCTG |
| hujh2 | CGATGGGCCCTTGGTGGAGGCTGAGGAGACAGTGACCAGGGT GCCACG |
| hujh3 | CGATGGGCCCTTGGTGGAGGCTGAAGAGACGGTGACCATTGT CCCTTG |
| hujh45 | CGATGGGCCCTTGGTGGAGGCTGAGGAGACGGTGACCAGGG TYCCYTG |
| hujh6a | CGATGGGCCCTTGGTGGAGGCTGAGGAGACGGTGACCGTGGT CCCTTG |
| hujh6b | CGATGGGCCCTTGGTGGAGGCTGAGGAGACGGTGACCGTGGT CCCTTT |
| *Vκ sense primers (12)* | |
| HUVK1A | GCTACCGTGGCCCAGGCGGCCGACATCCAGWTGACCCAGTCTCC |
| HUVK1B | GCTACCGTGGCCCAGGCGGCCGCCATCCRGWTGACCCAGTCTCC |
| HUVK1C | GCTACCGTGGCCCAGGCGGCCGTCATCTGGATGACCCAGTCTCC |
| HUVK2A | GCTACCGTGGCCCAGGCGGCCGATATTGTGATGACCCAGACTCC |
| HUVK2B | GCTACCGTGGCCCAGGCGGCCGATRTTGTGATGACTCAGTCTCC |
| HUVK3A | GCTACCGTGGCCCAGGCGGCCGAAATTGTGTTGACRCAGTCTCC |
| HUVK3B | GCTACCGTGGCCCAGGCGGCCGAAATAGTGATGAYGCAGTCTCC |
| HUVK3C | GCTACCGTGGCCCAGGCGGCCGAAATTGTAATGACACAGTCTCC |
| HUVK4 | GCTACCGTGGCCCAGGCGGCCGACATCGTGATGACCCAGTCTCC |
| HUVK5 | GCTACCGTGGCCCAGGCGGCCGAAACGACACTCACGCAGTCTCC |
| HUVK6A | GCTACCGTGGCCCAGGCGGCCGAAATTGTGCTGACTCAGTCTCC |
| HUVK6B | GCTACCGTGGCCCAGGCGGCCGATGTTGTGATGACACAGTCTCC |

(continued)

**Table 1 (continued)**

| Name | Sequence |
|---|---|
| *Vκ antisense primer (1)* | |
| huck | GACAGATGGTGCAGCCACAGTTCG |
| *Vλ sense primers (20)* | |
| HUVL1A | GCTACCGTGGCCCAGGCGGCCCAGTCTGTGCTGACTCAGCCACC |
| HUVL1B | GCTACCGTGGCCCAGGCGGCCCAGTCTGTSSTGACGCAGCCGCC |
| HUVL1C | GCTACCGTGGCCCAGGCGGCCCAGTCTGTGTTGACGCAGCCGCC |
| HUVL2A | GCTACCGTGGCCCAGGCGGCCCAGTCTGCCCTGACTCAGCCTCC |
| HUVL2B | GCTACCGTGGCCCAGGCGGCCCAGTCTGCCCTGACTCAGCCTCG |
| HUVL2C | GCTACCGTGGCCCAGGCGGCCCAGTCTGCCCTGACTCAGCCTGC |
| HUVL3A | GCTACCGTGGCCCAGGCGGCCTCCTATGWGCTGACTCAGCCACC |
| HUVL3B | GCTACCGTGGCCCAGGCGGCCTCCTATGAGCTGACTCAGCCACT |
| HUVL3C | GCTACCGTGGCCCAGGCGGCCTCTTCTGAGCTGACTCAGGACCC |
| HUVL3D | GCTACCGTGGCCCAGGCGGCCTCCTATGAGCTGACACAGCYAYC |
| HUVL3E | GCTACCGTGGCCCAGGCGGCCTCCTATGAGCTGATGCAGCCAC |
| HUVL4A | GCTACCGTGGCCCAGGCGGCCCTGCCTGTGCTGACTCAGCCC CCGT |
| HUVL4B | GCTACCGTGGCCCAGGCGGCCCAGCCTGTGCTGACTCAATCATC |
| HUVL4C | GCTACCGTGGCCCAGGCGGCCCAGCTTGTGCTGACTCAATCGCC |
| HUVL5A9 | GCTACCGTGGCCCAGGCGGCCCAGCCTGTGCTGACTCAGCCAYC |
| HUVL5B | GCTACCGTGGCCCAGGCGGCCCAGGCTGTGCTGACTCAGCCGKC |
| HUVL6 | GCTACCGTGGCCCAGGCGGCCAATTTTATGCTGACTCAGCCCCA |
| HUVL7 | GCTACCGTGGCCCAGGCGGCCCAGRCTGTGGTGACTCAGGAGCC |
| HUVL8 | GCTACCGTGGCCCAGGCGGCCCAGACTGTGGTGACCCAGGAGCC |
| HUVL10 | GCTACCGTGGCCCAGGCGGCCCAGGCAGGGCTGACTCAGCCACC |
| *Vλ antisense primers (3)* | |
| hujl1 | GAGGGGGCAGCCTTGGGCTGACCTAGGACGGTGACCTTGGTC CCAG |
| hujl23 | GAGGGGGCAGCCTTGGGCTGACCTAGGACGGTCAGCTTGGTC CCTC |
| hujl7 | GAGGGGGCAGCCTTGGGCTGACCGAGGACGGTCAGCTGGGT GCCTC |
| *Cκ-pelB and Cλ-pelB primers* | |
| HCK | CGAACTGTGGCTGCACCATCTGTC |
| HCL | GGTCAGCCCAAGGCTGCCCCCTC |
| pelb | GGCCATGGCTGGTTGGGCAGC |
| *Overlap extension PCR primers* | |
| C-5′SFIHUVL | CGCTACCGTGGCCCAGGCGGCC |
| c-3′sfivh | GAGGAGGAGGGCCGACGGGGCCAAGGGGAAGACCGATGGGCC CTTGGTGGAGGCTGA |
| *Sequencing primers* | |
| VLSEQ | GATAACAATTGAATTCAGGAG |
| vhseq | TGAGTTCCACGACACCGT |

Names of sense primers are in *uppercase letters*; names of antisense primers in *lowercase letters*
Nucleotide codes: M, A or C; R, A or G; S, C or G; Y, C or T

18. For 70% (vol/vol) ethanol, mix 15 mL ethanol with 35 mL water in a 50-mL centrifuge tube. Store at RT.
19. Qiagen MinElute Gel Extraction Kit (Qiagen, cat. no. 28606); store at RT.

#### 2.4. Assembly of Fab Expression Cassette

1. Plasmids pCκ and pCλ (4.3 kb), available from my laboratory through a Material Transfer Agreement. Store at −20°C.
2. Phagemid pC3C (4.7 kb), available from my laboratory through a Material Transfer Agreement. Store at −20°C.
3. Sense and antisense primers diluted to 20 μM in water (Table 1); store at −20°C.
4. Platinum Taq DNA Polymerase High Fidelity (Life Technologies cat. no. 11304-011) containing 5 U/μL Platinum Taq DNA Polymerase High Fidelity mixture, 10x High Fidelity PCR buffer, and 50 mM magnesium sulfate. Store at −20°C.
5. See Subheading 2.3.
6. 0.2-mL PCR tubes (see Subheading 2.3).
7. 6× Gel loading dye solution (see Subheading 2.3).
8. Model B1A EasyCast Mini Gel Electrophoresis System with B1A-10 and B1A-PREP combs (Owl Separation Systems).
9. Agarose (see Subheading 2.3).
10. TAE buffer (see Subheading 2.3).
11. SYBR Safe DNA gel stain (see Subheading 2.3).
12. 100-bp and 1-kb DNA ladders (Fermentas, cat. no. SM0243 and SM0314, respectively).
13. Safe Imager blue-light transilluminator (see Subheading 2.3).
14. 3 M Sodium acetate (pH 5.2) (see Subheading 2.3).
15. Ethanol (see Subheading 2.2).
16. 70% (vol/vol) ethanol (see Subheading 2.3).
17. Qiagen MinElute Gel Extraction Kit (see Subheading 2.3).

#### 2.5. Test Ligation and Transformation

1. 40 U/μL *Sfi*I and 10× SuRE/Cut buffer M (Roche Applied Science, Indianapolis, IN, USA, www.roche-applied-science.com, cat. no. 11288059001); store at −20°C.
2. 6× Gel loading dye solution (see Subheading 2.3).
3. Model B1A EasyCast Mini Gel Electrophoresis System with B1A-PREP combs (Owl Separation Systems).
4. Agarose (see Subheading 2.3).
5. TAE buffer (see Subheading 2.3).
6. SYBR Safe DNA gel stain (see Subheading 2.3).
7. 1-kb DNA ladder (see Subheading 2.4).
8. Safe Imager blue-light transilluminator (see Subheading 2.3).

9. Qiagen MinElute Gel Extraction Kit (see Subheading 2.3).
10. Isopropanol (see Subheading 2.1).
11. 2,000 U/μL T4 DNA ligase and 10× T4 DNA ligase buffer (New England Biolabs, cat. no. M0202M); store at −20°C.
12. Electrocompetent XL1-Blue with an efficiency of $\geq 1 \times 10^{10}$ colony forming units per microgram pUC18 plasmid (Agilent Technologies, www.genomics.agilent.com, cat. no. 200228); store at −80°C.
13. Eppendorf electroporator 2510 (Eppendorf, cat. no. 940000009).
14. Electroporation cuvettes with 1-mm electrode gap (e.g., Bulldog Bio, Portsmouth, NH, USA, www.bulldog-bio.com).
15. SOC medium (Invitrogen, cat. no. 15544-034); store at RT.
16. LB + 100 μg/mL carbenicillin plates (Teknova, Hollister, CA, www.teknova.com, cat. no. L1010); store at 4°C.

### 2.6. Phage Library Generation

1. 2,000 U/μL T4 DNA ligase and 10×T4 DNA ligase buffer (see Subheading 2.5).
2. Qiagen MinElute Gel Extraction Kit (see Subheading 2.3).
3. Isopropanol (see Subheading 2.1).
4. Electrocompetent XL1-Blue with an efficiency of $\geq 1 \times 10^{10}$ colony forming units per microgram pUC18 plasmid (see Subheading 2.5).
5. Eppendorf electroporator 2510 (see Subheading 2.5).
6. Electroporation cuvettes with 2-mm electrode gap (e.g., Bulldog Bio).
7. SOC medium (see Subheading 2.5).
8. SB medium: dissolve 20 g 3-(*N*-Morpholino)propanesulfonic acid (MOPS; Sigma-Aldrich, cat. no. M3183; store at RT), 60 g Bacto tryptone (BD Biosciences, www.bd.com, cat. no. 211705; store at RT), and 40 g Bacto yeast extract (BD Biosciences, cat. no. 212750; store at RT) in 1.9 L total volume with water. Bring to pH 7.0 with 1 N NaOH (Fisher Scientific, cat. no. AC12426-0010; store at RT). Bring to 2 L total volume with water. Sterilize by autoclaving in two 1 L or four 500-mL glass bottles. Store at RT.
9. 100 μg/μL Carbenicillin: dissolve 1 g carbenicillin disodium (Duchefa, www.duchefa.com, cat. no. C0109.0005; store at 4°C) in 10 mL water. Sterilize by filtration through 0.22 μm. Store 1-mL aliquots in 1.5-mL microfuge tubes at −20°C.
10. 5 μg/μL Tetracycline: dissolve 50 mg tetracycline hydrochloride (Sigma-Aldrich, cat. no. T7660; store at −20°C) in 10 mL ethanol. Store 1-mL aliquots in 1.5-mL microfuge tubes at −20°C.
11. LB + 100 μg/mL carbenicillin plates (see Subheading 2.5).

12. VCSM13 helper phage (Agilent Technologies, cat. no. 200251); store at −80°C.
13. 50 μg/μL Kanamycin: dissolve 500 mg kanamycin sulfate (Sigma-Aldrich, cat. no. K1377; store at RT) in 10 mL water. Sterilize by filtration through 0.22 μm. Store 1-mL aliquots in 1.5-mL microfuge tubes at −20°C.
14. QIAprep Spin Miniprep Kit (Qiagen, cat. no. 27106); store at RT.
15. PEG-8000 (Sigma-Aldrich, cat. no. P5413); store at RT.
16. NaCl (Mallinckrodt Baker, www.mallbaker.com, cat. no. 3624-01); store at RT.
17. Tris-buffered saline (TBS): 25 mM Tris–HCl, 137 mM NaCl, 3 mM KCl, pH 7.4; diluted in water from 10× TBS (Quality Biological, cat. no. 351-086-131); store at RT.
18. 1% (wt/vol) BSA in TBS: dissolve 0.5 g bovine serum albumin (BSA; Sigma-Aldrich, cat. no. A7906; store at 4°C) in 50 mL TBS, sterilize by filtration through 0.22 μm, and store at RT.
19. 2% (wt/vol) Sodium azide: dissolve 0.2 g sodium azide (Sigma-Aldrich, cat. no. S8032; store at RT) in 10 mL water. Store at RT.
20. Glycerol (Invitrogen, cat. no. 15514-011); store at RT.

### 2.7. Supplemental Protocol: Helper Phage Preparation

1. LB top agar (Teknova, cat. no. L5580); store at RT.
2. LB plates (Teknova, cat. no. L1100); store at 4°C.

## 3. Methods

### 3.1. PBMC and BMMC Preparation

This protocols takes about 2 h.

1. For PBMC, start with 50 mL whole blood in five 10-mL blood collection tubes with anticoagulant, e.g., heparin (vacutainer tubes with green top), citrate (light blue top), or EDTA (purple top). For BMMC, start with 20 mL aspirated bone marrow fluid and cells in a 20-mL syringe with anticoagulant. Perform steps 2–9 under sterile conditions in a laminar flow hood (see Note 1).
2. For PBMC, dilute 25 mL blood with 25 mL PBS in each of two 50-mL centrifuge tubes. For BMMC, dilute 20 mL aspirate with 30 mL PBS in a 50-mL centrifuge tube.
3. Slowly layer 25 mL of the diluted blood/diluted aspirate onto 14 mL Lymphocyte Separation Medium in each of four/two 50-mL centrifuge tubes, and centrifuge (no brake) at 800 × *g* for 20 min at RT to separate plasma/fluid in the upper phase, mononuclear cells (lymphocytes and monocytes) in the

interphase, polymorphonuclear cells (granulocytes) in the lower phase, and red cells (erythrocytes) at the bottom.

4. Carefully remove the upper phase without disturbing the interphase. Plasma with an endogenous antibody response of interest may be used for IgG purification and should be stored at –80°C. Using a 5-mL pipette, carefully transfer the interphase in a clean 50-mL centrifuge tube with 25 mL PBS, bring volume to 50 mL with PBS, and centrifuge at 300 × *g* for 10 min at 4°C.
5. *(Optional step)* Remove and discard the supernatant. To remove remaining erythrocytes, resuspend the cell pellet in 2 mL ACK Lysing Buffer, incubate for 2 min at RT, add PBS to 50 mL, and centrifuge at 300 × *g* for 10 min at 4°C.
6. Remove and discard the supernatant. Resuspend and combine the cell pellets in 50 mL PBS.
7. Determine the number of viable mononuclear cells by Trypan Blue staining using a hemocytometer or an electronic counting device. Expect a yield around $1–2 \times 10^6$ PBMC per milliliter of whole blood and $3–4 \times 10^6$ BMMC per milliliter bone marrow aspirate with a viability of >95%.
8. For proceeding with fresh mononuclear cells, centrifuge a volume corresponding to $2.5 \times 10^7$ mononuclear cells at 300 × *g* for 10 min at 4°C. Proceed to Subheading 3.2 step 1.
9. For cryopreservation, centrifuge at 300 × *g* for 10 min at 4°C and resuspend the cell pellet in cold Recovery Cell Culture Freezing Medium to a concentration of $1 \times 10^7$ cells/mL. Transfer each 1 mL of the cell preparation to a 2-mL cryovial. After securely tightening the caps, immediately place the cryovials in a freezing container with isopropanol. Store the container at –80°C overnight before transferring the cryovials to a cryobox in a liquid nitrogen tank (see Note 2).

### 3.2. Total RNA Preparation

This protocol takes about 2 h and is based on $2.5 \times 10^7$ human mononuclear cells and can be scaled up or down. Mononuclear cells that were freshly prepared from clinical specimens are preferred.

1. For cryopreserved mononuclear cells, partially thaw five 2-mL cryovial freezing tubes, each containing $1 \times 10^7$ cells in 1 mL, in a 37°C water bath. Add 1 mL PBS just before the cells are completely thawed. Determine the number of viable mononuclear cells by Trypan Blue staining using a hemocytometer or an electronic counting device. Transfer $2.5 \times 10^7$ viable mononuclear cells to a 15-mL centrifuge tube, add PBS to 15 mL, and centrifuge at 1,500 × *g* for 10 min at 4°C.
2. Remove the supernatant, add 2.5 mL TRI reagent (1 mL per $1 \times 10^7$ mononuclear cells), resuspend the cell pellet by repetitive pipetting, and incubate for 5 min at RT (see Note 3).

3. Transfer 1.25 mL to each of two RNase-free 1.5-mL microfuge tubes, add 125 μL (0.1 vol) BCP, vortex for 15 s, incubate for 10 min at RT, and centrifuge at 12,000 × *g* for 15 min at 4°C.
4. For each of the two samples, transfer the upper colorless aqueous phase to a clean RNase-free microfuge tube (discard the lower red organic phase), add 625 μL isopropanol, vortex for 15 s, incubate for 10 min at RT, and centrifuge at 12,000 × *g* for 10 min at 4°C.
5. For each of the two samples, carefully decant and discard the supernatant without disturbing the white pellet, add 1.25 mL 70% (vol/vol) ethanol, and centrifuge at 12,000 × *g* for 10 min at 4°C.
6. Carefully decant and discard the supernatant without disturbing the white pellet, air-dry in dust-free conditions for 10 min at RT, dissolve and pool the two samples in 100 μL RNA Storage Solution, and transfer to a clean RNase-free 1.5-mL microfuge tube.

   *Optional*: further purify RNA with the Qiagen RNeasy MinElute Cleanup Kit following the manufacturer's protocol or by precipitation with RNase-free 7.5 M LiCl as described (7).
7. Immediately remove a 2-μL aliquot and store the remaining sample on dry ice. Add 498 μL RNase-free water to the 2-μL aliquot and measure the absorbance at 260 and 280 nm in a UV photometer. Use the absorbance at 260 nm to calculate the total RNA concentration based on the assumption that 40 μg/mL RNA gives an absorbance of 1 (see Note 4; for troubleshooting see Table 2).
8. Total RNA in RNA Storage Solution may be stored for weeks at –80°C. For long-term storage (months to years), add 0.1 vol RNase-free 3 M sodium acetate (pH 5.2) and 2.2 vol ethanol, vortex, and store at –80°C.

### 3.3. RT-PCR Amplification of VH and VL cDNA

This step takes about 3 days and is depicted in Fig. 1a.

1. In an RNase-free 1.5-mL microfuge tube, dilute 20 μg of the total RNA with RNase-free water to 64 μL.
2. Add 8 μL 50 μM oligo(dT) and 8 μL 10 mM dNTP mix (Σ 80 μL), incubate for 5 min at 65°C, store on ice for at least 1 min, and collect by brief centrifugation (see Note 5).
3. Prepare reverse transcriptase reaction mixture by combining 16 μL 10× RT buffer, 32 μL 25 mM $MgCl_2$, 16 μL 100 mM DTT, 8 μL 40 U/μL RNaseOUT, and 8 μL 200 U/μL SuperScript III RT (Σ 80 μL) in another RNase-free 1.5-mL microfuge tube.
4. Add the prepared reverse transcriptase reaction mixture to the prepared RNA/oligo(dT)/dNTP sample (Σ 160 μL),

**Table 2**
**Troubleshooting**

| Step | Problem | Possible reason | Solution |
|---|---|---|---|
| Step 7 (Subheading 3.2) | Low RNA quantity or quality | RNase contamination | Start over with fresh reagents and clean equipment |
| Step 12 (Subheading 3.3) | Bands at ~400 bp not or only weakly visible | RNA is not pure | Further purify RNA with one of the two optional procedures mentioned in Subheading 3.2, step 6 and repeat RT-PCR amplification |
| Step 21 (Subheading 3.5) | Low number of independent transformants | The additional controls are designed to narrow down possible reasons: (1) Low numbers of colonies on all plates are indicative of an inefficient *Sfi*I-digested pC3C or a problem with one of the ligation or transformation reagents (2) A problem with the *Sfi*I-digested VL/CL/VH expression cassette is usually indicated if the re-ligation of *Sfi*I-digested pC3C vector and insert gives a high number of colonies, whereas the ligation of *Sfi*I-digested pC3C vector and VL/CL/VH expression cassette gives a low number of colonies. This can be due to poor quality of the prepared DNA or the *Sfi*I reagents and should be addressed accordingly | (1a) Prepare a new batch of *Sfi*I-digested pC3C with fresh reagents (*Sfi*I, agarose, Qiagen MinElute Gel Extraction Kit) (1b) Use fresh reagents (*Sfi*I, T4 DNA ligase, and electrocompetent XL1-Blue) (2) Prepare a new batch of *Sfi*I-digested VL/CL/VH expression cassette with fresh reagents (*Sfi*I, agarose, Qiagen MinElute Gel Extraction Kit) |

incubate for 50 min at 50°C, followed by 5 min at 85°C. Store on ice for at least 1 min and collect by brief centrifugation.

5. Add 8 μL 2 U/μL *E. coli* RNase H, incubate for 20 min at 37°C, collect by brief centrifugation, and pool first-strand cDNA from independent duplicates (Σ 336 μL). First-strand cDNA may be stored for weeks at –20°C. For long-term storage (months to years), add 0.1 vol 3 M sodium acetate (pH 5.2) and 2.2 vol ethanol, vortex, and store at –80°C.

6. For *VH amplification*, generate *114 primer combinations* for each sample by combining 1 μL of the first-strand cDNA with 3 μL 20 μM of the 19 human VH sense primers (Table 1) and 3 μL 20 μM of the six human VH antisense primers (Table 1) in 0.2-mL PCR tubes.
7. For *Vκ amplification*, generate *12 primer combinations* for each sample by combining 1 μL of the first-strand cDNA with 3 μL 20 μM of the 12 human Vκ sense primers (Table 1) and 3 μL 20 μM of the only human Vκ antisense primer (Table 1) in 0.2-mL PCR tubes.
8. For *Vλ amplification*, generate *60 primer combinations* for each sample by combining 1 μL of the first-strand cDNA with 3 μL 20 μM of the 20 human Vλ sense primers (Table 1) and 3 μL 20 μM of the three human Vλ antisense primers (Table 1) in 0.2-mL PCR tubes (see Note 6).
9. Prepare two PCR master mixes sufficient for a total of 186 reactions. These reactions can be run in parallel using two 96-well thermocyclers. In a 14-mL round-bottom tube, combine 1 mL 10× PCR buffer, 1 mL 25 mM $MgCl_2$, 800 μL 10 mM dNTP mix, 6.45 mL water, and 50 μL 5 U/μL Taq DNA polymerase (Σ 9.3 mL) (see Note 7).
10. Add 93 μL of the prepared PCR mixture to the prepared first-strand cDNA/sense primer/antisense primer samples (Σ 100 μL).
11. In a 96-well thermocycler, use these PCR parameters:

    95°C for 2 min.

    Followed by 35 cycles of 95°C for 30 s, 50°C for 30 s, and 72°C for 90 s.

    Followed by 72°C for 10 min.

    Followed by cooling to RT.
12. Remove a 10-μL aliquot from each sample, add 2 μL 6× gel loading dye solution, and separate by electrophoresis on a 1% (wt/vol) agarose gel in TAE buffer using a 100-bp DNA ladder as reference. The amplified VH, Vκ, and Vλ cDNA should be visible as bright band of approximately 400 bp (see Notes 8 and 9; for troubleshooting see Table 2).
13. Pool the remaining 90 μL of all amplified VH cDNA (114×90 μL=10.26 mL) in a 14-mL round-bottom tube. Divide pool in 28×360 μL-aliquots in 1.5-mL microfuge tubes, add 36 μL (0.1 vol) 3 M sodium acetate (pH 5.2) and 792 μL (2.2 vol) ethanol, vortex, and store at −20°C.
14. Pool the remaining 90 μL of all amplified Vκ cDNA (12×90 μL=1.08 mL) in a 14-mL round-bottom tube. Divide pool in 3×360-μL aliquots in 1.5-mL microfuge tubes, add 36 μL (0.1 vol) 3 M sodium acetate (pH 5.2) and 792 μL

(2.2 vol) ethanol, vortex, and store at −20°C. PCRs in ethanol may be stored for months to years at −20°C.

15. Pool the remaining 90 μL of all amplified Vλ cDNA (60 × 90 μL = 5.4 mL) in a 14-mL round-bottom tube. Divide pool in 16 × 360-μL aliquots in 1.5-mL microfuge tubes, add 36 μL (0.1 vol) 3 M sodium acetate (pH 5.2) and 792 μL (2.2 vol) ethanol, vortex, and store at −20°C.
16. Proceed with two aliquots of the VH cDNA. Precipitate VH cDNA by centrifugation at 16,000 × *g* for 15 min at 4°C, decant and discard the supernatant, rinse pellet with 1 mL 70% (vol/vol) ethanol (RT), and briefly dry in a Savant SpeedVac concentrator. Dissolve and pool the pellet of the two aliquots in 200 μL water, add 40 μL 6× gel loading dye solution, and separate by electrophoresis on a 1% (wt/vol) agarose gel in TAE buffer using a preparative comb and a 100-bp DNA ladder as reference.
17. Cut out the ~400 bp band with a razor blade, dissect it further into smaller pieces, and transfer ~0.3 g portions into 1.5-mL microfuge tubes. Purify VH cDNA using reagents and protocols supplied by the Qiagen MinElute Gel Extraction Kit. Elute VH cDNA in 100 μL water and measure the absorbance at 260 nm in a UV photometer. Use the absorbance at 260 nm to calculate the cDNA concentration based on the assumption that 50 μg/mL DNA gives an absorbance of 1.
18. Dilute the purified VH cDNA with water to a final concentration of 100 ng/μL and store at −20°C.
19. Repeat the procedure described in steps 16–18 to purify Vκ and Vλ cDNA. Purified VH, Vκ, and Vλ cDNA may be stored for weeks at −20°C.

### 3.4. Assembly of the Fab Expression Cassette

This step is illustrated in Fig. 1b and takes about 3 days.

For assembly of the Fab expression cassette in phagemid pC3C, a human Cκ-pelB DNA fragment and a human Cλ-pelB DNA fragment are required in addition to VH, Vκ, and Vλ cDNA (Fig. 1b).

1. For Cκ-pelB amplification, prepare a PCR master mix sufficient for ten reactions. In a 1.5-mL microfuge tube, mix 10 μL 100 ng/μL plasmid pCκ (5) with 30 μL 20 μM HCK (sense primer; Table 1), 30 μL 20 μM pelb (antisense primer; Table 1), 100 μL 10× High Fidelity PCR buffer, 80 μL 10 mM dNTP mix, 40 μL 50 mM magnesium sulfate, 706 μL water, and 4 μL 5 U/μL Platinum Taq DNA Polymerase High Fidelity mixture (Σ 1 mL).
2. In a 96-well thermocycler, run ten 100 μL reactions in 0.2-mL PCR tubes using these PCR parameters:

   94°C for 2 min.

Followed by 20 cycles of 94°C for 30 s, 55°C for 30 s, and 72°C for 30 s.

Followed by 72°C for 10 min.

Followed by cooling to RT.

3. Pool all ten reactions.
4. Remove a 10-μL aliquot from the pool in step 3, add 2 μL 6× gel loading dye solution, and separate by electrophoresis on a 1% (wt/vol) agarose gel in TAE buffer using a 100-bp DNA ladder as reference. The amplified Cκ-pelB DNA fragment should be visible as bright band of approximately 400 bp.
5. Precipitate and purify the amplified Cκ-pelB DNA fragment as described in Subheading 3.3 steps 13, 16–18 for VH cDNA, and dilute with water to a final concentration of 100 ng/μL. Store at −20°C.
6. Repeat the procedure described in steps 1–5 to amplify and purify a human Cλ-pelB DNA fragment, using plasmid pCλ (8) and sense primer HCL (Table 1) in place of pCκ and HCK, respectively.
7. For assembly of the Vκ/Cκ/VH cassette by overlap extension PCR, prepare two master mixes, each sufficient for 10 reactions. *Master Mix I* (without primers): In a 1.5 mL microfuge tube, mix 10 μL 100 ng/μL VH cDNA with 10 μL 100 ng/μL Vk cDNA and 10 μL 100 ng/μL Ck-pelB DNA. Add 50 μL 10× High Fidelity PCR buffer, 40 μL 10 mM dNTP mix, 20 μL 50 mM magnesium sulfate, 358 μL water, and 2 μL 5 U/μL Platinum Taq DNA Polymerase High Fidelity mixture (Σ 500 μL). *Master Mix II* (with primers): In a 1.5 mL microfuge tube, mix 30 μL 20 μM C-5'SFIHUVL (sense primer; Table 1), 30 μL 20 μM c-3'sfivh (antisense primer; Table 1), 50 μL 10× High Fidelity PCR buffer, 40 μL 10 mM dNTP mix, 20 μL 50 mM magnesium sulfate, 328 μL water, and 2 μL 5 U/μL Platinum Taq DNA Polymerase High Fidelity mixture (Σ 500 μL).
8. In a 96-well thermocycler, run ten 50 μL reactions of *Master Mix I* in 0.2-mL PCR tubes using these PCR parameters (see Note 10):

94°C for 2 min.

Followed by 30 cycles of 94°C for 30 s, 55°C for 30 s, and 72°C for 90 s.

Followed by 72°C for 10 min.

After cooling to RT, add 50 μL of *Master Mix II* to each reaction and run 20 additional cycles using the same PCR parameters.

9. Pool all ten reactions, remove a 10-μL aliquot, add 2 μL 6× gel loading dye solution, and separate by electrophoresis on a 1% (wt/vol) agarose gel in TAE buffer using 100-bp and 1-kb

DNA ladders as reference. The fused Vκ/Cκ/VH expression cassette should be visible as bright 1.2-kb band.

10. Precipitate and purify the fused Vκ/Cκ/VH expression cassette as described in Subheading 3.3, steps 13, 16–18 for VH cDNA. Expect a yield of at least 30 μg DNA. Dilute with water to a final concentration of 150 ng/μL and store at −20°C.
11. Repeat the procedure described in steps 7–10 to assemble and purify the Vλ/Cλ/VH expression cassette. Use Vλ cDNA and Cλ-pelB DNA in place of Vκ cDNA and Cκ-pelB DNA, respectively. Purified Vκ/Cκ/VH and Vλ/Cλ/VH expression cassettes may be stored for months at −20°C.

### 3.5. Test Ligation and Transformation

For the generation of phagemid libraries, Vκ/Cκ/VH and Vλ/Cλ/VH expression cassettes may be kept separate or combined depending on whether separate Fab libraries with only κ or λ light chains are desired. This step takes about 3 days (Fig. 1c).

1. For *Sfi*I digestion of the assembled Vκ/Cκ/VH and Vλ/Cλ/VH expression cassettes, combine 200 μL 150 ng/μL (30 μg) DNA with 30 μL 10× SuRE/Cut buffer M, 60 μL water, and 10 μL 40 U/μL *Sfi*I. Incubate at 50°C for 3 h.
2. After cooling to RT, directly add 60 μL 6× gel loading dye solution, and separate by electrophoresis on a 1% (wt/vol) agarose gel in TAE buffer using a preparative comb and a 1-kb DNA ladder as reference.
3. Cut out the 1.2-kb band with a razor blade, dissect it further into smaller pieces, and transfer ~0.3 g portions to 1.5-mL microfuge tubes.
4. Purify the *Sfi*I-digested Vκ/Cκ/VH and Vλ/Cλ/VH expression cassettes using reagents and protocols supplied by the Qiagen MinElute Gel Extraction Kit.
5. Pool the DNA in 100 μL water and measure the absorbance at 260 nm. Use the absorbance at 260 nm to calculate the DNA concentration based on the assumption that 50 μL/mL DNA gives an absorbance of 1.
6. Dilute with water to a final concentration of 50 ng/μL and store at −20°C.
7. For *Sfi*I digestion of phagemid pC3C (5), combine 50 μL 1 μg/μL (50 μg) DNA with 30 μL 10× SuRE/Cut buffer M, 208 μL water, and 12 μL 40 U/μL *Sfi*I. Incubate at 50°C for 2 h.
8. After cooling to RT, directly add 60 μL 6× gel loading dye solution, and separate by electrophoresis on a 1% (wt/vol) agarose gel in TAE buffer using a preparative comb and a 1-kb DNA ladder as reference.
9. Purify both the 3.5 kb band (vector) and the 1.2 kb band (insert) as described for the *Sfi*I-digested Vκ/Cκ/VH and Vλ/Cλ/VH expression cassettes in steps 3–5.

10. Dilute with water to a final concentration of 100 ng/μL (vector) or 50 ng/μL (insert). Store at −20°C.
11. For test ligation, combine 1.5 μL 100 ng/μL *Sfi*I-digested pC3C vector (150 ng) with 2 μL 50 ng/μL *Sfi*I-digested Vκ/Cκ/VH and Vλ/Cλ/VH expression cassettes (100 ng; ~1:2 molar ratio of vector–insert), 2 μL 10× T4 DNA ligase buffer, 13.5 μL water, and 1 μL 2,000 U/μL T4 DNA ligase in a 1.5-mL microfuge tube (Σ 20 μL).
12. Prepare a test ligation mixture in parallel with *Sfi*I-digested pC3C vector alone as *background control*. Prepare another test ligation mixture in parallel by combining *Sfi*I-digested pC3C vector with *Sfi*I-digested pC3C insert as *re-ligation control*. Incubate at RT for 3 h.
13. For *E. coli* transformation, these instructions assume the use of an Eppendorf electroporator 2510 with a 10 μF capacitor, a fixed time constant of 5 ms, and a voltage range from 200 to 2,500 V. Each test ligation requires 50 μL electrocompetent XL1-Blue and one 1-mm cuvette. Thaw electrocompetent XL-1 Blue on ice for 10 min. Cool required number of cuvettes on ice.
14. Transfer 1 μL of the test ligation mixture to a 1.5-mL microfuge tube and cool on ice.
15. Add 50 μL of the thawed electrocompetent XL-1 Blue to the 1-μL test ligation mixture, transfer immediately to a cuvette, and store on ice for 1 min.
16. Electroporate at 1,500 V. Expect $\tau$ to be approximately 4.5 ms.
17. Flush the cuvette immediately with a total of 3 mL (twice 1.5 mL) SOC medium at RT.
18. Transfer to a 14-mL round-bottom tube with snap cap.
19. Shake at 37°C and 250 rpm for 1 h.
20. Of this culture, plate 1 and 10 μL, each diluted in 100 μL SOC medium, on LB + 100 μg/mL carbenicillin plates. Incubate at 37°C overnight.
21. Calculate the number of independent transformants that can be expected from one library ligation from the number of colonies times 300 or 3,000 (dilution factor) times 20 (fraction of test ligation that was transformed) times 10 (library ligation scale). For example, 50 colonies on the 1 μL plate predict $3 \times 10^7$ independent transformants per library ligation. The *background control* should give a much lower number of colonies, whereas the *re-ligation control* typically gives a higher number of colonies. To proceed with library ligation, the number of predicted transformants per library ligation should be at least $1 \times 10^7$ with a background <10% (see Note 11; for troubleshooting see Table 2).

### 3.6. Phage Library Generation

This step takes 2 days. Figure 1c, d depict phagemid and phage assembly.

1. For each library ligation, combine 15 μL 100 ng/μL *Sfi*I-digested pC3C vector (1.5 μg) with 20 μL 50 ng/μL *Sfi*I-digested Vκ/Cκ/VH and Vλ/Cλ/VH expression cassettes (1 μg), 20 μL 10× T4 DNA ligase buffer, 135 μL water, and 10 μL 2,000 U/μL T4 DNA ligase in a 1.5-mL microfuge tube (Σ 200 μL). Incubate at RT for 3 h (see Note 12).
2. Add 600 μL Qiagen buffer QG from the Qiagen MinElute Gel Extraction Kit to the library ligation, incubate for 10 min at RT.
3. Add 200 μL isopropanol, and proceed with DNA purification using reagents and protocols supplied by the Qiagen MinElute Gel Extraction Kit. Elute DNA with 20 μL water and store on ice.
4. As before for the *E. coli* transformation of the test ligations, these instructions assume the use of an Eppendorf electroporator 2510. Each library ligation requires 300 μL electrocompetent XL1-Blue and one 2-mm cuvette. Thaw electrocompetent XL-1 Blue on ice for 10 min. Cool required number of cuvettes on ice.
5. Transfer purified DNA from library ligation (~19 μL) to a 1.5-mL microfuge tube and cool on ice.
6. Using a 1-mL pipette tip with a snipped-off end, add 300 μL of the thawed electrocompetent XL-1 Blue to the ~19 μL sample, transfer immediately to a cuvette, and store on ice for 1 min.
7. Electroporate at 2,500 V. Expect τ to be approximately 3.5 ms.
8. Flush the cuvette immediately with a total of 5 mL (1 mL and twice 2 mL) SOC medium at RT and transfer to a 50-mL centrifuge tube. Shake at 37°C and 250 rpm for 1 h (see Note 13).
9. Add 10 mL SB, 3 μL 100 μg/μL carbenicillin, and 30 μL 5 μg/μL tetracycline. Shake at 37°C and 250 rpm for 1 h.
10. To determine the number of independent transformants, remove a 2-μL aliquot, add to 198 μL SB medium in a 1.5-mL microfuge tube, and plate 10 μL on an LB + 100 μg/mL carbenicillin plate. Incubate at 37°C overnight (see Note 14).
11. Add 4.5 μL 100 μg/μL carbenicillin to the culture in the 50-mL centrifuge tube and continue shaking at 37°C and 250 rpm for 1 h.
12. Add 2 mL VCSM13 helper phage [$10^{11}$–$10^{12}$ plaque forming units (pfu)/mL; see Subheading 3.7] and combine two samples derived from identical library ligations in a 500-mL centrifuge bottle. Add 166 mL SB, 85 μL 100 μg/μL carbenicillin, and 340 μL 5 μg/μL tetracycline (Σ 200 mL). Shake at 37°C and 275 rpm for 90 min.
13. Add 280 μL 50 μg/μL kanamycin and continue shaking at 37°C and 275 rpm overnight (12–16 h) (see Note 15).

14. Centrifuge at 3,000 ×*g* for 15 min at 4°C. Save both pellet and supernatant.
15. For phagemid preparation, resuspend the pellet in 5 mL Qiagen buffer P1 from the QIAprep Spin Miniprep Kit and process 4×250 μL using reagents and protocols supplied by the QIAprep Spin Miniprep Kit. Pool in 80 μL water and store at −20°C. This phagemid library stock serves as a backup from which the VL/CL/VH expression cassette can be retrieved by *Sfi*I digestion.
16. For phage precipitation, transfer the supernatant to a clean 500-mL centrifuge tube with 8 g PEG-8000 and 6 g NaCl and dissolve by shaking at 37°C and 300 rpm for 5 min.
17. Incubate on ice for 30 min. Centrifuge at 15,000 ×*g* for 15 min at 4°C.
18. Discard the supernatant, drain the bottle by inverting on a paper towel for 10 min, and carefully wipe off remaining liquid with a paper towel.
19. Resuspend the phage pellet in 2 mL 1% (wt/vol) BSA in TBS by pipetting up and down along the side of the centrifuge tube.
20. Transfer to a 2-mL microfuge tube, pipette up and down in a 1-mL pipette tip.
21. Centrifuge at 16,000 ×*g* for 5 min at 4°C.
22. Pass the supernatant through a 0.22 μm filter into a clean 2-mL microfuge tube.
23. Store on ice for panning on the same day or add 0.01 vol 2% (wt/vol) sodium azide for storage at 4°C. For long-term storage, add 1 vol glycerol and store at −20°C (see Note 16).

### 3.7. Supplemental Protocol: Helper Phage Preparation

Phage display selection of phagemid libraries requires the addition of helper phage (Subheading 3.6, step 12) to provide all genes needed for production of infectious phage particles. This protocol uses helper phage VCSM13 which includes a gene for kanamycin resistance and a mutated origin of replication that, in the presence of phagemid with unmutated origin of replication, favors the production of infectious phage particles with phagemid phenotype and genotype. This protocol takes about 3 days.

1. Inoculate 2 mL SB medium in 50-mL centrifuge tubes with 4 μL XL1-Blue (from a single electrocompetent XL1-Blue aliquot that can be thawed from and frozen at −80°C multiple times), add 4 μL 5 μg/μL tetracycline, and shake at 37°C and 275 rpm for approximately 2 h.
2. Prepare $10^{-6}$, $10^{-7}$, and $10^{-8}$ dilutions of commercial helper phage VCSM13 in SB medium.
3. Add 1 μL of each of these dilutions to 50 μL of the XL1-Blue culture and incubate at RT for 15 min.

4. Add 3 mL of LB top agar liquefied in a microwave oven and cooled to below 50°C and pour onto plain LB agar plates prewarmed to 37°C. Incubate at 37°C overnight. Proceed with a plate from which a single plaque can be picked. Plaques are XL1-Blue colonies that grow slower due to helper phage infection. Plates with plaques can be stored for up to 1 week at 4°C.
5. In a 50-mL centrifuge tube, inoculate 10 mL SB prewarmed to 37°C with 20 μL of XL1-Blue, add 20 μL 5 μg/μL tetracycline, and shake at 37°C and 275 rpm for approximately 2 h.
6. Use a 20 μL pipette tip to transfer a single plaque to the culture and shake at 37°C and 275 rpm for approximately 2 h.
7. Transfer the infected culture to a 2-L Erlenmeyer flask with 500 mL SB prewarmed to at 37°C and 275 rpm, add 1 mL 5 μg/μL tetracycline and 700 μL 50 μg/μL kanamycin, and continue shaking overnight (12–16 h) at 37°C and 250 rpm.
8. Transfer the culture to ten 50-mL centrifuge tubes and centrifuge at 2,500 × *g* for 15 min at RT.
9. Transfer the supernatants to clean 50-mL centrifuge tubes and discard the pellets. Incubate in a water bath at 70°C for 20 min.
10. Centrifuge at 2,500 × *g* for 15 min at RT, transfer the supernatants to clean 50-mL centrifuge tubes, and discard the pellets. Store at 4°C.
11. To determine the titer of the helper phage preparation, repeat steps 1–4. Count the number of plaques on the plates. The number of plaques (e.g., 50) times dilution factor (e.g., $1 \times 10^7$) times 1,000 gives the titer of the helper phage preparation in pfu/mL (e.g., $5 \times 10^{11}$). Expect the titer to be in a range from $10^{11}$ to $10^{12}$ pfu/mL. Although the titer will drop over time, helper phage preparations can be stored for several months at 4°C.

### *3.8. Supplemental Protocol: Phage Reamplification*

It is recommended to use original rather than reamplified phage for library selection where practically possible. Phage reamplification is likely to further bias the library toward Fab sequences that are transcribed, translated, and folded at higher rates. On the other hand, phage should be used for library selection only if they have been prepared on the same day because Fab displayed on phage are susceptible to trace amounts of proteases that cleave the physical linkage of phenotype and genotype. Thus, phage reamplification is often necessary. To minimize biases in the library selection, only use original phage obtained from library ligation and transformation or phage obtained from the third, fourth, or subsequent panning rounds for reamplification.

1. Inoculate 50 mL SB medium in a 250-mL Erlenmeyer flask with 50 μL XL1-Blue (from a single electrocompetent XL1-Blue aliquot), add 100 μL 5 μg/μL tetracycline, and shake at

37°C and 250 rpm for approximately 1.5–2.5 h to an optical density at 600 nm of approximately 1 (see Note 13).

2. Add 10 μL of the stored original phage preparation to the XL1-Blue culture and incubate at RT without shaking for 15 min.
3. Add 10 μL 100 μg/μL carbenicillin, remove a 1-μL aliquot, and shake at 37°C and 275 rpm for 1 h.
4. To determine the number of independently reamplified phage, add the 1-μL aliquot to 10 mL SB medium in a 14-mL round-bottom tube and plate 10 μL on an LB + 100 μg/mL carbenicillin plate. Incubate at 37°C overnight. The number of colonies (e.g., 50) times 50,000 (culture volume) times 1,000 (dilution factor) gives the number of independently reamplified phage (e.g., $2.5 \times 10^9$). For reamplification of a phage library or already selected phage, this number should be factor 5–10 higher than the number of independent transformants or the output titer, respectively.
5. Add 15 μL 100 μg/μL carbenicillin to the culture in the 250 mL Erlenmeyer flask and continue shaking at 37°C and 275 rpm for 1 h.
6. Add 2 mL VCSM13 helper phage ($10^{11}$–$10^{12}$ pfu/mL; see Subheading 3.7) and transfer to a 500-mL centrifuge bottle with 148 mL SB, 75 μL 100 μg/μL carbenicillin, and 300 μL 5 μg/μL tetracycline (Σ 200 mL).
7. After shaking at 37°C and 275 rpm for 90 min, add 280 μL 50 μg/μL kanamycin and continue shaking at 37°C and 275 rpm overnight (12–16 h) (see Note 15). Proceed with phage precipitation as described in Subheading 3.6, steps 16–23.

## 4. Notes

1. The collection and processing of clinical specimens from human subjects must be approved by an institutional review board. Clinical specimens should be treated as potentially infectious and appropriate safety precautions should be taken.
2. Protect hands and eyes when handling liquid nitrogen. Cryopreserved PBMC and BMMC may be stored for years in liquid nitrogen.
3. Wear gloves and safety glasses. Keep all reagents RNase-free by changing gloves frequently and working with clean equipment in dust-free conditions. TRI reagent contains a poison (phenol) and an irritant (guanidine thiocyanate). Wear appropriate protection and handle with care.

4. The ratio of the absorbance at 260 and 280 nm is typically in a range from 1.6 to 1.9. The yield of total RNA from $2.5 \times 10^7$ mononuclear cells is expected to be ~100 μg. RNA can be separated by electrophoresis under denaturing conditions in an agarose-formaldehyde gel (9). Two sharp bands of ~4.7 and ~1.9 kb corresponding to 28S and 18S ribosomal RNA should be visible in addition to a ~0.1–0.15 kb smear corresponding to 5S ribosomal RNA and transfer RNA (9). Total RNA in RNA Storage Solution may be stored for weeks at −80°C. For long-term storage (months to years), add 0.1 vol RNase-free 3 M sodium acetate (pH 5.2) and 2.2 vol ethanol, vortex, and store at −80°C.
5. For first-strand cDNA synthesis, process total RNA from different human tissues (e.g., PBMC and BMMC) or different human subjects in parallel and each in independent duplicates.
6. For PCR, process first-strand cDNA from different human tissues (e.g., PBMC and BMMC) or different human subjects in parallel. Each sample will be subjected to 186 primer combinations in separate reactions. Take precautions to avoid the amplification of VH, Vκ, and Vλ cDNA from contaminating sources in the laboratory, such as phagemids and phage, and include negative controls without first-strand cDNA. Consider using a PCR workstation.
7. Taq DNA polymerase has an error rate range from $10^{-4}$ to $10^{-5}$ depending on the PCR conditions. If higher fidelity is desired, use other thermostable DNA polymerases such as Platinum Taq DNA Polymerase High Fidelity mixture which is used for the subsequent overlap extension PCR in Subheading 3.4.
8. For both DNA analysis and preparation by agarose gel electrophoresis, the use of SYBR Safe stain and blue light illumination rather than the hazardous combination of ethidium bromide and UV illumination is strongly recommended.
9. Not all primer combinations are expected to work. For normal and post-alloHSCT PBMC our success rate was 89% (166/186) and 71% (132/186), respectively (6).
10. To make sure that the overlap extension PCR is not contaminated with an already assembled Fab expression cassette that would get amplified rapidly and diminish library complexity, it is recommended to carry out pilot experiment with VH cDNA, Vκ (Vλ) cDNA, and Cκ-pelB (Cλ-pelb) DNA alone and in combination.
11. Based on the test ligation results, calculate the number of library ligations that are necessary to generate a library consisting of $10^8$–$10^9$ independent transformants. This complexity can be achieved with eight or less library ligations. To confirm that the library contains functional and diverse human Fab sequences,

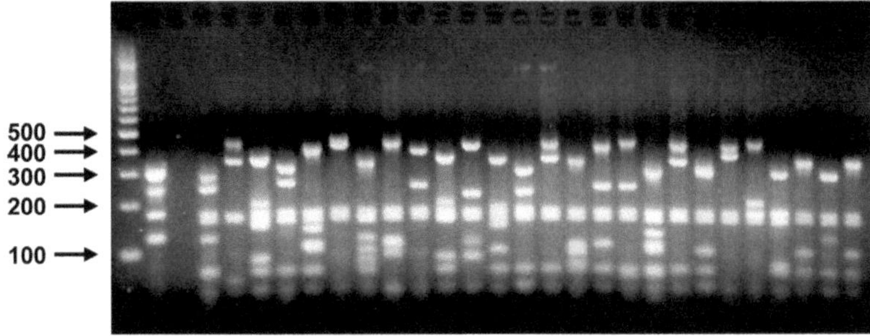


Fig. 2. *Alu*I fingerprinting. PCR-amplified VL/CL/VH expression cassettes of phagemid clones before and after library selection are analyzed by DNA fingerprinting using restriction enzyme *Alu*I with the abundant 4 bp recognition sequence 5′-AG/CT-3′. Shown here is a 4% (wt/vol) agarose gel for 28 *Alu*I-digested 1.2 kb VL/CL/VH expression cassettes of phagemid clones that were randomly picked from a human Fab library before selection. All but one (*lane 3*) gave a readable and unique *Alu*I fingerprint. A 100-bp DNA ladder was run as reference in *lane 1*.

analyze 20 colonies from the test ligation first by Fab ELISA using goat anti-human kappa light chain pAbs and goat anti-human lambda light chain pAbs as capturing antibodies and rat anti-HA mAb 3F10 conjugated to HRP as detecting antibody (see Chapter 5). Expect ≥75% positive clones. Subsequently, analyze positive clones by DNA fingerprinting with *Alu*I (see Subheading 3.9 in Chapter 5). Each positive clone is expected to give a unique DNA fingerprint (Fig. 2).

12. Up to eight library ligations and transformations can be processed in parallel.

13. Take precautions to avoid contaminating the *E. coli* culture with phage including helper phage. Use a separate area and filtered pipette tips for pipetting and a phage-free shaker for growth. This is important because the wild-type pIII protein of helper phage (unlike the C-terminal pIII protein domain encoded by the phagemid) renders *E. coli* immune to superinfection (10).

14. The number of colonies (e.g., 200) times 15,000 (culture volume) times 10 (dilution factor) gives the number of independent transformants for each library ligation (e.g., $3 \times 10^7$).

15. Other protocols based on bacterial strains (e.g., TG1) that grow faster than XL1-Blue typically use lower temperatures (e.g., 30°C) in this step (11). This may help to increase the diversity of selected clones by limiting the advantage of faster growth.

16. Only fresh phage prepared on the same day should be used for library panning because the covalent linkage of Fab (phenotype) and phage (genotype) (Fig. 1d) is susceptible to cleavage by contaminating proteases. Fresh phage can be reamplified from the stored phage library as described in Subheading 3.7.

## Acknowledgments

This work was supported by the Intramural Research Program of the Center for Cancer Research, National Cancer Institute, National Institutes of Health. I thank current and former members of my laboratory, in particular Dr. Ka Yin Kwong, Dr. Jiahui Yang, Dr. Sivasubramanian Baskar, and Jessica M. Suschak, for their contributions to this protocol.

## References

1. Beerli RR, Rader C (2010) Mining human antibody repertoires. MAbs 2:365–378
2. Webster R (2001) Filamentous phage biology. In: Barbas CF III, Burton DR, Scott JK, Silverman GJ (eds) Phage display, a laboratory manual. Cold Spring Harbor Laboratory, Cold Spring Harbor, NY
3. Sidhu SS (2001) Engineering M13 for phage display. Biomol Eng 18:57–63
4. Barbas CF III, Kang AS, Lerner RA, Benkovic SJ (1991) Assembly of combinatorial antibody libraries on phage surfaces: the gene III site. Proc Natl Acad Sci USA 88:7978–7982
5. Hofer T, Tangkeangsirisin W, Kennedy MG, Mage RG, Raiker SJ, Venkatesh K, Lee H, Giger RJ, Rader C (2007) Chimeric rabbit/human Fab and IgG specific for members of the Nogo-66 receptor family selected for species cross-reactivity with an improved phage display vector. J Immunol Methods 318:75–87
6. Baskar S, Suschak JM, Samija I, Srinivasan R, Childs RW, Pavletic SZ, Bishop MR, Rader C (2009) A human monoclonal antibody drug and target discovery platform for B-cell chronic lymphocytic leukemia based on allogeneic hematopoietic stem cell transplantation and phage display. Blood 114:4494–4502
7. Andris-Widhopf J, Rader C, Barbas CF III (2001) Generation of antibody libraries: immunization, RNA preparation, and cDNA synthesis. In: Barbas CF III, Burton DR, Scott JK, Silverman GJ (eds) Phage display, a laboratory manual. Cold Spring Harbor Laboratory, Cold Spring Harbor, NY
8. Kwong KY, Baskar S, Zhang H, Mackall CL, Rader C (2008) Generation, affinity maturation, and characterization of a human anti-human NKG2D monoclonal antibody with dual antagonistic and agonistic activity. J Mol Biol 384:1143–1156
9. Brown T, Mackey K, Du T (2004) Analysis of RNA by northern and slot blot hybridization. Curr Protoc Mol Biol chapter 4:unit 4 9
10. Scott JK, Barbas CF III (2001) Phage-display vectors. In: Barbas CF III, Burton DR, Scott JK, Silverman GJ (eds) Phage display, a laboratory manual. Cold Spring Harbor Laboratory, Cold Spring Harbor, NY
11. Zhu Z, Dimitrov DS (2009) Construction of a large naive human phage-displayed Fab library through one-step cloning. Methods Mol Biol 525:129–142, xv
12. Andris-Widhopf J, Rader C, Steinberger P, Fuller R, Barbas CF III (2000) Methods for the generation of chicken monoclonal antibody fragments by phage display. J Immunol Methods 242:159–181

# Chapter 5

# Selection of Human Fab Libraries by Phage Display

Christoph Rader

## Abstract

This protocol describes the selection of human antibody libraries in Fab format by phage display. It includes panning against immobilized antigens, biotinylated antigens in solution, and cell surface antigens.

**Key words:** Immune antibody repertoires, Antibody libraries, Fab, Human monoclonal antibodies

## 1. Introduction

This protocol describes the selection of human Fab libraries generated in phagemid pC3C as described in Chap. 4. We describe methods for library selection with immobilized and soluble purified antigens as well as whole cells. To determine whether the library selection was successful, a phage ELISA is carried out designed to analyze the binding of each phage preparation acquired over the course of the panning experiment. Subsequently, positive clones are identified in a crude Fab ELISA and further analyzed by DNA fingerprinting and sequencing following phagemid preparation.

## 2. Materials

All steps in this protocol can be successfully executed in a laboratory with standard molecular and cell biology equipment, including autoclave, digital balance with 0.01 g readability, freezers (−20 and −80°C), ELISA microplate reader (e.g., VersaMax, Molecular

Gabriele Proetzel and Hilmar Ebersbach (eds.), *Antibody Methods and Protocols*, Methods in Molecular Biology, vol. 901, DOI 10.1007/978-1-61779-931-0_5, © Springer Science+Business Media, LLC 2012

Devices, www.moleculardevices.com), power supply for agarose gel electrophoresis (e.g., EC 105 Compact Power Supply, Owl Separation Systems, www.owlsci.com), refrigerated floor centrifuge (e.g., Sorvall Evolution RC, Thermo Scientific, www.thermoscientific.com) with fixed-angle rotor (e.g., Sorvall SLA-3000 Super-Lite, Thermo Scientific) for 500-mL centrifuge bottles (e.g., Sorvall Dry-Spin Polypropylene Bottles, Fisher Scientific, www.fishersci.com, cat. no. 50-866-922), refrigerator (4°C), rocking platform, single-channel and multichannel micropipettes (1–1,000 μL), shaker (e.g., Innova 4000 Benchtop Incubator Shaker, New Brunswick Scientific, www.nbsc.com; two separate shakers, one for phage-free conditions and one for phage are required), and 96-well thermocyclers (e.g., GeneAmp PCR System 9700; Applied Biosystems, www.appliedbiosystems.com). General disposables such as centrifuge tubes (50 mL), filtered 10-μL, 20-μL, 100-μL, 200-μL, 1-mL pipette tips (e.g., ART, Molecular BioProducts, www.mbpinc.com), 0.22-μm filters (e.g., Millex GP from Millipore, www.millipore), microfuge tubes (1.5 and 2 mL), pipettes (5 mL), round-bottom tubes with snap caps (14 mL), and screw cap tubes (2 mL) are not specially listed. It is recommended to use highly purified water from, e.g., a Picopure 2 UV Plus system (Hydro Service and Supplies, www.hydroservice.com) sterilized by filtration (e.g., Millipore Steriflip Filter Units, cat. no. SCGP00525) and stored at room temperature (RT).

### *2.1. Library Selection with Immobilized Antigen*

1. Purified antigen, at least 10 μg.
2. Phage preparation.
3. 96-Well half-area ELISA plate (Costar 3690, Fisher Scientific, cat. no. 07-200-37).
4. Tris-buffered saline (TBS): 25 mM Tris–HCl, 137 mM NaCl, 3 mM KCl, pH 7.4; diluted in water from 10× TBS (Quality Biological, www.qualitybiological.com, cat. no. 351-086-131); store at RT.
5. Plate sealer (SealPlate, Excel Scientific, www.excelscientific.com, cat. no. 100-SEAL-PLT).
6. 3% (w/v) Bovine serum albumin (BSA) in TBS: Dissolve 1.5 g BSA (Sigma–Aldrich, www.sigmaaldrich.com, cat. no. A7906; store at 4°C) in 50 mL TBS, sterilize by filtration through 0.22 μm, and store at RT (blocking solution).
7. 1% (w/v) BSA in TBS: Dissolve 1.5 g BSA in 50 mL TBS, sterilize by filtration through 0.22 μm, and store at RT.
8. SB medium: Dissolve 20 g 3-(*N*-Morpholino)propanesulfonic acid (MOPS; Sigma–Aldrich, cat. no. M3183; store at RT), 60 g Bacto tryptone (BD Biosciences, www.bd.com, cat. no. 211705; store at RT), and 40 g Bacto yeast extract (BD Biosciences, cat. no. 212750; store at RT) in 1.9 L total volume

with water. Bring to pH 7.0 with 1 N NaOH (Fisher Scientific, cat. no. AC12426-0010; store at RT). Bring to 2 L total volume with water. Sterilize by autoclaving in two 1-L or four 500-mL glass bottles. Store at RT.

9. Electrocompetent XL1-Blue (Agilent Technologies, www.genomics.agilent.com, cat. no. 200228); store at −80°C.
10. 5 μg/μL Tetracycline: Dissolve 50 mg tetracycline hydrochloride (Sigma–Aldrich, cat. no. T7660; store at −20°C) in 10 mL ethanol. Store 1-mL aliquots in 1.5-mL microfuge tubes at −20°C.
11. 0.05% (v/v) Tween 20 in TBS: Dilute 25 μL Tween 20 (Sigma–Aldrich, cat. no. P1379; store at RT) in 50 mL TBS, sterilize by filtration through 0.22 μm, and store at RT (washing solution).
12. 10 mg/mL Trypsin in TBS: Dissolve 50 mg Difco trypsin 1:250 (BD Biosciences, cat. no. 215240; store at RT) in 5 mL TBS and sterilize by filtration through 0.22 μm; use freshly.
13. 100 μg/μL Carbenicillin: Dissolve 1 g carbenicillin disodium (Duchefa, www.duchefa.com, cat. no. C0109.0005; store at 4°C) in 10 mL water. Sterilize by filtration through 0.22 μm. Store 1-mL aliquots in 1.5-mL microfuge tubes at −20°C.
14. LB + 100 μg/mL carbenicillin plates (Teknova, www.teknova.com, cat. no. L1010); store at 4°C.
15. VCSM13 helper phage (Agilent Technologies, cat. no. 200251); store at −80°C.
16. 50 μg/μL Kanamycin: Dissolve 500 mg kanamycin sulfate (Sigma–Aldrich, cat. no. K1377; store at RT) in 10 mL water. Sterilize by filtration through 0.22 μm. Store 1-mL aliquots in 1.5-mL microfuge tubes at −20°C.
17. PEG-8000 (Sigma–Aldrich, cat. no. P5413); store at RT.
18. NaCl (Mallinckrodt Baker, www.mallbaker.com, cat. no. 3624-01); store at RT.

### 2.2. Library Selection with Biotinylated Antigen in Solution

1. Phage preparation.
2. Biotinylated antigen at a concentration of 1 μg/μL.
3. 1% (w/v) BSA in TBS: Dissolve 1.5 g BSA in 50 mL TBS, sterilize by filtration through 0.22 μm, and store at RT.
4. SB medium (see Subheading 2.1).
5. XL-1 Blue cells (see Subheading 2.1).
6. Tetracycline (see Subheading 2.1).
7. Mini rotator (e.g., Glas-Col, www.glascol.com).
8. Dynabeads MyOne Streptavidin C1 (Invitrogen, www.invitrogen.com, cat. no. 650.01); store at 4°C.
9. Dynal MPC-S magnetic particle concentrator (Invitrogen, cat. no. 120.20D).

10. 0.05% (v/v) Tween 20 in TBS.
11. 10 mg/mL Trypsin in PBS: Dissolve 50 mg Difco trypsin 1:250 (see Subheading 2.1) in 5 mL PBS and sterilize by filtration through 0.22 μm; use freshly.

***2.3. Library Selection with Soluble or Suspended Human Cells***

1. Phage preparation.
2. Rat-anti-HA mAb 3F10 (Roche Applied Science, www.roche-applied-science.com, cat. no. 11867423001); store at 4°C.
3. SB medium (see Subheading 2.1).
4. XL1-Blue cells (see Subheading 2.1).
5. 5 μg/μL Tetracycline (see Subheading 2.1).
6. Human serum or fetal bovine serum (FBS; e.g., Invitrogen); store at −20°C.
7. Phosphate-buffered saline (PBS): 5.6 mM $Na_2HPO_4$, 154 mM NaCl, 1.06 mM $KH_2PO_4$, pH 7.4; diluted in water from 10× PBS (Quality Biological, cat. no. 119-069-101); store at RT.
8. 5% (v/v) human serum or FBS in PBS.
9. 1% (w/v) BSA in PBS: Dissolve 0.5 g BSA (see Subheading 2.1) in 50 mL PBS, sterilize by filtration through 0.22 μm, and store at RT.
10. 2% (w/v) sodium azide: Dissolve 0.2 g sodium azide (Sigma–Aldrich, cat. no. S8032; store at RT) in 10 mL water. Store at RT.
11. 10 mg/mL Trypsin in PBS: (see Subheading 2.2).

***2.4. Phage ELISA with Immobilized Antigen***

1. 96-Well half-area ELISA plate (see Subheading 2.1).
2. TBS (see Subheading 2.1).
3. Plate sealer (see Subheading 2.1).
4. 3% (w/v) BSA in TBS (see Subheading 2.1).
5. 1% (w/v) BSA in TBS (see Subheading 2.1).
6. 0.05% (v/v) Tween 20 in TBS (see Subheading 2.1).
7. Mouse anti-M13 mAb conjugated to horse radish peroxidase (HRP) (GE Healthcare, www.gelifesciences.com, cat. no. 27-9421-01), store at −20°C.
8. HRP substrate solution: Prepare a 50× (100 mM) 2,2′-azino-bis(3-ethylbenzthiazoline-6-sulfonic acid) (ABTS) solution by dissolving 549 mg ABTS (Roche Applied Science, cat. no. 10102946001; store at 4°C) in 10 mL water. Store in 1-mL aliquots at −20°C. Prepare 10× (500 mM) sodium citrate (pH 4.0) buffer by dissolving 48.025 g citric acid (Sigma–Aldrich, cat. no. C0759; store at RT) in 450 mL water; adjust to pH 4.0 with 1 N NaOH (Fisher Scientific, cat. no. AC12426-0010; store at RT) and adjust the volume to 500 mL with water; autoclave and store at RT. Prepare the HRP substrate solution

freshly by mixing 5.3 mL water, 120 μL 50× ABTS solution, 600 μL 10× sodium citrate (pH 4.0) buffer, and 2 μL 30% (w/w) hydrogen peroxide (Fisher Scientific, cat. no. H325-100; store at 4°C) in a 14-mL round-bottom tube.

#### 2.5. Phage ELISA with Soluble or Suspended Human Cells

1. Phage preparation.
2. PBS (see Subheading 2.3).
3. Soluble or suspended human cells.
4. 96-Well V-bottom tissue-culture plate (Costar 3894, Fisher Scientific, cat. no. 07-200-96).
5. Mouse anti-M13 mAb conjugated to HRP (see Subheading 2.4).
6. HRP substrate (see Subheading 2.4).

#### 2.6. Crude Fab Preparation

1. SB medium (see Subheading 2.1).
2. 100 μg/μL Carbenicillin (see Subheading 2.1).
3. LB + 100 μg/mL carbenicillin plates (see Subheading 2.1).
4. 0.5 M IPTG: Dissolve 6 g isopropyl-β-d-thiogalactoside (IPTG, Gold Biotechnology, www.goldbio.com, cat. no. I2481C25; store at −20°C) in 50 mL water. Sterilize by filtration through 0.22 μm. Store 1-mL aliquots in 1.5-mL microfuge tubes at −20°C.

#### 2.7. Crude Fab ELISA with Immobilized Antigen

1. 96-Well half-area ELISA plates (see Subheading 2.1).
2. TBS (see Subheading 2.1).
3. Goat anti-human kappa light chain polyclonal antibodies (pAbs) (SouthernBiotech, www.southernbiotech.com, cat. no. 2060-01); store at 4°C.
4. Goat anti-human lambda light chain pAbs (SouthernBiotech, cat. no. 2070-01); store at 4°C.
5. Plate sealer (see Subheading 2.1).
6. 3% (w/v) BSA in TBS (see Subheading 2.1).
7. 1% (w/v) BSA in TBS (see Subheading 2.1).
8. Water.
9. Rat-anti-HA mAb 3F10 conjugated to HRP (Roche Applied Science, cat. no. 12013819001); store at 4°C.
10. HRP substrate solution (see Subheading 2.4).

#### 2.8. Crude Fab ELISA with Soluble or Suspended Human Cells

1. Soluble or suspended human cells.
2. PBS (see Subheading 2.3).
3. 96-Well V-bottom tissue-culture plate (see Subheading 2.3).
4. Rat-anti-HA mAb 3F10 conjugated to HRP (see Subheading 2.7).

5. HRP substrate solution (see Subheading 2.4).
6. ELISA microplate reader.

#### 2.9. DNA Fingerprinting and Sequencing

1. SB medium (see Subheading 2.1).
2. 100 μg/μL Carbenicillin (see Subheading 2.1).
3. QIAprep Spin Miniprep Kit (Qiagen, www.qiagen.com, cat. no. 27106); store at RT.
4. 0.2-mL PCR tubes (e.g., Eppendorf, cat. no. 951010022).
5. Sense and antisense primers diluted to 20 μM in water (see Table 1 in Chap. 4).
6. 10 mM dNTP mix: 2.5 mM of each dATP, dCTP, dGTP, and dTTP diluted in water from 100 mM stock concentrations (GE Healthcare, cat. no. 28-4065-52); store at −20°C.
7. 5 U/μL Taq DNA polymerase, 10× Taq buffer with $(NH_4)_2SO_4$, and 25 mM $MgCl_2$ (Fermentas, www.fermentas.com, cat. no. EP0072); store at −20°C.
8. 10 U/μL *Alu*I and 10× Tango buffer (Fermentas, cat. no. ER0011); store at −20°C.
9. 6× Gel loading dye solution (Fermentas, cat. no. R0611); store at RT.
10. Model D2 Spider Wide Gel Electrophoresis System with two D1-20C combs (Owl Separation Systems).
11. Agarose (Invitrogen, cat. no. 16500500); store at RT.
12. TAE buffer (40 mM Tris–acetate (pH 8.0), 1 mM EDTA; diluted in water from 50× TAE) (Quality Biological, cat. no. 351-008-131); store at RT.
13. SYBR Safe DNA gel stain (Invitrogen, cat. no. S33102); store at RT.
14. 100-bp DNA ladder (Fermentas, cat. no. SM0243); store at RT.
15. Safe Imager blue-light transilluminator (Invitrogen).

## 3. Methods

#### 3.1. Library Selection with Immobilized Antigen

This step outlined in Fig. 1 takes about 5 days. The selection can be performed using three different options depending on the type of antigen the library is panned against. If purified stable antigen is available, it can be used immobilized (Subheading 3.1) or, following biotinylation, in solution (Subheading 3.2). Subheading 3.3 provides a protocol for panning the library against soluble or

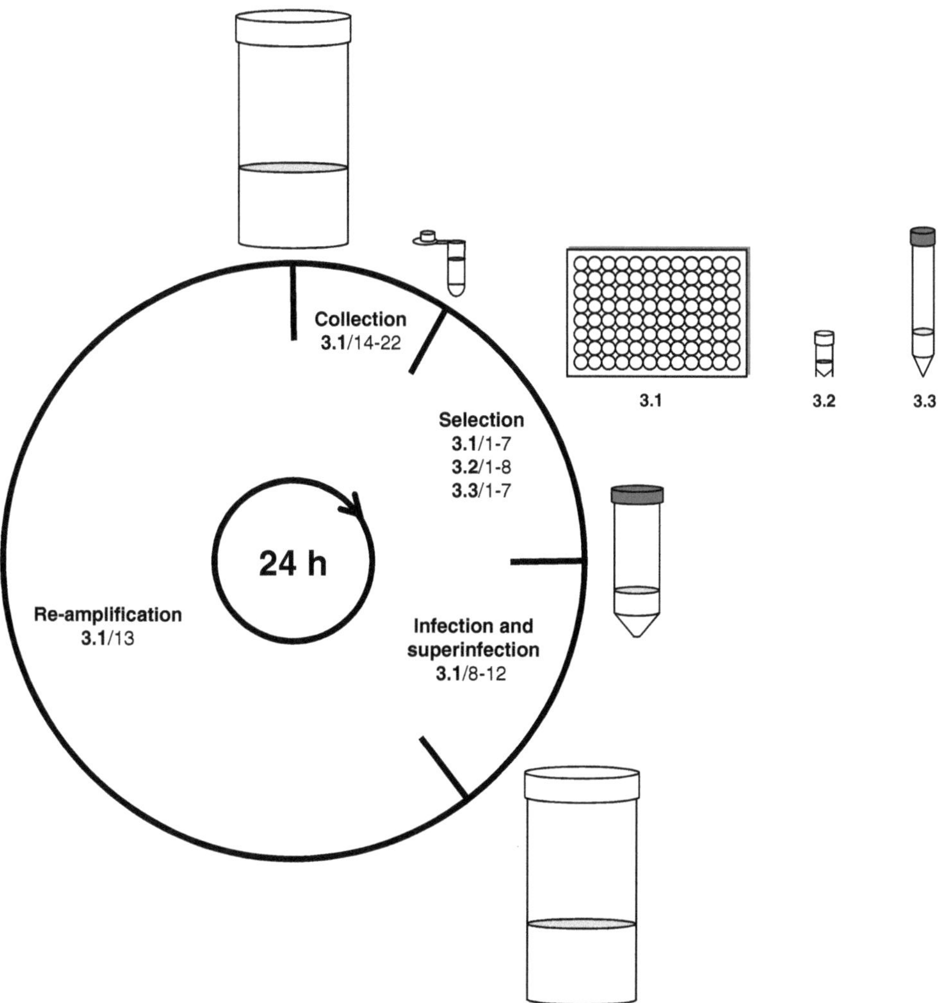


Fig. 1. Library selection. Each panning round consists of a 24-h cycle of phage collection (Subheading 3.1, steps 14–22), phage selection (with options 3.1, 3.2, or 3.3), phage infection followed by helper phage superinfection (Subheading 3.1, steps 8–12), and re-amplification (Subheading 3.1, step 13). Plasticware used for collection (500-mL centrifuge tube and 2-mL microfuge tube), selection (96-well half-area ELISA plate, 2-mL screw cap tube, or 15-mL conical centrifuge tube depending on option 3.1, 3.2, or 3.3), and infection, superinfection, and re-amplification (50- and 500-mL centrifuge tubes) are shown.

suspended human cells which may be the option of choice if the antigen is unknown or purified stable antigen is unavailable. Using different libraries or different antigens, up to four panning experiments for Subheading 3.1 and 3.2 and two panning experiments for Subheading 3.3 can be carried out in parallel.

In the first panning round, carry out steps 1 and 2 in parallel to Subheading 3.6, steps 14–23, described in Chap. 4. In subsequent panning rounds, carry out steps 1 and 2 in parallel to steps 14–22. In the first panning round, coat two wells for each library to be selected. One well is sufficient in each of all subsequent panning rounds.

1. Coat 1–2 wells of a 96-well half-area ELISA plate with 0.1–1 μg of antigen in 25 μL TBS, cover the wells with plate sealer, and incubate at 37°C for 1 h.
2. Shake out the coating solution, add 150 μL 3% (w/v) BSA in TBS for blocking to each coated well, cover with plate sealer, and incubate at 37°C for 1 h.
3. Shake out the blocking solution, add 50 μL of the phage preparation in 1% (w/v) BSA in TBS to each blocked well, cover with plate sealer, and incubate at 37°C for 2 h.
4. In the meantime, inoculate 2 mL SB medium in a 50-mL centrifuge tube with 4 μL XL1-Blue (from a single electrocompetent XL1-Blue aliquot that can be thawed from and frozen at -80°C multiple times), add 4 μL 5 μg/μL tetracycline, and shake at 37°C and 275 rpm for approximately 2 h. Grow one culture for each parallel panning experiment and one additional culture for input titering (see Note 1).
5. Shake out the phage solution, add 150 μL 0.05% (v/v) Tween 20 in TBS to each prepared well, pipette five times vigorously up and down, and incubate for 5 min at RT (a multichannel pipette may be used to wash two or more wells at the same time). Shake out the washing solution and repeat this washing step 5 times (first panning round), 5–10 times (second and third panning rounds), and 10–15 times (fourth and all subsequent panning rounds).
6. Shake out the final washing solution, add 50 μL of freshly prepared 10 mg/mL trypsin in TBS to each prepared well, cover with plate sealer, and incubate at 37°C for 30 min.
7. Pipette ten times vigorously up and down and transfer the combined trypsin solution (2× 50 μL in the first panning round, 1× 50 μL in all subsequent panning rounds) to the prepared 2-mL XL1-Blue culture. Incubate at RT for 15 min.
8. To each phage-infected 2-mL XL1-Blue culture, add 6 mL SB, 1.6 μL 100 μg/μL carbenicillin, and 12 μL 5 μg/μL tetracycline. Shake at 37°C and 250 rpm for 1 h. Carry out steps 9 and 10 during this incubation.
9. For output titering, remove a 2-μL aliquot, add to 198 μL SB medium in a 1.5-mL microfuge tube, and plate 100 μL on an LB + 100 μg/mL carbenicillin plate. Incubate at 37°C overnight (see Note 2; for troubleshooting see Table 1).
10. For input titering, prepare a $10^{-8}$ dilution of the phage preparation by serial dilutions in SB medium. Transfer 150 μL of the XL1-Blue culture that was prepared for input titering into a 1.5-mL microfuge tube, add 1 μL of the $10^{-8}$ dilution, incubate for 15 min at RT, and plate the entire volume on an

**Table 1**
**Troubleshooting**

| Step | Problem | Possible reason | Solution |
|---|---|---|---|
| Subheading 3.1, steps 9, 10, and 13 | (1) No colonies on input and output plates | (1) Contamination of XL1-Blue cultures with helper phage | (1) Repeat panning round with fresh reagents and clean equipment for growing XL1-Blue cultures in phage-free conditions as discussed in Note 1 |
| | (2) No colonies on output plates and no growth in overnight culture | (2) Selection conditions are too stringent | (2a) Increase the amount of antigen used for panning and reduce the number of washing steps<br>(2b) Consider other options for library selection (Subheadings 3.1, 3.2, or 3.3) |
| Subheading 3.4, step 7 | (1) Only weak specific antigen reactivity after four rounds of panning | (1a) Selection conditions are not optimal<br>(1b) Selected phage have weak affinity | (1) Carry out two additional panning rounds |
| | (2) No specific antigen reactivity after four rounds of panning | (2) Selection failed | (2) Consider other options for library selection (Subheadings 3.1, 3.2, or 3.3) |
| Subheadings 3.7, step 7 and 3.8, step 6 | (1) Percentage of positive clones is low | (1) Selection conditions are not optimal | (1) Carry out two additional panning rounds |
| | (2) Only weak specific antigen reactivity | (2a) Selected Fab are expressed at low levels | (2a) Repeat with purified Fab (see Note 15) |
| | | (2b) Selected Fab have weak affinity | (2b (1)) Convert Fab to IgG (see Note 15)<br>(2b (2)) Increase the stringency of selection by reducing the amount of antigen used for panning and increasing the number of washing steps<br>(2b (3)) Consider other options for library selection (Subheadings 3.1, 3.2, or 3.3) |

(continued)

**Table 1 (continued)**

| Step | Problem | Possible reason | Solution |
|---|---|---|---|
| Subheading 3.9, steps 6 and 7 | (1) No distinct *Alu*I fingerprints and DNA sequences | (1) Selection conditions are too stringent | (1a) Analyze positive clones from the previous panning round<br>(1b) Reduce stringency of selection by increasing the amount of antigen used for panning and reducing the number of washing steps |
| | (2) No repeated *Alu*I fingerprints and DNA sequences | (2) Selection conditions are not optimal | (2a) Carry out two additional panning rounds with increased stringency of selection through reducing the amount of antigen and increasing the number of washing steps<br>(2b) Consider other options for library selection (Subheadings 3.1, 3.2, or 3.3) |

LB + 100 μg/mL carbenicillin plate. Incubate at 37°C overnight (see Note 2; for troubleshooting see Table 1).

11. Add 2.4 μL 100 μg/μL carbenicillin to the culture in the 50-mL centrifuge tube and continue shaking at 37°C and 250 rpm for 1 h.
12. Add 1 mL VCSM13 helper phage ($10^{11}$–$10^{12}$ pfu/mL) and transfer into a 500-mL centrifuge bottle. Add 91 mL SB, 46 μL 100 μg/μL carbenicillin, and 184 μL 5 μg/μL tetracycline (Σ 100 mL). Shake at 37°C and 275 rpm for 90 min.
13. Add 140 μL 50 μg/μL kanamycin and continue shaking at 37°C and 275 rpm overnight (12–16 h) (see Note 3; for troubleshooting see Table 1).
14. Centrifuge at 3,000 × *g* for 15 min at 4°C.
15. For phage precipitation, transfer the supernatant to a clean 500-mL centrifuge tube with 4 g PEG-8000 and 3 g NaCl and dissolve by shaking at 37°C and 300 rpm for 5 min.
16. Incubate on ice for 30 min. Centrifuge at 15,000 × *g* for 15 min at 4°C.
17. Discard the supernatant, drain the bottle by inverting on a paper towel for 10 min, and carefully wipe off the remaining liquid with a paper towel.

18. Resuspend the phage pellet in 2 mL 1% (w/v) BSA in TBS by pipetting up and down along the side of the centrifuge tube.
19. Transfer to a 2-mL microfuge tube, and pipette up and down in a 1-mL pipette tip.
20. Centrifuge at 16,000 × $g$ for 5 min at 4°C.
21. Pass the supernatant through a 0.22-μm filter into a clean 2-mL microfuge tube.
22. Store on ice and continue with the next panning round (go back to step 1) (see Notes 4 and 5).

### 3.2. Library Selection with Biotinylated Antigen in Solution

1. Transfer 1 mL of the phage preparation in 1% (w/v) BSA in TBS to a 2-mL screw cap tube. Add 5 μL of 1 μg/μL biotinylated antigen in TBS. Using a mini rotator, rotate the mixture at 37°C and 10 rpm for 1 h (see Note 6).
2. In the meantime, inoculate 2 mL SB medium in a 50-mL centrifuge tube with 4 μL XL1-Blue (from a single electrocompetent XL1-Blue aliquot that can be thawed from and frozen at −80°C multiple times), add 4 μL 5 μg/μL tetracycline, and shake at 37°C and 275 rpm for approximately 2 h. Grow one culture for each parallel panning experiment and one additional culture for input titering (see Note 1).
3. Wash 50 μL Dynabeads MyOne Streptavidin C1 with 1 mL TBS according to the manufacturer's protocol and add to the incubation mixture. Rotate at 37°C and 10 rpm for 30 min.
4. Place the sample on a Dynal MPC-S magnetic particle concentrator for 2 min. Keep the sample on the magnet while removing the supernatant with a pipette.
5. Remove the sample from the magnet and resuspend the beads in 1 mL 0.05% (v/v) Tween 20 in TBS. Rotate at 37°C and 10 rpm for 5 min. Place the sample on the magnet for 2 min. Keep the sample on the magnet while removing the supernatant with a pipette. Repeat this washing step 5 times (first panning round), 5–10 times (second and third panning rounds), and 10–15 times (fourth and all subsequent panning rounds).
6. After removing the final supernatant, resuspend the beads in 50 μL of freshly prepared 10 mg/mL trypsin in TBS and incubate at 37°C for 30 min.
7. Add the prepared 2-mL XL1-Blue culture directly to the trypsinized beads. Incubate at RT for 15 min.
8. Pipette ten times vigorously up and down and transfer the combined trypsin solution (2× 50 μL in the first panning round, 1× 50 μL in all subsequent panning rounds) to the prepared 2-mL XL1-Blue culture. Incubate at RT for 15 min. Continue as described in Subheading 3.1, steps 8–22.

### 3.3. Library Selection with Soluble or Suspended Human Cells

1. Carry out one panning round against 500 ng immobilized rat anti-hemagglutinin (HA) mAb 3F10 (Roche) in each of the two wells as described in Subheading 3.1, steps 1–22 (see Note 7).
2. Inoculate 2 mL SB medium in 50-mL centrifuge tubes with 4 μL XL1-Blue (from a single electrocompetent XL1-Blue aliquot that can be thawed from and frozen at −80°C multiple times), add 4 μL 5 μg/μL tetracycline, and shake at 37°C and 275 rpm for approximately 2 h. Grow two cultures for each parallel panning experiment and one additional culture for input titering (see Note 1).
3. Mix 0.5 mL of the phage preparation with 0.5 mL 5% (v/v) human serum or FBS in PBS and 0.5 mL 1% (w/v) BSA in PBS in a 15-mL conical centrifuge tube. Add 15 μL (0.01 vol) 2% (w/v) sodium azide and incubate for 30 min at RT (see Note 8).
4. Collect $1–5 \times 10^7$ soluble or suspended human cells in 1.5 mL 5% (v/v) human serum or FBS in PBS, add to the 1.5 mL phage preparation, and incubate for 30 min at RT with gentle agitation every 5 min.
5. Add 12 mL PBS, centrifuge at $300 \times g$ for 10 min at RT, and decant and discard the supernatant. Repeat this washing step twice more with 15 mL PBS.
6. Resuspend the cells in 0.6 mL freshly prepared 10 mg/mL trypsin in PBS and shake at 37°C and 250 rpm for 30 min.
7. Pipette ten times vigorously up and down and transfer half of the trypsin solution to each of the two prepared 2-mL XL1-Blue cultures. Incubate at RT for 15 min. Continue as described in Subheading 3.1, steps 8–22 (see Note 9).

### 3.4. Phage ELISA with Immobilized Antigen

To determine whether the library selection was successful, a phage ELISA is carried out designed to analyze the binding of each phage preparation acquired over the course of the panning experiment. For example, four panning rounds yield five phage preparations. This step takes about 6 h and can be performed with purified antigen as described here or with soluble or suspended human cells as described under Subheading 3.5.

1. For each phage preparation, coat two wells in row A of a 96-well half-area ELISA plate with 0.1–1 μg of antigen in 25 μL TBS, cover the wells with plate sealer, and incubate at 37°C for 1 h or overnight at 4°C.
2. Shake out the coating solution, add 150 μL 3% (w/v) BSA in TBS for blocking to each coated well and to a corresponding empty well in row B, cover with plate sealer, and incubate at 37°C for 1 h.
3. Shake out the blocking solution, add 50 μL of the phage preparations diluted 1:5 in 1% (w/v) BSA in TBS to the

appropriate blocked wells, cover with plate sealer, and incubate at 37°C for 2 h.

4. Shake out the phage solution. Use a multichannel pipette to wash each well ten times with 150 μL 0.05% (v/v) Tween 20 in TBS.
5. Shake out the final washing solution, add 50 μL of a 1:1,000 dilution of mouse anti-M13 mAb conjugated to HRP in 1% (w/v) BSA in TBS to each well, cover with plate sealer, and incubate at 37°C for 1 h.
6. Shake out the detecting antibody solution. Use a multichannel pipette to wash each well ten times with 150 μL water.
7. Shake out the final washing solution, add 50 μL HRP substrate solution to each well, and incubate at RT for 5 min to 1 h. Determine the absorbance at 405 nm with an ELISA microplate reader (see Note 10; for troubleshooting see Table 1).

### 3.5. Phage ELISA with Soluble or Suspended Human Cells

1. On the basis of input titers determined during library selection, dilute phage preparations to approximately $10^{11}$ phage in 75 μL PBS and store on ice.
2. Add $5 \times 10^5$ soluble or suspended human cells that were washed twice with PBS and brought in 100 μL PBS to each well of a 96-well V-bottom tissue-culture plate. For each phage preparation to be tested, prepare one well in row A and one well in row B.
3. Centrifuge the plate at $300 \times g$ for 10 min at RT, decant and discard the supernatant, and resuspend the cells in 75 μL prepared phage preparation (row A) or 75 μL PBS (row B). Incubate the covered plate at RT for 1 h with gentle rocking.
4. Centrifuge the plate at $300 \times g$ for 10 min at RT, decant and discard the supernatant, and resuspend the cells in 100 μL PBS with a multichannel pipette. Repeat this washing step once more.
5. Decant and discard the final washing solution and resuspend the cells in 100 μL of a 1:1,000 dilution of mouse anti-M13 mAb conjugated to HRP in PBS. Incubate the covered plate at RT.
6. Centrifuge the plate at $300 \times g$ for 10 min at RT, decant and discard the supernatant, and resuspend the cells in 100 μL PBS with a multichannel pipette. Repeat this washing step once more.
7. Decant and discard the final washing solution and resuspend the cells in 50 μL HRP substrate solution. Incubate the covered plate at RT for 5 min to 1 h. Determine the absorbance at 405 nm with an ELISA microplate reader (see Note 10; for troubleshooting see Table 1).

### 3.6. Crude Fab Preparation

If the phage ELISA revealed reactive phage preparations from the third, fourth, or any subsequent panning round, crude Fab prepared from colonies of the output plate that corresponds to the most reactive phage preparation should be analyzed next (see Note 11).

1. Prepare thirty-two 14-mL round-bottom tubes with snap cap, each containing 3 mL SB medium supplemented with 100 μg/mL carbenicillin, and inoculate with 31 colonies from the output plate of interest. Use the remaining tube as negative control for both culture growth and ELISA. Shake at 37°C and 300 rpm for 8 h.
2. Transfer a 2-μL aliquot of each culture to a labeled grid on a prewarmed LB + 100 μg/mL carbenicillin plate. Incubate at 37°C overnight. This backup plate will be used in Subheading 3.9, steps 1 and 2, for phagemid preparation.
3. Add 12 μL 0.5 M IPTG to each culture (to a final concentration of 2 mM). Continue shaking at 37°C and 300 rpm overnight (12–16 h) (see Note 12).
4. Centrifuge at 3,000 × *g* for 15 min at 4°C. Transfer 1 mL of the supernatant to 1.5-mL microfuge tubes and discard the remaining supernatant and pellet. Store on ice.

The next step can be performed with purified antigen (Subheading 3.7) or with soluble or suspended human cells (Subheading 3.8).

### 3.7. Crude Fab ELISA with Immobilized Antigen

1. Use two 96-well half-area ELISA plates. On the first plate, coat each of 32 wells with 0.1–1 μg of antigen in 25 μL TBS, each of 32 wells with 200 ng goat anti-human kappa light chain pAbs in 25 μL TBS, and leave the remaining 32 wells empty. On the second plate, coat each of 32 wells with 0.1–1 μg of antigen in 25 μL TBS, each of 32 wells with 200 ng goat anti-human lambda light chain pAbs in 25 μL TBS, and leave the remaining 32 wells empty. Cover the wells with plate sealer, and incubate at 37°C for 1 h or overnight at 4°C.
2. Shake out the coating solution, add 150 μL 3% (w/v) BSA in TBS for blocking to each coated or empty well, cover with plate sealer, and incubate at 37°C for 1 h.
3. Shake out the blocking solution, and add 50 μL of the supernatant prepared in Subheading 3.6, step 4, to each well so that each of the 32 samples is incubated with BSA-blocked antigen (on both plates), BSA-blocked goat anti-human kappa light chain pAbs (on the first plate), BSA-blocked goat anti-lambda light chain pAbs (on the second plate), and BSA alone (on both plates). Cover with plate sealer, and incubate at 37°C for 2 h.
4. Shake out the supernatant. Use a multichannel pipette to wash each well ten times with 150 μL water.
5. Shake out the final washing solution, add 50 μL of a 1:1,000 dilution of rat-anti-HA mAb 3F10 conjugated to HRP in 1%

(w/v) BSA in TBS to each well, cover with plate sealer, and incubate at 37°C for 1 h.

6. Shake out the detecting antibody solution. Use a multichannel pipette to wash each well ten times with 150 μL water.
7. Shake out the final washing solution, add 50 μL of HRP substrate solution to each well, and incubate at RT for 5 min to 1 h. Determine the absorbance at 405 nm with an ELISA microplate reader (see Note 13; for troubleshooting see Table 1).

### 3.8. Crude Fab ELISA with Soluble or Suspended Human Cells

1. Add $5 \times 10^5$ soluble or suspended human cells that were washed twice with PBS and brought in 100 μL PBS to each of 32 wells of a 96-well V-bottom tissue-culture plate.
2. Centrifuge the plate at 300 × *g* for 10 min at RT, decant and discard the supernatant, and resuspend the cells in 75 μL of the supernatant prepared in Subheading 3.6, step 4. Incubate the covered plate at RT for 1 h with gentle rocking.
3. Centrifuge the plate at 300 × *g* for 10 min at RT, decant and discard the supernatant, and resuspend the cells in 100 μL PBS with a multichannel pipette. Repeat this washing step once more.
4. Decant and discard the final washing solution and resuspend the cells in 100 μL of a 1:1,000 dilution of rat-anti-HA mAb 3F10 conjugated to HRP in PBS. Incubate the covered plate at RT.
5. Centrifuge the plate at 300 × *g* for 10 min at RT, decant and discard the supernatant, and resuspend the cells in 100 μL PBS with a multichannel pipette. Repeat this washing step once more.
6. Decant and discard the final washing solution and resuspend the cells in 50 μL HRP substrate solution. Incubate the covered plate at RT for 5 min to 1 h. Determine the absorbance at 405 nm with an ELISA microplate reader (see Note 13; for troubleshooting see Table 1).

### 3.9. DNA Fingerprinting and Sequencing

If the crude Fab ELISA revealed positive clones, these should be analyzed by DNA fingerprinting and sequencing following phagemid preparation. The following steps take about 3 days and are based on the analysis of 20 positive clones.

1. Prepare twenty 14-mL round-bottom tubes with snap cap, each containing 2 mL SB medium supplemented with 100 μg/mL carbenicillin, and inoculate each with a colony from the backup plate prepared in Subheading 3.6, step 2, that corresponds to a positive clone. Shake at 37°C and 300 rpm overnight (12–16 h).
2. Centrifuge at 3,000 × *g* for 15 min at 4°C. Discard the supernatant and resuspend the pellet in 250 μL Qiagen buffer P1 from the QIAprep Spin Miniprep Kit. Continue the phagemid

preparation using reagents and protocols supplied by the QIAprep Spin Miniprep Kit. Store phagemid preparations in 20 μL water at –20°C.

3. For PCR amplification of the VL/CL/VH expression cassette, transfer 1 μL of each sample into 0.2-mL PCR tubes. Prepare a PCR master mix sufficient for 20 reactions. In a 1.5-mL microfuge tube, combine 75 μL 10× PCR buffer, 75 μL 25 mM $MgCl_2$, 60 μL 10 mM dNTP mix, 22.5 μL 20 μM C-5′SFIHUVL (sense primer; Table 1 in Chap. 4), 22.5 μL 20 μM c-3′sfivh (antisense primer; Table 1 in Chap. 4), 466 μL water, and 4 μL 5 U/μL Taq DNA polymerase (Σ 725 μL). Add 29 μL of the PCR master mix to each prepared 1 μL sample.
4. In a 96-well thermocycler, use these PCR parameters:

   95°C for 2 min, followed by 30 cycles of 95°C for 30 s, 52°C for 30 s, and 72°C for 90 s.

   Followed by 72°C for 10 min, followed by cooling to RT.

   Transfer a 10-μL aliquot from each sample to 1.5-mL microfuge tubes.
5. Prepare an *Alu*I master mix sufficient for 20 reactions. In a 1.5-mL microfuge tube, combine 90 μL 10× Tango buffer, 495 μL water, and 15 μL 10 U/μL *Alu*I (Σ 600 μL). Add 20 μL of the *Alu*I master mix to each prepared 10 μL sample and incubate at 37°C for 2 h.
6. Add 3 μL 6× gel loading dye solution, and separate by electrophoresis on a 4% (w/v) agarose gel in TAE buffer using a 100-bp DNA ladder as reference. For troubleshooting see Table 1.
7. Further analyze the phagemid preparations of clones that look different by DNA fingerprinting by custom DNA sequencing. Use sense primer VLSEQ (a sense primer located around the *Eco*RI site in pC3C; see Fig. 1 and Table 1 in Chap. 4) and vhseq (an antisense primer located downstream of the *Sfi*I (b) site in pC3C; see Fig. 1 and Table 1 in Chap. 4) to determine the DNA and deduced amino acid sequences of light- and heavy-chain variable domains (see Notes 14 and 15; for troubleshooting see Table 1).

## 4. Notes

1. Take precautions to avoid contaminating the *E. coli* culture with phage including helper phage. Use a separate area and filtered pipette tips for pipetting and a phage-free shaker for growth. This is important because the wild-type pIII protein

of helper phage (unlike the C-terminal pIII protein domain encoded by the phagemid) renders *E. coli* immune to superinfection (1).

2. *Output titering.* The number of colonies (e.g., 50) times 8,000 (volume of output solution) determines the output number for each panning round (e.g., $4 \times 10^5$). *Input titering*: The number of colonies (e.g., 50) times $1 \times 10^8$ (dilution factor) times 50 or 100 (volume of input phage preparation) determines the input number for each panning round (e.g., $5 \times 10^{11}$). Output numbers can range anywhere from $1 \times 10^4$ to $1 \times 10^7$. They are typically low in the second panning round and sometimes increase by factor 10–100 from second to third or third to fourth panning rounds, indicating a successful library selection. Input numbers vary less with a typical range from $1 \times 10^{11}$ to $1 \times 10^{12}$.
3. Other protocols based on bacterial strains (e.g., TG1) that grow faster than XL1-Blue typically use lower temperatures (e.g., 30°C) in this step (2). This may help to increase the diversity of selected clones by limiting the advantage of faster growth.
4. Typically, four panning rounds are sufficient to select a panel of human Fab that bind with high affinity and specificity. If the panning experiment needs to be interrupted, add 0.01 volume 2% (w/v) sodium azide to the phage preparation, store at 4°C, and resume the panning experiment by first re-amplifying phage as described in Subheading 3.8 in Chap. 4.
5. Before proceeding with the analysis of library selection as described in Subheadings 3.4 and 3.5, phage preparations and output plates from each panning round can be stored for up to 1 week at 4°C.
6. Recommended biotinylation reagents and protocols are supplied by the BiotinTag Micro Biotinylation Kit which is based on an *N*-hydroxysuccinimide derivative of biotin that reacts with primary amino groups provided in protein or peptide antigens by the ε-amino group of lysine or the N-terminus. Note that this modification may remove natural epitopes or add artificial epitopes.
7. Panning against immobilized rat anti-HA mAb 3F10 eliminates phage that do not display functional human Fab with HA tag (see Fig. 1 in Chap. 4). Including this cleaning step before and at some point during panning against human cells was found to be critical for the selection of functional human Fab (3).
8. In this blocking step, use serum the human cells have been exposed to, e.g., human serum for primary human cells and FBS for human cell lines. Sodium azide is added to prevent internalization of phage.

9. The provided basic protocol (Subheading 3.3) uses a simple strategy that is based on positive selection only. Depending on the outcome of this basic protocol, the library, the antigen of interest, and the available cells, it may be advisable to include consecutive or simultaneous negative and positive selection with antigen-negative (or antigen-masked (4)) and antigen-positive cells (5, 6). These advanced protocols may avoid the selection of both phage that stick to cells nonspecifically and phage that bind to common cell surface antigens.
10. A successful panning experiment typically reveals strong antigen (but not background) reactivity in phage preparations from the third and/or fourth panning round.
11. The term "crude Fab" refers to unpurified Fab-HA-pIII fusion protein and its proteolytic fragments.
12. Lower temperatures (e.g., 30°C) in this step may increase the quality and quantity of crude Fab from some clones.
13. The detecting antibody, rat anti-HA mAb 3F10 conjugated to HRP, binds to the hemagglutinin (HA) decapeptide tag that is located between the human CH1 domain and the C-terminal pIII protein domain (see Fig. 1 in Chap. 4). Although the Fab-HA-pIII fusion protein is assembled in the *E. coli* periplasm, detectable quantities of Fab-HA-pIII fusion protein and its proteolytic fragments are found in the supernatant due to outer membrane leakage and cell death. The crude Fab ELISA with immobilized antigen is designed to (1) identify clones with antigen (but not background) reactivity and (2) compare the expression level of positive (and, possibly, negative) clones through capturing with the goat anti-human kappa light-chain pAbs and the goat anti-human lambda light-chain pAbs. If the phage ELISA revealed strong antigen reactivity, typically ≥90% clones in the crude Fab ELISA are positive.
14. Expect to identify distinct repeated *Alu*I fingerprints. Each unique *Alu*I fingerprint indicates a different DNA sequence. However, identical *Alu*I fingerprints may still have slightly different DNA and amino acid sequences that are only detectable by DNA sequencing. In general, a small panel of selected human Fab that reveals strong antigen reactivity and reasonable expression levels in the crude Fab ELISA as well as a unique amino acid sequence should be pursued.
15. Selected human Fab can be expressed and purified in milligram quantities, facilitating a variety of downstream applications. For this, the C-terminal pIII protein domain encoded by pC3C is first removed by *Spe*I/*Nhe*I self-ligation (see Fig. 1 in Chap. 4). Subsequently, soluble Fab can be purified from supernatants of IPTG-induced *E. coli* cultures by affinity chromatography (7). In addition to a variety of functional

assays, purified human Fab are typically subjected to extensive specificity analyses by Western blotting, ELISA, flow cytometry, and immunofluorescence microscopy as well as to affinity measurements by surface plasmon resonance (8). Depending on the application, promising candidates can subsequently be converted to a variety of alternative antibody formats, including monovalent scFv or bivalent scFv-Fc and IgG. For the cloning, expression, and purification of mAbs in scFv-Fc format, see Chap. 14.

## Acknowledgments

This work was supported by the Intramural Research Program of the Center for Cancer Research, National Cancer Institute, National Institutes of Health. I thank the current and former members of my laboratory, in particular Dr. Ka Yin Kwong, Dr. Jiahui Yang, and Jessica M. Suschak, for their contributions to this protocol.

### References

1. Scott JK, Barbas CF III (2001) Phage-display vectors. In: Barbas CF III, Burton DR, Scott JK, Silverman GJ (eds) Phage display, a laboratory manual. Cold Spring Harbor Laboratory, Cold Spring Harbor, NY
2. Zhu Z, Dimitrov DS (2009) Construction of a large naive human phage-displayed Fab library through one-step cloning. Methods Mol Biol 525:129–142, xv
3. Baskar S, Suschak JM, Samija I et al (2009) A human monoclonal antibody drug and target discovery platform for B-cell chronic lymphocytic leukemia based on allogeneic hematopoietic stem cell transplantation and phage display. Blood 114:4494–4502
4. Popkov M, Rader C, Barbas CF 3rd (2004) Isolation of human prostate cancer cell reactive antibodies using phage display technology. J Immunol Methods 291:137–151
5. Siegel DL (2002) Selecting antibodies to cell-surface antigens using magnetic sorting techniques. Methods Mol Biol 178: 219–226
6. Siva AC, Kirkland RE, Lin B et al (2008) Selection of anti-cancer antibodies from combinatorial libraries by whole-cell panning and stringent subtraction with human blood cells. J Immunol Methods 330:109–119
7. Kwong KY, Rader C (2009) *E. coli* expression and purification of Fab antibody fragments. Curr Protoc Protein Sci. Chapter 6, Unit 6, 10
8. Kwong KY, Baskar S, Zhang H et al (2008) Generation, affinity maturation, and characterization of a human anti-human NKG2D monoclonal antibody with dual antagonistic and agonistic activity. J Mol Biol 384: 1143–1156

# Chapter 6

# Ribosome Display

George Thom and Maria Groves

## Abstract

Ribosome display is a powerful polymerase chain reaction-based in vitro display technology that is well suited to the selection and evolution of proteins. This technology exploits cell-free translation to achieve coupling of phenotype and genotype by the production of stabilized ribosome complexes, whereby translated protein and their cognate mRNA remain attached to the ribosome. The *Escherichia coli* S30 extract for in vitro display of an mRNA library has proven to be very successful for the evolution of high-affinity antibodies and the optimization of defined protein characteristics. These methodologies will enable the end user to successfully perform ribosome display selections.

**Key words:** Ribosome display, *Escherichia coli* S30 lysates, scFv, In vitro selection

## 1. Introduction

Ribosome display is a powerful in vitro display technology for the selection of proteins with specific function and as such has been demonstrated for the discovery of high-affinity monoclonal antibodies and peptides along with the optimization of defined protein attributes by directed evolution (1–8).

The development of ribosome display provides a complementary polymerase chain reaction (PCR)-based in vitro technology to phage or yeast display. However, ribosome display does offer certain advantages over other selection technologies, for example, phage or yeast display, that have limited library sizes ($10^7$–$10^{10}$/μg DNA; (9)) due to the in vitro transformation steps required for these technologies. In general, the probability of finding a given antibody becomes higher as the size of the library increases (10). Ribosome display allows selection from much larger libraries ($10^{14}$) whilst permitting Darwinian evolution of the displayed protein due to introduction of PCR-based mutations throughout the selection cascade.

Gabriele Proetzel and Hilmar Ebersbach (eds.), *Antibody Methods and Protocols*, Methods in Molecular Biology, vol. 901, DOI 10.1007/978-1-61779-931-0_6, © Springer Science+Business Media, LLC 2012

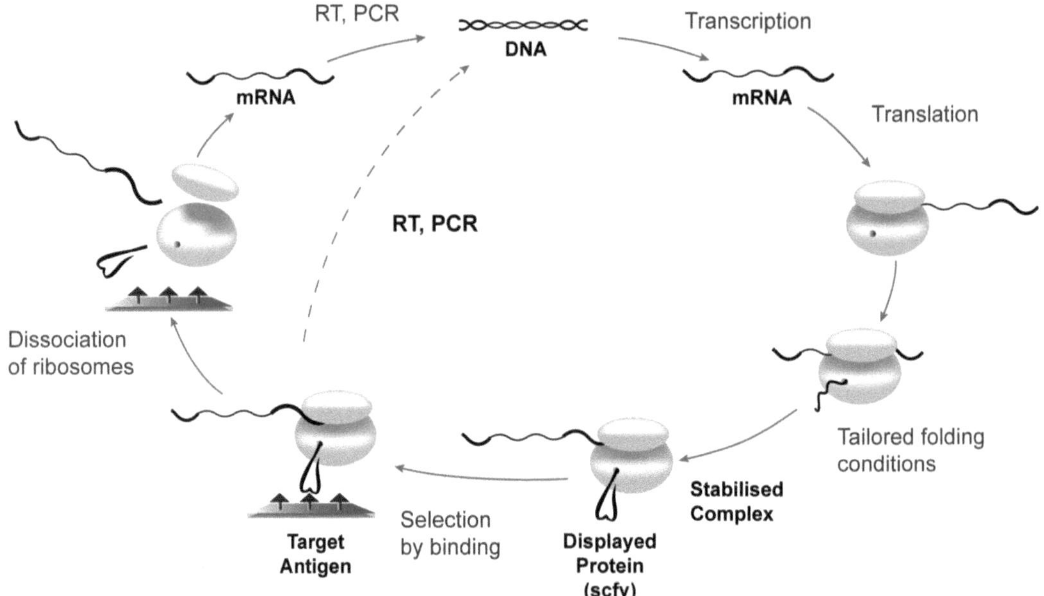


Fig. 1. The ribosome display cycle. A construct or library of constructs containing all features necessary for ribosome display is transcribed to mRNA. After its purification, mRNA is translated in vitro. The mRNA–scFv–ribosome ternary complexes are chilled and stabilized by increasing the magnesium concentration. Ribosomal complexes are affinity selected from the translation mixture. Selection can be performed on either immobilized ligand (panning) or biotinylated ligand in solution. Ribosome complexes partially displaying peptide or displaying peptides with no or nonspecific interaction with the ligand are removed by extensive wash steps. mRNA encoding ligand-bound peptide is isolated from the ribosomal complexes, reverse transcribed to cDNA, and then amplified by a separate PCR. Processing of selected ribosome complexes directly into RT-PCR is also illustrated. The next round of selection is ready to initiate.

The ribosome display process contains a series of steps that may be performed in an iterative manner as required (Fig. 1). First, mRNA is transcribed in vitro from DNA encoding a ligand-binding molecule or a library of molecules. This is then transcribed in vitro under conditions to produce stable tertiary mRNA–ribosome–protein complexes (ribosomal complexes) to achieve coupling of phenotype and genotype via a non-covalent link. Recovery of the selected mRNA is achieved by dissociation of ribosomal complexes, and subsequent reverse transcription (RT) and PCR to generate DNA for subsequent rounds of selection or for expression and screening. Recovery of sequence in this way does not require the breakdown of the interaction between ligand and its binding partner; therefore, higher affinity interactions can be selected more efficiently, thus conferring an additional advantage of ribosome display over other in vitro display technologies, such as covalent mRNA display.

Ribosome display uses an *Escherichia coli* S30 cell extract for in vitro translation and display of an mRNA library. This is a relatively crude cell extract that contains all enzymes and factors required for translation as described in Zubay and Jermutus (11, 12).

The DNA construct used for ribosome display and its assembly by PCR has been described in detail previously (2). On the DNA level, the construct requires a T7 RNA polymerase promoter for strong in vitro transcription to generate mRNA. On the mRNA level, the construct possesses a ribosome-binding site (Shine–Dalgarno sequence) for prokaryotic translational initiation. Immediately following is an open reading frame encoding the peptide or peptide library without a stop codon to avoid dissociation of synthesized peptide and its cognate mRNA from the ribosome. The protein of interest is followed by a spacer/tether sequence fused in-frame to the protein. The mRNA contains 5′ and 3′ stem loop structures for increased mRNA stability against RNases. The presence of stem loops is important, especially in the *E. coli* ribosome display system, because at least 5 of the 20 or so *E. coli* RNases have been shown to contribute to mRNA degradation (13), and they are most likely all present in the S30 extract used for in vitro translation. In one of the most frequently used ribosome display constructs the 5′-untranslated region of the mRNA, including the 5′ stem loop and the ribosome-binding site, is derived from gene 10 of phage T7 (14) and the 3′ stem loop is derived from the early terminator of phage T3 (15). One successful spacer/tether sequence is derived from the geneIII sequence of filamentous phage M13, spanning amino acids 130–204 (SwissProt P03622). Alternatively, spacers derived from other *E. coli* genes can be used.

## 2. Materials

All solutions are prepared using ultrapure water (prepared by purifying deionized water to attain a sensitivity of 18 MΩ cm at 25°C) and molecular biology-grade reagents. Prepare and store all reagents at 4°C (unless indicated otherwise). General, good laboratory practice guidelines when performing ribosome display selections are provided in Notes 1–6.

### 2.1. Generation of Ribosome Display Construct

1. Plasmid midiprep kit (Qiagen, Hildesheim, Germany).
2. pCANTAB6 plasmid (16).
3. SDCAT forward primer (**AGACCACAACGGTTTCCC**TCTAGAAATAATTTTGTTTAACTTTAAG<u>AAGGAG</u>ATATATCC***ATG***NNNNNNNNN), where N is target-specific sequence. The first 18 bases (shown in bold) are part of the 5′ mRNA stem-loop; the underlined region is the Shine–Dalgarno sequence and the ATG in bold italics is the start codon for the displayed peptide (e.g., scFv).

4. Myc-Restore reverse primer (ATTCAGATCCTCTTCTGAGATGAG) is generic, and recognizes the myc-tag that is common to all pCANTAB6 scFv sequences.
5. Myc-Forward primer binds to the generic myc-tag (ATCTCAGAAGAGGATCTGAATGGTGGCGGCTCCGGTTCCGGTGAT) and is complementary to the reverse primer described above (Myc-restore).
6. GeneIII-Reverse primer (CCGTCACCGACTTGAGCC) is complementary to a nucleotide sequence within the geneIII bacteriophage coat protein.
7. T7B forward primer has the sequence (ATACGAAATTAATACGACTCACTATA**GGGAGACCACAACGG**), the underlined region indicating the T7 RNA polymerase promoter. It recognizes and completes the 5′ stem-loop of the SDCAT primer (bold).
8. T6te reverse primer has the sequence (CCGCACACCAGTAAGGTGTGCGG**TATCACCAGTAGCACCATTACCATTAGCAAG**). It recognizes the 3′ end of the geneIII tether sequence (bold) and contains a stem-loop (underlined) to help prevent degradation of the mRNA transcripts.
9. T7te reverse primer (GTAGCACCATTACCATTAGCAAG). The T7te reverse primer is a short form of the T6te primer (above) and is used when the stem-loop is not required, since it generally results in better yields and a higher purity PCR product.
10. Nuclease-free water (Promega, Madison, WI, USA).
11. Quantitative DNA ladder (1 kb+). Store at 4°C (Invitrogen, Life Technologies, Carlsbad, CA, USA).
12. DNA gel extraction kit (Qiagen).
13. PCR elution buffer: 10 mM Tris–HCl pH 8.0.
14. 2× ABI universal PCR master mix (Applied Biosystems, Life Technologies); or separate *Taq* polymerase with suitable reaction buffer and dNTPs.
15. Agarose gel electrophoresis sample loading buffer. Store at 4°C.
16. TAE gel running buffer: 40 mM Tris–base, 1.14% (v/v) glacial acetic acid, 1 mM EDTA, pH 7.6. Store at room temperature.
17. Agarose gels: 1% (w/v) agarose (electrophoresis grade) is weighed out and added to the appropriate volume of 1× TAE. The solution is swirled before microwaving for 1-min pulses with mixing between pulses until all the agarose is dissolved. 1/1,000th volume of 1,000× DNA gel stain SYBRsafe (Invitrogen) is added and mixed before pouring into a gel casting tray (see Note 7). These should be freshly made on the day of use as the SYBRsafe stain is light sensitive.

### 2.2. Transcription of Ribosome Display Libraries

1. T7B–T6te amplified linear PCR product (linear DNA template).
2. Non-stick, RNAse-free 1.5-mL microcentrifuge tubes (Sarstedt, Nümbrecht, Germany) (see Note 8).
3. Ribomax™ Large Scale RNA production system-T7 (Promega).
4. Illustra ProbeQuant™ G-50 Micro Columns (GE Healthcare, UK) or equivalent.
5. Nuclease-free water.

### 2.3. Ribosome Display Selection

1. Heparin at 200 mg/mL (Sigma).
2. 10× *E. coli* wash buffer: 0.5 M Tris–acetate pH 7.5, 1.5 M NaCl, 0.5 M magnesium acetate, 1% (v/v) Tween-20. Can be prepared in bulk, aliquoted, and stored at 4°C.
3. Heparin-block (HB) buffer on ice: 5 mL of 10× *E. coli* wash buffer, 45 mL of sterile, filtered milliQ water, and 625 μL of heparin at 200 mg/mL in a 50-mL Falcon tube.
4. Non-stick, RNAse-free 1.5-mL microcentrifuge tubes (Sarstedt, Nümbrecht, Germany) (see Note 8).
5. 10% (w/v) nonfat dried milk in water, mix thoroughly before autoclaving on a liquids cycle.
6. Streptavidin coated magnetic beads, 280 Dynabeads® (Invitrogen).
7. Biotinylated target protein.
8. PD-10 columns (GE Healthcare, UK).
9. High Pure RNA Isolation Kit (Roche, Indianapolis, IN, USA).
10. *Saccharomyces cerevisiae* RNA at 10 μg/mL.
11. EB20 buffer: 50 mM Tris–acetate pH 7.5, 150 mM NaCl, 20 mM EDTA. Can be prepared in bulk, aliquoted, and stored at 4°C.
12. Nuclease-free water.
13. 2 M potassium glutamate.
14. 0.1 M magnesium acetate.
15. 5 mg/mL protein disulfide isomerase (PDI) (17).
16. Premix X: 250 mM Tris–acetate pH 7.5, 1.75 mM of each standard amino acid, 10 mM ATP, 2.5 mM GTP, 5 mM cAMP, 150 mM acetylphosphate (usually cloudy white), 2.5 mg/mL *E. coli* tRNA, 0.1 mg/mL folinic acid, 7.5% (w/v) PEG-8000. Can be prepared in bulk and stored at –20°C (see Note 9).
17. S30 *E. coli* extract (see Note 10).
18. Magnetic device Dynal MPC-S (Invitrogen).
19. Superscript II reverse transcription kit (Invitrogen).

20. RNase-free DNase I (Roche).
21. 100 mM DTT.
22. dNTP mix containing 25 mM each of dATP, dTTP, dCTP, and dGTP.
23. RNasin® at 40 U/μL (Promega).
24. 2× TaqMan® Universal PCR Master Mix (Applied Biosystems).
25. Thin-walled 0.2-mL PCR tubes.

## 3. Methods

These methods use antibody single chain (scFv) sequences as a reference (see Note 11). However, these methods can equally be applied to any peptide sequence or libraries being displayed. Libraries can also be built from this initial template DNA. These libraries can be created for directed evolution, for example, NNS libraries directed to the complementarity-determining regions (CDRs) of the variable regions of an IgG or a binding region of any protein wishing to be displayed. Alternatively, libraries can be generated in a nondirected approach, for example, using error-prone PCR and/or non-proofreading Taq polymerase during PCR steps of the process.

### *3.1. Generation of Ribosome Display Construct*

1. For the amplification of scFv sequences obtain purified plasmid DNA preparation of pCANTAB6 (16) by performing a plasmid midiprep isolation.
2. Set up the following PCR in PCR amplification tubes or 8-well strips: 50 μL of 2× PCR master mix, 2 μL of Myc-Restore primer (10 μM), 2 μL of SDCAT-DP47 primer (10 μM), 1 μL of template DNA (100 ng/μL), and 45 μL of nuclease-free water. Also include a no-template control.
3. Amplify the sequences using the following PCR conditions: 94°C for 3 min; 25 cycles of 94°C for 30 s, 55°C for 30 s, and 72°C for 105 s; 72°C for 5 min; 10°C hold.
4. 90 μL of each PCR product is added to 10 μL of 10× PCR loading dye before loading onto a preparative 1% agarose/TAE gel containing SYBRsafe stain (from 10,000× stock solution). 10 μL of the 1 kb + DNA ladder is run on each agarose gel to allow the identification of the correct PCR product. The PCR products are separated by electrophoresis (see Note 4). The stain is light sensitive and must be visualized under blue light. Subsequently, the correct PCR product is cut from the gel and purified from the matrix using a DNA gel extraction kit

according to the manufacturer's instructions. The DNA is eluted into PCR elution buffer or nuclease-free water.

5. Store the purified scFv DNA library at –20°C.
6. For production of the geneIII tether (see Note 12) the following PCR is set up to amplify the tether from pCANTAB6: 50 μL of 2× PCR master mix, 2 μL of GeneIII-Reverse primer (10 μM), 2 μL of Myc-Forward primer (10 μM), 1 μL of pCANTAB6 vector (10 ng/μL), and 45 μL of nuclease-free water. Also include a no-template control.
7. Amplify the sequences using the regime of step 3.
8. Gel-purify the PCR product as described in step 4.
9. Store the purified tether DNA at –20°C.
10. The next steps will link the geneIII tether to the scFv library.
11. Run a 5 μL sample of both the purified scFv and tether products on the same analytical 1% agarose/TAE gel containing SYBRsafe dye (see Note 13). Verify their relative sizes using blue light and determine the DNA concentrations by measuring the absorbance at 260 nm. If both products look pure, then set up the following PCR for each library: 50 μL of 2× PCR master mix, 10 μL of purified scFv library (10–20 ng/μL), 3 μL of purified geneIII tether (50 ng/μL), and 35 μL of nuclease-free water.
12. Generate the full-length sequences using the following PCR regime: 94°C for 3 min; 5 cycles of 94°C for 30 s, 50°C for 30 s, and 72°C for 105 s.
13. During the fifth annealing step (i.e., at 50°C), pause the PCR block and add 2 μL of mixed primers (SDCAT-DP47 and T7te, each at 10 μM) to the reactions.
14. Resume the PCR program and, once the 72°C extension step is complete, proceed with the following regime: 3 cycles of 94°C for 30 s, 35°C for 30 s, and 72°C for 105 s; 15 cycles of 94°C for 30 s, 50°C for 30 s, and 72°C for 105 s; 72°C for 5 min.
15. Run a 5 μL sample of each pull-through product on a 1% agarose/TAE gel containing SYBRsafe dye and compare to 2 μL of the initial purified scFv library. The pull-through product should be noticeably larger at ~1,100 bp.
16. Gel-purify the PCR product as described in step 4 (see Note 14).
17. Store the full-length construct at –20°C.
18. To amplify the full-length transcription template the following PCR for each sample is set up: 50 μL of 2× PCR master mix, 2 μL of T7B forward primer (10 μM), 2 μL of T6te reverse primer (10 μM), 10 μL of purified pull-through product (10–20 ng/μL), and 36 μL of nuclease-free water.

19. Amplify the sequences using the following PCR conditions: 94°C for 3 min; 20 cycles of 94°C for 30 s, 55°C for 30 s, and 72°C for 105 s; 72°C for 5 min.
20. Check 5 μL of each PCR sample on a 1% agarose/TAE gel for size and purity (see Note 15). If the size is correct, and there are no nonspecific products visible, then the DNA is ready for transcription (see Subheading 3.2). Do not gel-purify the product at this stage!
21. Store the transcription template at −20°C.

### 3.2. Transcription of Ribosome Display Libraries

This protocol describes how mRNA transcripts are produced from a T7B–T6te-amplified linear PCR product (see Note 16). Briefly, the reaction components are mixed and are then incubated at 37°C for 2 h. The mRNA is purified, quantified, and stored at −80°C or used immediately for selections.

1. Thaw the Ribomax large scale RNA production components at room temperature. Use quickly, and refreeze immediately. Keep the T7 RNA polymerase at −20°C until required.
2. Assemble the transcription components in the order listed in a nonstick nuclease-free microcentrifuge tube: 10 μL of 5× transcription buffer, 15 μL of rNTP mix (25 mM ATP, CTP, GTP, UTP), 20 μL of linear DNA template (T7B–T6te PCR), 5 μL of T7 polymerase. Prepare a master mix if performing multiple reactions.
3. Mix well by pipetting or gentle vortexing. If necessary, pulse-spin to ensure that all liquid has collected at the bottom of the tube.
4. Incubate at 37°C for at least 2 h and no more than 3 h.
5. Pulse-spin to collect condensation from the tube lid.
6. Purify mRNA using a ProbeQuant G50 microcolumn. Vortex column to resuspend the matrix. Loosen cap, add to a 2-mL RNAse-free tube, and spin for 1 min at 1,000×*g* to remove storage buffer. Discard the flow through. Add 50 μL transcription reaction per column. Loosen cap, and spin for 2 min at 1,000×*g* into a fresh 1.5-mL RNAse-free microcentrifuge tube. Transfer purified mRNA immediately onto ice.
7. Quantify the mRNA sample by measuring the $A_{260}$, in a spectrophotometer, of a 1 in 50 dilution in nuclease-free water. This should be done twice to ensure accuracy in the spectrophotometric reading (see Note 17).
8. Use the mRNA immediately for ribosome display selection, or snap freeze in aliquots on dry ice and store at −70°C until needed.

### 3.3. Ribosome Display Selection

This protocol details a single round of ribosome display selection that can be repeated as often as required. A standard affinity optimization campaign could consist of between 2 and 10 cycles of ribosome display selection, with the target antigen concentration being reduced at each round of selection (see Note 18). It is strongly advised to perform a positive control selection in parallel. This can be a single scFv clone that is known to bind to another suitable antigen.

Firstly, the mRNA is translated in vitro and the resulting scFv–ribosome–mRNA ternary complexes are stabilized. These ternary complexes are incubated with a biotin-tagged target antigen at 4°C for several hours, and bound individuals are captured using streptavidin-coated magnetic beads (although this protocol is amenable to other methods of tagging and capture as required). Any nonspecific binders are washed away. The output mRNA is eluted, purified, and amplified by RT-PCR, and then used as a template for both real-time PCR and end-point PCR. This final cDNA output is gel-purified and re-amplified for subsequent rounds of selection, or for sub-cloning into an appropriate expression vector.

1. Prechill a benchtop microcentrifuge to 4°C.
2. Prepare heparin-block (HB) buffer on ice by combining the following in a 50-mL Falcon tube: 5 mL of 10× *E. coli* wash buffer, 45 mL of sterile, filtered milliQ water, and 625 μL of heparin at 200 mg/mL. Prepare sufficient buffer for the number of selections being performed (~15 mL per translation reaction). Store on ice at all times and prepare fresh buffer each day.
3. For each translation, prechill four 1.5-mL RNAse-free microcentrifuge tubes on ice (one for the translation reaction, three for the selections) and prepare an additional 2-mL RNAse-free microcentrifuge tube on ice, containing 1,320 μL of ice-cold HB buffer.
4. Prepare the strepatavidin-coated magnetic beads. Use 50 μL of beads per selection (plus an extra 100 μL of beads if blocking the selections). Wash the beads four times with chilled HB buffer in RNAse-free microcentrifuge tubes, and resuspend in HB buffer to the original volume. Store on ice until required.
5. Prepare biotinylated antigen by body labeling with biotin with an average of 2–4 fold molar excess of biotin for 2 min. Biotinylation success is observed via mass spectrometry, achieving an average of 1–2 biotinylation events per antigen molecule. Buffer exchange biotinylated antigen with PBS using PD-10 columns and test for activity, before selection takes place.
6. *Optional*: If blocking the selections, prepare de-biotinylated, sterile skimmed milk. Add 100 μL of streptavidin-coated magnetic beads to 1 mL of autoclaved 10% (w/v) skimmed milk powder in water in an RNAse-free microcentrifuge tube. Incubate with end-over-end rotation for at least 10 min. Collect the beads using a magnetic particle separator and transfer the milk to a fresh tube. Store on ice until required.

7. Thaw premix X buffer, PDI, and S30 extract on ice and start the following procedure immediately. These components must be used as soon as possible once thawed!
8. The following steps are to be performed *on ice* unless otherwise specified.
9. A 300 μL in vitro translation reaction is performed for each library, population, or single clone to be selected. This reaction is then split between three selections: two with antigen and one without as a negative control. All reactions are performed in RNAse-free nonstick microcentrifuge tubes.
10. Prepare a translation master mix for the total number of translation reactions required (plus one extra volume to account for pipetting errors) as follows. For one translation reaction, combine the following reagents in the order listed in an RNAse-free microcentrifuge tube: 60.9 μL of nuclease-free water, 38.5 μL of potassium glutamate (2 M), 26.6 μL of magnesium acetate (0.1 M), 7 μL of PDI (5 mg/mL), and 77 μL of premix X. Mix gently by pipetting up and down several times. *Do not vortex.*
11. If mRNA has been produced on a previous day and stored at −70°C, thaw quickly by holding between fingertips and place immediately on ice when thawed.
12. For each translation of library, control, or scFv add 30 μL of diluted mRNA at 1 μg/mL (approximately $6 \times 10^{13}$ molecules) to the bottom of a prechilled 1.5-mL RNAse-free microcentrifuge tube on ice (from step 3).
13. Very gently mix the thawed S30 extract by pipetting, but do not vortex or mix vigorously. Add 140 μL per translation to the master mix, and mix all reagents by pipetting up and down five times. Proceed to the next step *immediately.*
14. Add 300 μL of translation master mix to each 30 μL stock of mRNA, and mix gently by pipetting up and down five times. Immediately transfer one of the tubes to a 37°C heat-block for exactly 9 min (see Note 19).
15. Repeat for all other selections at suitable intervals (10–30 s). The timing needs to be accurate; therefore, use a timing device to space each reaction.
16. After translation, immediately pipette each 330 μL translation reaction into a prechilled 2-mL microcentrifuge tube containing 1,320 μL of chilled HB buffer (from step 3) and mix by gentle pipetting. This buffer stabilizes the ternary scFv–ribosome–mRNA complexes.
17. Once all samples have been removed from the hot-block and stabilized, centrifuge at 17,000 × *g* for 5 min at 4°C in a prechilled benchtop centrifuge (from step 1) and place on ice. The samples are now ready for selection and capture.

18. For each translation reaction, transfer 500 μL of supernatant to three of the prechilled 1.5-mL RNAse-free selection tubes (from step 3). If required, add 50 μL of chilled, de-biotinylated, sterile milk (from step 6) to each tube. Cap the negative selection to prevent accidental addition of antigen.
19. For each positive selection, add the appropriate biotinylated antigen, at the required concentration. Do not exceed 30 μL total volume for antigen addition.
20. Incubate all selections at 4°C for between 2 and 24 h with gentle end-over-end rotation.
21. Capture the selected complexes by the addition of 50 μL HB-washed streptavidin-coated magnetic beads (from step 4) to each selection. Incubate for 5 min at 4°C with gentle end-over-end rotation.
22. Wash each selection five times with 800 μL prechilled HB buffer and transfer the beads to 220 μL of EB20 containing a 1/1,000 dilution of *S. cerevisiae* mRNA stock and mix well. Allow 10 min for the ternary complexes to dissociate and then remove the magnetic beads from the elution buffer (see Note 20).
23. For each selection, prechill a fresh RNAse-free microcentrifuge tube on ice and add 400 μL of lysis buffer from the High Pure RNA Isolation Kit (the volume may vary depending on the kit used). This step should be performed during the 10-min mRNA elution.
24. Transfer 200 μL of the EB20 solutions (containing the eluted mRNA) into the prechilled RNAse-free microcentrifuge tubes containing lysis buffer. Vortex each tube immediately to mix.
25. The eluted RNA can be isolated using the High Pure RNA Isolation Kit, and a benchtop microcentrifuge prechilled to 4°C according to the manufacturer's instructions; however, elute in 40 μL of nuclease-free water. Then proceed immediately to the next step.
26. Prepare a master mix for the required number of reverse transcription (RT) reactions (include two extra reaction volumes to allow for a no-template control and for pipetting error). For one sample, mix the following components in a fresh RNAse-free microcentrifuge tube on ice: 4 μL of 5× First-Strand buffer, 2 μL of 0.1 M DTT, 0.25 μL of T7te reverse primer (100 μM), 0.5 μL of dNTP mix (25 mM each oligonucleotide), 0.5 μL of RNasin® (40 U/μL), and 0.5 μL of Superscript II Reverse Transcriptase (200 U/μL).
27. Mix the RT master mix well and for each sample (plus the no-template control) aliquot 7.75 μL into the bottom of a thin-walled 0.2-mL PCR tube. Keep on ice.

28. Mix the eluted mRNA from step 1 by pipetting up and down five times, and add 12.25 μL of each sample to the 7.75 μL of RT mix. Mix well, but gently, by pipetting up and down five times. Immediately freeze any unused mRNA and store at −80°C.
29. Incubate the reactions in a PCR block at 50°C from 30 min. Prepare the PCR master mix during this time (see step 31).
30. Transfer completed RT reactions onto ice until used in the end-point PCR in the following steps. The end-point PCR is performed to visualize amplification of the selected mRNA. Real-time PCR can also be performed to provide relative quantification of selection outputs (protocol not provided).
31. Prepare a master mix for the required number of PCRs to be performed (include three extra reaction volumes to allow for the RT no-template control and a PCR no-template control and to account for pipetting error). For one reaction, mix the following components in a fresh RNase-free microcentrifuge tube on ice: 34.5 μL of nuclease-free water, 50 μL of PCR master mix (2×), 0.25 μL of T7te reverse primer (100 μM), 0.25 μL of SDCAT $V_H$-specific forward primer (100 μM), and 5 μL of DMSO.
32. Mix well by pipetting. For each sample (plus the RT no-template control and the PCR no-template control), aliquot 90 μL of master mix into the bottom of a thin-walled 0.2-mL PCR tube. Keep on ice.
33. Add 10 μL of each cDNA (step 30) to a separate PCR tube. Mix well, but gently, by pipetting up and down five times. Freeze any unused cDNA and store at −20°C.
34. Amplify the cDNA samples using the following conditions: 94°C for 3 min; 25–35 cycles (see Note 21) of 94°C for 30 s, 55°C for 30 s, 72°C for 105 s; 72°C for 5 min.
35. Run 5 μL of each PCR sample on a 1% agarose/TAE gel alongside a quantitative DNA ladder. The two positive selections should be similar, and should yield clearly more DNA than the selection without antigen (see Note 22). If this is the case, then the selection appears successful, and the positive outputs can be re-amplified for further processing.

## 4. Notes

1. Ensure that all consumables are RNAse-free. Clean working area with detergent and 70% ethanol and irradiate pipettes with UV before commencing experiments each day. Use filter pipette

tips at all times. Avoid sharing of reagents and equipment with scientists working on other ribosome display constructs.

2. Prepare all PCRs in a clean environment to prevent DNA contamination.
3. Always grow clones from different samples in separate plates.
4. Leave one lane free between samples when running PCR products on agarose gels. Use separate blades for each band being excised from an agarose gel.
5. For gel extraction, always spin down the dissolved band before opening the Eppendorf lid.
6. Use Tris-based buffers to elute DNA from purification columns for greater long-term storage stability (e.g., 10 mM Tris, pH 8.0).
7. For DNA visualization, we use SYBR® Safe from Invitrogen. This stain is excited with blue light, and is therefore much safer than alternative stains that require excitation with ultraviolet light. In addition, the blue light is less destructive to the DNA samples and gives better ligation of selection outputs.
8. The preference is for Sarstedt microcentrifuge tubes, since they are nonstick and produce the best selection windows. In addition, their lids are less prone to snapping when eluting from mRNA purification columns.
9. Premix X is a complicated reagent to prepare. Start by making M2 mix, where 1 mL contains the following: 40 μL ATP (1 M), 50 μL GTP (0.2 M), 50 μL cAMP (0.4 M), 300 μL acetylphosphate (2 M) (ACP—gives a turbid solution), 560 μL nuclease-free water. Then all 20 amino acids are separately weighed out and stock solutions prepared at 0.2 M. Care is needed as many of the amino acids will take a long time to dissolve and may require heating to 37°C or above to improve solubility. Once all amino acids are prepared then take 100 μL of each to make a working stock amino acid solution, whereby each amino acid is at 10 mM. This solution is subsequently used to prepare premix X. Any unused amino acid working stock solution can be stored at –20°C for future use. *E. coli* tRNA is also very difficult to dissolve and may take >1 h to dissolve at 37°C. Always vortex before pipetting. Premix X (5×) is prepared by adding the following together: 125 μL M2 mix, 50 μL *E. coli* tRNA (25 mg/mL), 62.5 μL Tris–acetate pH 7.5 (2 M), 75 μL PEG 8000 (50%), 87.5 μL amino acid complete mix (10 mM each), 3 μL Folinic acid (10 mg/mL), and 95 μL nuclease-free water.
10. S30 extract can be prepared as homemade extract as described in Zubay and Jermutus (11, 12) or can be bought commercially. Be sure to purchase systems that are free of DTT when

displaying peptides with disulfide bonds as the reducing conditions will not allow these bonds to form, and therefore will prevent correct folding of displayed peptides.

11. The antibody format used for ribosome display (RD) selections is predominantly scFv, and this protocol describes the conversion of scFv phage display construct to scFv ribosome display construct. When converting an scFv from the pCANTAB6 vector, the $V_H$ and $V_L$ domains are already concatenated and can be amplified together using the SDCAT-specific and Myc-Restore primers.
12. For ribosome display, a tether sequence (polypeptide spacer) is necessary. This tether occupies the ribosome tunnel in the stalled ribosome complex and thereby allows the scFv library sequences to protrude from the ribosome and fold. In our constructs, the tether is produced from the pCANTAB6 vector using the Myc-Forward and GeneIII-Reverse primers. However, this particular tether can be substituted for other nucleotide sequences of ~300 bp, provided that the 5′ tether primer contains a sequence that is complementary to the 3′ scFv primer.
13. If an scFv construct is being amplified, the PCR product should be approximately 850 bp in length. The tether should be approximately 300 bp.
14. When separating the PCR products on a preparative 1% agarose/TAE gel, make sure that the gel is run for sufficient time so that the full-length construct is clearly separated from any un-recombined scFv that may be present.
15. Following T7B–T6te amplification, there should only be one strong band at ~1,200 bp. Nonspecific bands of lower molecular weight will be amplified preferentially at the next PCR and will thus eliminate the specific product. Lower molecular weight smears suggest degradation of the specific product. In either case, the conversion has not been successful and should be repeated.
16. We prepare mRNA in vitro from ribosome display constructs under the control of the T7 promoter using the Ribomax Large Scale RNA production system (T7) from Promega. The resulting mRNA can (and should) be used immediately for ribosome display selections. The template for transcription should be a non-purified PCR product (i.e., a T7B–T6te re-amplification reaction) as we have previously found that the use of purified PCR products can compromise translation efficiency. The template can be a single scFv sequence, or a population such as an error-prone library or a previous selection output.
17. If the $A_{260}$ spectrophotometric reading does not lie within the range 0.1–1.0 then repeat the analysis with a more suitable

dilution. The concentration should be higher than 2 μg/μL. If the concentration is lower than this value, the transcription should be repeated.

18. The first round of ribosome display selection is typically performed at an antigen concentration of 100 nM. This concentration is typically reduced tenfold with each subsequent round of RD selection. However, if the selection outputs contain clones with lower affinity than the selection input, or if there is no discernable difference between selections with and without antigen, then the concentration drops may be too severe. In these cases, return to the last successful output and try dropping the antigen concentration two- to fivefold instead.
19. Although we have found between 7 and 9 min to be the best for our in-house translation system, alternative systems may require optimization of this incubation step.
20. For the wash and elution steps we strongly recommend the use of an automated system (e.g., a Kingfisher mL) that has been prechilled to 4°C.
21. The number of amplification cycles used in the end-point PCR depends on the parent, the library type, and the degree of enrichment that has occurred. Typically, 25 cycles are required for our "model" selections, whilst 30 cycles is standard for a parent test selection. Early rounds of ribosome display selection typically require 35 cycles, whereas later rounds require fewer (~30) cycles of amplification. Too few cycles will result in DNA yields that are too low to be quantified/purified, whereas too many cycles will reduce the selection window between the +ve and −ve antigen runs and will favor the generation of nonspecific PCR products. Guidance can be obtained by performing real-time PCR before the end-point PCR.
22. There should only be one strong band at ~1,100 bp, and an absence of nonspecific bands of lower molecular weight. If present, these smaller products will be preferentially amplified in the next PCR step, causing deterioration in input quality and leading to selection failure. If the positive runs produce weak bands, with insufficient DNA for subsequent processing, the number of cycles in the end-point PCR can be increased up to a maximum of 35 cycles.

## References

1. Hanes J, Plückthun A (1997) In vitro selection and evolution of functional proteins by using ribosome display. Proc Natl Acad Sci U S A 94: 4937–4942
2. Hanes J, Schaffitzel C, Knappik A, Plückthun A (2000) Picomolar affinity antibodies from a fully synthetic naïve library selected and evolved by ribosome display. Nat Biotechnol 18:1287–1292
3. Lamla T, Erdmann V (2001) In vitro selection of other proteins than antibodies by means of ribosome display. FEBS Lett 502:35–40

4. Jermutus L, Honeggar A, Schwesinger F, Hanes J, Plückthun A (2001) Tailoring in vitro evolution for protein affinity or stability. Proc Natl Acad Sci U S A 98:75–80
5. Amstutz P, Pelletier JN, Guggisberg A (2002) In vitro selection for catalytic activity with ribosome display. J Am Chem Soc 124: 9396–9403
6. Matsuura T, Plückthun A (2004) Strategies for selection from protein libraries composed of de novo designed secondary structure modules. Orig Life Evol Biosph 34:151–157
7. Thom G, Cockroft AC, Buchanan AG et al (2006) Probing a protein–protein interaction by in vitro evolution. Proc Natl Acad Sci U S A 103:7619–7624
8. Zahnd C, Wyler E, Schwenk JM et al (2007) A designed ankyrin repeat protein evolved to picomolar affinity to Her2. J Mol Biol 369: 1015–1028
9. Dower WJ, Cwirla SE (1992) Creating vast peptide expression libraries: electroporation as a tool to construct plasmid libraries of greater than 109 recombinants. In: Chang DC et al (eds) Guide to electroporation and electrofusion. Academic, San Diego, CA, pp 291–301
10. Vaughan TJ, Williams AJ, Pritchard K et al (1996) Human antibodies with sub-nanomolar affinities isolated from a large nonimmunized phage display library. Nat Biotechnol 14: 309–314
11. Zubay G (1973) In vitro synthesis of protein in microbial systems. Annu Rev Genet 7: 267–287
12. Jermutus L, Ryabova LA, Plückthun A (1998) Recent advances in producing and selecting functional proteins by using cell-free translation. Curr Opin Biotechnol 9:534–548
13. Hajnsdorf E, Braun F, Haugel-Nielsen J et al (1996) Multiple degradation pathways of the rpsO mRNA of *Escherichia coli* RNase E interacts with the 5′ and 3′ extremities of the primary transcript. Biochemie 78:416–424
14. Studier FW, Rosenberg AH, Dunn JJ, Dubendorff JW (1990) Use of T7 RNA polymerase to direct expression of cloned genes. Methods Enzymol 185:60–89
15. Reynolds R, Bermudez-Cruz RM, Chamberlin MJ (1992) Parameters affecting transcription termination by Escherichia coli RNA polymerase. I. Analysis of 13 rho independent terminators. J Mol Biol 224:31–51
16. McCafferty J, Fitzgerald KJ, Earnshaw J et al (1994) Selection and rapid purification of murine antibody fragments that bind a transition-state analog by phage display. Appl Biochem Biotechnol 47:157–171
17. Freedman RB, Hawkins HC, McLaughlin SH (1995) Protein disulfide-isomerase. Methods Enzymol 251:397–406

# Chapter 7

# Hybridoma Technology for the Generation of Monoclonal Antibodies

Chonghui Zhang


## Abstract

Hybridoma technology has long been a remarkable and indispensable platform for generating high-quality monoclonal antibodies (mAbs). Hybridoma-derived mAbs have not only served as powerful tool reagents but also have emerged as the most rapidly expanding class of therapeutic biologics. With the establishment of mAb humanization and with the development of transgenic-humanized mice, hybridoma technology has opened new avenues for effectively generating humanized or fully human mAbs as therapeutics. In this chapter, an overview of hybridoma technology and the laboratory procedures used routinely for hybridoma generation are discussed and detailed in the following sections: cell fusion for hybridoma generation, antibody screening and characterization, hybridoma subcloning and mAb isotyping, as well as production of mAbs from hybridoma cells.


**Key words:** Cell fusion, ELISA, Flow cytometry, Hybridoma technology, Immunohistochemistry, Immunization, Monoclonal antibody, Myeloma cells, Therapeutic antibody, Screening

## 1. Introduction

The invention of hybridoma technology by Georges Köhler and César Milstein in 1975 is a significant milestone in immunology and biomedicine (1). This technology has enabled scientists for the first time to generate unlimited quantities of pure, monospecific antibodies directed against virtually any antigen. A monoclonal antibody (mAb) is a highly specific and homogeneous species of immunoglobulin molecule produced by a single hybridoma clone that has been generated by the fusion of a myeloma cell with a B lymphocyte from a donor or from an immunized animal. Hybridoma technology has thus revolutionized discovery research and therapeutic development in such diverse fields as immunology, biology, oncology, and infectious diseases (2–4). The mAbs generated from

Gabriele Proetzel and Hilmar Ebersbach (eds.), *Antibody Methods and Protocols*, Methods in Molecular Biology, vol. 901, DOI 10.1007/978-1-61779-931-0_7, 

this technology have served as reagents for the identification and characterization of cell surface antigens (5, 6), for classification and isolation of hematopoietic cell subsets (7–9), and for the development of biomarkers to distinguish aberrant or cancerous cells from normal cells (10–13). Hybridoma technology has long been a powerful tool for investigators to make discoveries in the biological sciences and has led to many important advances in medicine.

With the breakthrough in molecular engineering and antibody humanization (14, 15), mAbs have emerged as the most rapidly expanding category of biopharmaceuticals for a large variety of clinical scenarios. For example, mAbs have been used to aid in successful organ transplantation (16, 17), as well as being used to treat inflammatory diseases (18, 19), cancer, and infectious diseases (20–22). Based on published data, nearly 30 FDA-approved antibody drugs are on the US market today (Fig. 1) and it is estimated that hundreds of mAbs are currently in various phases of clinical trials worldwide (23).

mAbs can be produced from an immune or nonimmune resource using a range of recently developed antibody technologies, including methods such as display technologies (24, 25) or memory B-cell immortalization and cloning (26, 27). However, since hybridoma technology is so well established, it will continue to provide a powerful and indispensable platform for generating high-quality mAbs to meet unmet needs. It is important to note that mAbs generated from immune hosts by the hybridoma approach often exhibit good binding affinity due to in vivo secondary immune responses. These mAbs routinely obviate the requirements for subsequent in vitro affinity maturation or other modifications to improve antibody potency by additional technologies (28, 29). Furthermore, the primary production of the whole Ig molecule from hybridomas allows investigators to screen directly for the desired biological function of mAbs from the very beginning. Therefore, it is not surprising that 26 out of the 28 therapeutic mAbs that have been approved by the FDA in the United States today have originated from hybridomas, with or without chimerization or humanization (Fig. 1). With the recent development of transgenic humanized mouse strains that are capable of natural recombination and affinity maturation in vivo and which have a large repertoire of high-affinity antibodies to any antigen (30–32), the "old-fashioned" hybridoma technology will open up new avenues for more effectively generating large panels of high-quality and fully human mAbs. These fully human mAbs generated from transgenic humanized mice will accelerate the development and application of mAbs as therapeutics for human cancer and disease (29, 33).

Hybridoma technology is composed of several technical aspects, including antigen preparation, animal immunization, cell fusion, hybridoma screening and subcloning, as well as characterization and production of specific antibodies (Fig. 2). mAb generation by

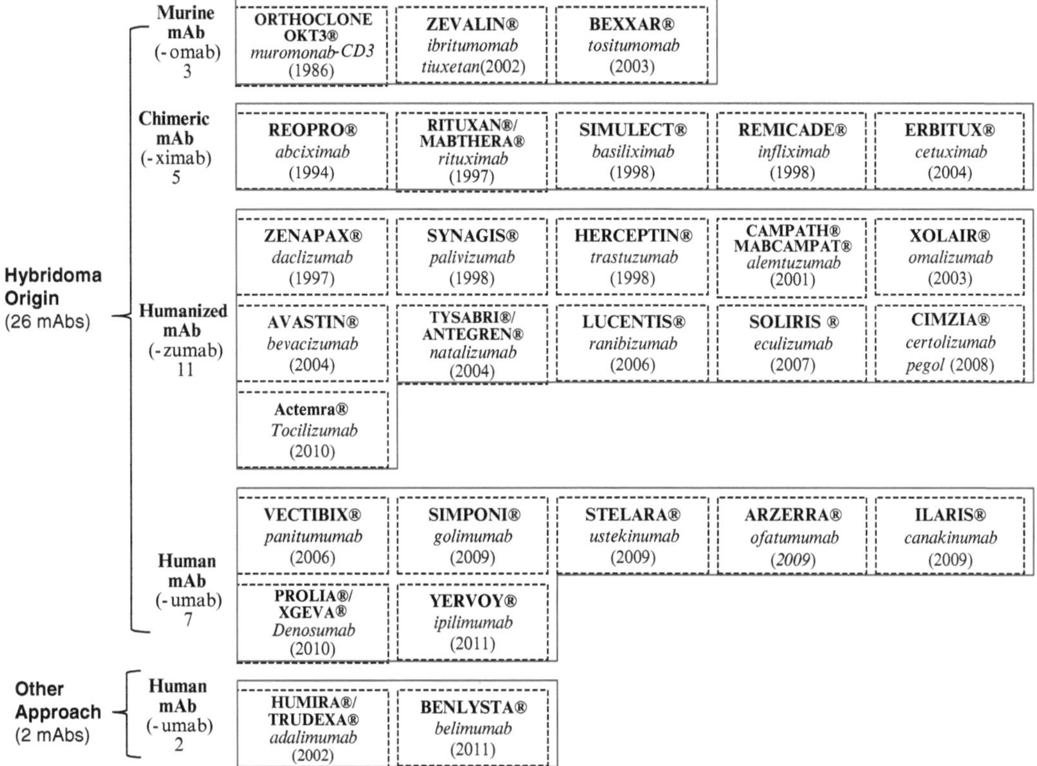


Fig. 1. A list of FDA-approved therapeutic mAbs currently on the market. Over 30 therapeutic mAbs have been approved by the FDA for marketing in the United States to date, whereas a small number of the mAb drugs, such as Mylotarg (*Gumtuzumab ozogamicin*) and Raptiva (*Efalizumab*), have been withdrawn from the market due to their side effects and/or poor clinical benefits. Most of the FDA-approved therapeutic mAbs currently on the market have originated from hybridomas and are in the full-length antibody molecular format, including the murine (suffixed with *-omab*), chimeric (*-ximab*), humanized (*-zumab*), and human (*-umab*) antibody category. All human mAbs of hybridoma origin are generated from the XenoMouse® or HuMAb-Mouse® transgenic strain, both of which have nearly the entire human Ig loci introduced into the germ line with inactivation of the mouse Ig machinery. For each antibody drug, its trade name, generic mAb name and the year of FDA approval are indicated in the figure. The digit shown represents the number of therapeutic mAbs in the antibody category.

the hybridoma approach requires knowledge of multiple disciplines and practice of versatile technical skills, ranging from animal handling (immunization and sample collection), immunology (immunoassays and antibody characterization) to cellular and molecular biology (cell fusion for hybridoma generation, protein sequencing analysis for antigen preparation, and flow cytometry or other cell-based assays for screening hybridomas). Generation and identification of high-quality hybridoma clones is a comprehensive and labor-intensive process, and requires months of work during the time frame from immunization to specific hybridoma identification. The key aspect of hybridoma generation is the screening procedure used to identify and select the desired hybridoma clones from the fusion plates. As shown in Fig. 3, cell fusion

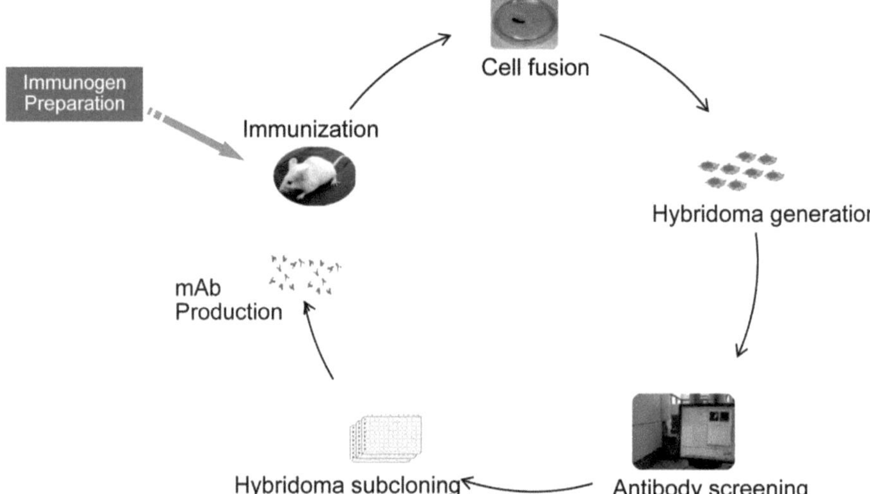


Fig. 2. A diagram of mAb generation by the hybridoma approach. Generation and identification of high-quality mAbs by the hybridoma approach requires months of work during the time frame from immunization to establishment of specific hybridoma clones. The work involves stages of antigen preparation, animal immunization, cell fusion for hybridoma generation, hybridoma screening and subcloning, as well as characterization and production of specific mAbs.

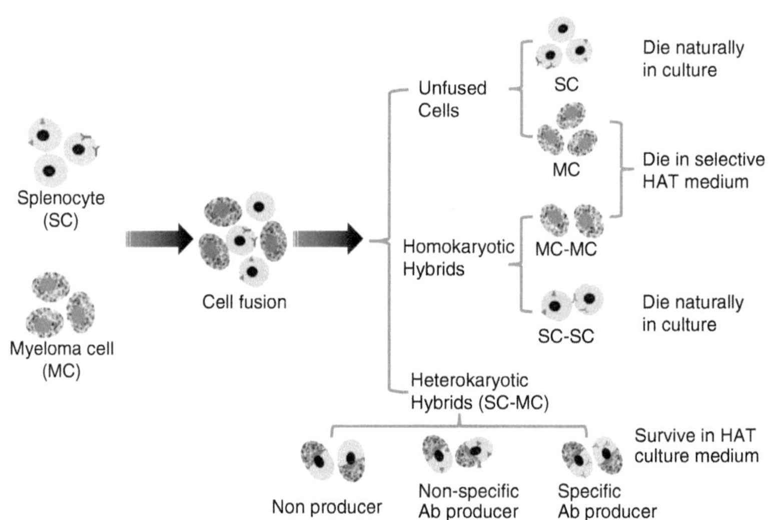


Fig. 3. Multiple cell types generated from fusion of splenocytes (SC) and myeloma cells (MC). PEG-mediated cell fusion is likely to result in a mixed population of cells consisting of nonproducing hybridomas, antibody-producing hybridomas and unfused cells. In the presence of aminopterin in HAT-selective medium, cells are dependent on another pathway that needs the enzyme hypoxanthine-guanine phosphoribosyl transferase (HGPRT) for survival. Under this culture condition, unfused myeloma cells or hybrids of myeloma cells with myeloma cells will die because of the absence of HGPRT, whereas unfused splenocytes or hybrids of splenocytes with splenocytes also die because of their lack of immortal growth potential. Only hybridomas from fusion of splenocytes with myeloma cells will inherit the HGPRT gene from splenocytes and the immortal growth property from myeloma cells, and can thus grow in HAT medium. By hybridoma screening and subcloning, specific hybridoma clones will be identified and isolated from nonspecific antibody producers or nonproducers of myeloma-splenocyte hybridomas.

mediated either by PEG or electrofusion typically generates a mixture of cells within the culture, which is composed of unfused splenocytes or myeloma cells, heterokaryotic hybrids (hybridomas) of splenocytes and myelomas with or without the secretion of specific antibodies, and the homokaryotic hybrids of either myeloma–myeloma cells or splenocytes–splenocytes. However, only the hybridomas from the fusion between splenocytes and myeloma cells are able to survive in the HAT medium. It is important to note that the myeloma–splenocyte hybridoma cells may turn out to be a specific antibody producer, nonspecific antibody producer or nonproducer. Development of appropriate antibody screening assays is thus required to efficiently identify the subpopulation of hybridoma cells in the fusion plates. The screening assays of choice should be specific, reliable, and effective. In general, the identification and selection process of antibody-secreting hybridomas comprises an initial screening of antibodies in polyclonal cultures and a secondary, more sophisticated characterization of mAbs afterwards. With the initial screening, antibody-secreting hybridomas are identified from the well of fusion plates, of which positive hybridomas are selected and then subcloned into monoclonals. A more sophisticated characterization of the mAbs generated will further determine their specificity, binding affinity, molecular features, and the functional activity of the mAbs, if any. Culture supernatants from the fusion plates are initially screened for positive hybridoma clones by a number of different immunoassays. While immunofluorescence flow cytometry is often applied to particulate antigens such as whole cells, an enzyme-linked immunosorbent assay (ELISA) is used for soluble antigens such as proteins or polypeptides, and immunohistochemistry (IHC) is developed for tissue antigens. Lastly, the hybridoma clones selected from the initial screens often require more testing for biochemical features of the mAb by immunoprecipitation and/or immunoblots, and further testing for biological activity by in vitro functional assays, such as blocking of the ligand binding to its receptor, detection of protein phosphorylation or signaling pathway, mediating agonistic or antagonistic activity, inhibiting cell proliferation, or interfering with the potency to mediate cell killing (34–36). In general, the functional screening assays are complex to perform and construe, and therefore are only carried out as necessary.

In this chapter, the strategy and laboratory methods for hybridoma generation are described and detailed in the following sections: cell fusion for hybridoma generation, antibody screening and characterization, hybridoma subcloning, cryopreservation and antibody isotyping, as well as production and purification of mAbs from hybridoma cells.

## 2. Materials

*2.1. Preparation of Splenocytes*

1. Spleens from immunized mice.
2. RPMI-1640 medium.
3. Petri dishes.
4. Sterile surgical instruments, including microdissecting scissors and forceps, for collecting animal samples.
5. Sterile microscope glass slides with frosted ends.
6. 15-mL conical tubes.

*2.2. Preparation of Myeloma Cells as the Fusion Partner*

1. Murine myeloma P3X63Ag8.653 cell or other fusion partner (ATCC, Manassas, Virginia, USA).
2. RPMI-1640 medium supplemented with 10% fetal bovine serum (FBS).
3. RPMI-1640 medium supplemented with 10% FBS and 130 μM 8-azaguanine.
4. 50-mL conical tube.

*2.3. Cell Fusion*

1. Splenocytes from immunized mice.
2. Myeloma cells.
3. Sterile polyethylene glycol-1500 (PEG-1500), i.e., 50% PEG-1500 solution (w/v) in 75 mM HEPES buffer, pH 8.0 as fusogen.
4. Serum-free RPMI-1640 medium.
5. Hybridoma culture medium: RPMI-1640 medium supplemented with 20% FBS, 1× MEM nonessential amino acid solution, 2 mM L-glutamine, 0.5 mM sodium pyruvate, 50 μM beta-mercaptoethanol, penicillin (100 U/mL), and streptomycin (100 μg/mL).
6. Hypoxanthine–aminopterin–thymidine (HAT) medium: hybridoma culture medium (above) supplemented with 100 μM hypoxanthine, 0.4 μM aminopterin, and 16 μM thymidine.
7. HT medium: hybridoma culture medium (above) supplemented with 100 μM hypoxanthine, and 16 μM thymidine.
8. 96-Well flat-bottom culture plates.

*2.4. Hybridoma Screening by FACS*

1. Phosphate buffered saline (PBS), pH 7.4.
2. F buffer: PBS containing 0.1% bovine serum albumin and 0.01% sodium azide.
3. Fixation buffer: PBS containing 1% formalin (i.e., 37% formaldehyde solution).

4. Fluorescein-conjugated anti-mouse IgG antibody.
5. 96-Well microtest U-bottom plates.
6. Centrifuge with plate carriers.
7. Flow cytometer.

#### 2.5. Hybridoma Screening by ELISA

1. 96-Well ELISA plates, e.g., Immulon 2HB plates.
2. 0.2 M carbonate–bicarbonate buffer, pH 9.4.
3. Tris buffered saline (TBS): 25 mM Tris and 0.15 M sodium chloride, pH 7.2.
4. Wash buffer: 0.05% Tween-20 in TBS.
5. Sealing tape for 96-well plates.
6. Blocking buffer: 3% normal goat serum and 0.05% Tween-20 in TBS.
7. TMB (3,3′,5,5′-tetramethylbenzidine) or other substrate solution.
8. Stop solution: 2.5 M sulfuric acid in $H_2O$.
9. Purified protein or polypeptides as antigen.
10. Hybridoma culture supernatants.
11. Peroxidase-conjugated anti-mouse IgG antibody.
12. ELISA plate reader with an appropriate analysis software.

#### 2.6. Hybridoma Screening by IHC

1. Tissue section slides.
2. Tissue-Tek* OCT Compound (Sakura* Finetek).
3. Antibody supernatant samples.
4. 50 mM Tris–HCl buffer saline (TBS-50), pH 7.6.
5. 1% Hydrogen peroxide in 50% methanol solution.
6. 10% Normal goat serum in TBS-50.
7. Peroxidase-conjugated anti-mouse IgG antibody.
8. AEC substrate solution consisting of 5 mg of 3-amino-9-ethylcarbazole dissolved in 3 mL dimethyl sulfoxide, 2.5 mL of 200 mM acetate buffer, pH 5.5, 22.5 mL of 150 mM NaCl, and 200 μL of 0.3% hydrogen peroxide.
9. Gill’s hematoxylin solution.
10. Scott’s water: Tap water containing 0.2% sodium carbonate and 1% magnesium sulfate.
11. Glycergel mounting medium (Dako, Denmark).
12. Humid chamber.
13. Microscope slides and cover.
14. Microscope.

### 2.7. Hybridoma Subcloning

1. Hybridoma culture medium (see Subheading 2.3).
2. HT medium (see Subheading 2.3).
3. 96-Well flat-bottom culture plates.
4. Cell counter.
5. Sterile cryogenic vials.
6. Multichannel pipettes.

### 2.8. Hybridoma Cryopreservation

1. Cells to be frozen.
2. Centrifuge tubes.
3. Freezing medium: RPMI-1640 medium supplemented with 20% FBS, 2 mM L-glutamine, 0.5 mM sodium pyruvate, penicillin (100 U/mL), streptomycin (100 μg/mL), and 5% dimethyl sulfoxide (DMSO).
4. Cryogenic vials.
5. Liquid nitrogen freezer.

### 2.9. Antibody Isotyping

1. Isotyping strips.
2. Hybridoma supernatant.

### 2.10. Thawing and Growth of Hybridoma Cells

1. Water bath at 37°C.
2. 70% Ethanol.
3. 15-mL conical tube.
4. Hybridoma culture medium (see Subheading 2.3).
5. Tissue culture flasks, e.g., T-25 or T-75.
6. 5% $CO_2$ tissue culture incubator at 37°C.

## 3. Methods

The following protocol describes the method by which splenocytes from the immunized mouse are fused with a BALB/c mouse myeloma line using polyethylene glycol-1500 (PEG-1500) as a fusogen to generate hybridoma cells. Upon fusion, cells are suspended in an HAT-selective medium and then cultured in 96-well flat-bottom plates for the growth of hybridoma clones.

### 3.1. Preparation of Splenocytes from the Immunized Mouse

1. Three days before cell fusion, boost mice with the antigen. On the day of the fusion, sacrifice mice for spleen collection according to the IACUC-approved standard animal use protocol.
2. Autoclave surgical instruments and perform all experiments under sterile conditions.
3. Prepare and warm serum-free RPMI-1640 medium in a water-bath at 37°C.

4. Collect spleen from the euthanized mouse under tissue culture conditions and place the spleen in a conical tube containing approximately 10 mL RPMI-1640 medium.
5. Rinse spleen twice in sterile Petri dishes with RPMI-1640 medium.
6. In a Petri dish with 10 mL of RPMI-1640 medium, grind the spleen tissue between the frosted ends of two sterile microscope glass slides.
7. Pipette cell clumps vigorously and transfer the suspension into a 15 mL conical tube.
8. Allow debris to settle for 5 min onto the bottom of the tube and gently transfer the cell suspension into another conical tube, leaving the debris behind.
9. Spin down cells at 300×*g* for 5 min and discard the supernatant.
10. Suspend cells in RPMI-1640 medium and count the lymphocytes using a cell counter.
11. Wash cells twice in RPMI-1640 medium by centrifugation.

### 3.2. Preparation of Myeloma Cells

1. Mouse myeloma cell P3X63Ag8.653 as the fusion partner (37), is thawed from a stock stored in liquid nitrogen a week prior to the fusion.
2. The myeloma cells are first cultured in medium containing 10% FBS and 130 μM 8-azaguanine to select for clones that are HAT-sensitive and thus unable to survive in the presence of aminopterin (see Note 1).
3. After a few days, transfer and culture the myeloma cells in RPMI-1640 medium supplemented with 10% FBS.
4. Check culture microscopically to assess the status of the cells, and harvest the cells from culture flasks in the logarithmic phase of growth.
5. Spin down cells at 300×*g* for 5 min and discard the supernatant.
6. Suspend myeloma cell pellets in serum-free RPMI-1640 medium.
7. Count and calculate the number of cells needed for fusion. Typically, splenocytes from the immunized mouse are fused with the myeloma cells at a ratio of 2:1 or 3:1.
8. Wash myeloma cells once more with RPMI-1640 medium by centrifugation and discard the supernatant.
9. Suspend cell pellet in a small volume of RPMI-1640 medium and then mix the myeloma cells with splenocytes in a 50-mL conical tube for cell fusion.

### 3.3. Cell Fusion

1. Spin down the mixture of splenocytes and myeloma cells at 300×*g* for 5 min, and aspirate all supernatant from the cell pellet.
2. Suspend cell pellet by running the bottom of the conical tube over the air-grill of the biosafety cabinet.
3. Keep fusion tube in a beaker of warm water at 37°C for all of the following steps during cell fusion.
4. Using a 2-mL pipette, gradually add 1.5 mL of PEG-1500 over 90 s to the mixture of splenocytes and myeloma cells in the bottom of the fusion tube, and then allow the cells to stand for 1 min with occasional stirring.
5. Add 10 mL of warm RPMI-1640 medium gradually over 3 min to dilute the PEG-1500 fusogen (see Note 2).
6. Fill the fusion tube up to 45 mL with warm RPMI-1640 medium and allow the suspension to incubate in a water-bath at 37°C for 5 min.
7. Spin down cells at 300×*g* for 5 min and discard the supernatant.
8. Suspend cell pellets in warm HAT medium at a concentration of approximately $5 \times 10^5$ splenocytes/mL.
9. Plate out cells in 96-well flat-bottom culture plates by adding 200 μL of cell suspension per well (see Note 3).
10. Incubate fusion plates in a 5% $CO_2$, 37°C incubator to grow hybridomas (see Note 4).
11. On day 5 post-fusion, remove half the volume (100 μL/well) of HAT medium from the fusion plates and replace with 100 μL of HT medium (i.e., HAT medium without aminopterin).
12. Sample culture supernatants from the fusion plates for antibody screening between days 10 and 14 when hybridomas have grown to be half-confluent and the medium has changed to an orange color.

### 3.4. Hybridoma Screening Using Flow Cytometry

Flow cytometry is one of the most powerful techniques for screening antibodies against cell surface antigens. It not only enables one to determine the presence of a specific mAb in the hybridoma culture supernatant but also allows one to measure the binding profile of the mAb. Flow cytometry in a high-throughput mode is much more rapid and suitable for the quantitative screening of a large number of samples in a short amount of time. The flow cytometric procedure includes cell labeling with antibodies, acquiring data with a flow cytometer, and analyzing the data with the appropriate software (see Notes 5 and 6).

1. Harvest antigen–expressing cells from culture flasks or isolate cells from tissue samples according to the standard cell isolation protocol.

2. Wash cells twice in PBS, followed by F buffer and by centrifugation at $300 \times g$ for 5 min.
3. Count and calculate the number of cells needed, which is usually $0.25–0.5 \times 10^6$ cells per labeling sample.
4. Place 50–100 μL of hybridoma culture supernatant or control antibody in each well of a 96-well microtest U-bottom plate.
5. Suspend cell pellets in F buffer at a concentration of $1 \times 10^7$ cells/mL, and add 25–50 μL of cell suspension to each plate well containing the appropriate antibody supernatant.
6. Mix reaction plate by shaking gently and incubate at 4°C for 30–45 min.
7. Wash plate three times in 250 μL of F buffer per well by centrifugation at $400 \times g$ for 5 min using plate carriers. Flick supernatant off the cell pellet in each of the plates between washes.
8. Suspend and incubate cells in 100 μL of fluorescein-conjugated anti-mouse IgG antibody at an appropriate dilution in F buffer.
9. Incubate plate at 4°C for 30–45 min.
10. Wash labeling plate twice with F buffer as above, and then once with fixation buffer.
11. Suspend cell pellets in an appropriate volume of fixation buffer. Typically, 30–50 μL sample volumes are required for high-throughput flow cytometric analysis.
12. Analyze samples by flow cytometry immediately, or store the samples at 4°C covered with foil to analyze at a later time.

### 3.5. Hybridoma Screening by ELISA

To detect protein- or polypeptide-reactive antibodies in the hybridoma supernatant, a standard ELISA protocol is commonly used. The ELISA procedure consists of an antigen pre-coating onto ELISA plates, an incubation with the antibody supernatant followed by another incubation with the enzyme-conjugated antibody, which is an enzymatic reaction for color development, and a final reading and subsequent analysis of the ELISA data.

1. On day 1, coat plates with purified protein or polypeptides as antigen. Dilute the antigen to a concentration of 0.5–1 μg/mL in carbonate–bicarbonate buffer, pH 9.4.
2. Add 100 μL of antigen solution (0.05–0.1 μg antigen) to each well of ELISA plates.
3. Seal plates with sealing tape and incubate the plates at 4°C overnight.
4. On day 2 after incubation overnight, empty all solution from the antigen-coated plates.
5. Rinse plates once with 250 μL of wash buffer.

6. Add 250 μL of blocking buffer to each well on all the plates and incubate at room temperature for 20 min to block nonspecific-binding sites.
7. Empty plates and rinse once with 250 μL of wash buffer.
8. Add 25–50 μL of hybridoma supernatant to each well of the antigen-coated plates, together with the appropriate negative and positive controls. Cover plates with sealing tape and incubate by rocking at room temperature for 45–60 min.
9. Empty and then rinse plates with 250 μL of wash buffer three times.
10. Fill plate wells with 250 μL of blocking buffer, and incubate at room temperature for 15–20 min.
11. Empty liquid from plates and add 50 μL of peroxidase-conjugated anti-mouse IgG antibody diluted in blocking buffer, and incubate plates at room temperature for 45–60 min.
12. Empty and rinse plates with wash buffer three times, followed by one wash with TBS.
13. Remove all liquid from ELISA plates.
14. Prepare substrate solution immediately before use. Add 100 μL of TMB substrate solution to each well of all the plates, and incubate at room temperature for 15–30 min or until the desired color develops. Peroxidase substrate solution is prepared according to the manufacturer's instructions.
15. Measure the absorbance (optical density) of each well at 450 nm immediately with an ELISA plate reader, or add 50 μL of stop solution to each plate well before reading.
16. Analysis of data (optional): a standard curve from the serial dilutions is prepared with concentration on the *X*-axis (log scale) versus absorbance on the *Y*-axis (linear). Interpolate the concentration of the hybridoma supernatant sample from this standard curve.

### 3.6. Hybridoma Screening by IHC

The reactivity of antibodies to the tissue antigen is often tested by IHC assays on slides of freshly frozen tissues or renatured paraffin-embedded sections. For the latter, specific antigen-retrieval techniques are commonly used to improve staining by modifying the molecular conformation of target antigens through an exposure of sectioned tissue to a heated buffer solution (38, 39). In general, mAbs selected by IHC assay may recognize denatured epitopes or intracellular antigens in addition to the native antigens on the cell surface.

Fresh tissue specimens are either snap-frozen in OCT medium in liquid nitrogen or embedded in paraffin. Frozen tissue sections are usually cut 4–8 μm thick on a cryostat and coated onto microscope slides. Tissue sections are fixed in acetone at 4°C and stored at −80°C until use. Paraffin-embedded sections in the form of tissue microarrays have become commercially available in recent years for antibody screening and characterization. The IHC assay is a very valuable tool for localization of the antigen defined by mAbs. A detailed protocol is described below to screen antibodies in the hybridoma supernatant.

1. For frozen tissue sections, thaw tissue slides at room temperature and then place the samples in a humid chamber.
2. Apply 50–100 μL of hybridoma culture supernatant to the section slide and incubate at room temperature for 30 min.
3. Rinse slides with TBS-50 three times for 5 min each.
4. For tissue sections with highly endogenous peroxidase activity (e.g., thymus tissue sections), slides are submerged in 1% hydrogen peroxide in 50% methanol solution for 20 min on an ice bath to inactivate the endogenous enzyme after the first incubation with antibody supernatant.
5. Incubate slides with 10% normal goat serum in TBS-50 for 15 min to block nonspecific binding.
6. After draining the slides, apply 300 μL of peroxidase-conjugated anti-mouse IgG antibody at an appropriate dilution to each slide and incubate for 30 min at room temperature. The antibody conjugate reagent used at this concentration should yield an optimal reaction based upon previous titrations.
7. Following three washes in TBS-50, the color reaction is developed by incubating the slides for 40 min with AEC substrate solution.
8. After rinsing, counterstain the sections with Gill's hematoxylin for 1 min.
9. Wash slides and then submerge them in tap water or Scott's water for 2 min for better background staining.
10. Mount the slides with heated glycergel and examine the slides microscopically.

### 3.7. Hybridoma Subcloning

Hybridoma cells from fusion plates require subcloning to achieve a truly monoclonal population that produces a monospecific antibody. Under the initial plating conditions of cells in the fusion plates, a plate well probably contains no hybridoma clone or more than one hybridoma with or without the ability to produce antibodies (Fig. 3). While some hybridomas may be genetically unstable at an early stage, the stable clones must be identified and selected as soon as possible. Hybridoma cloning is a time-consuming step in the generation of mAbs; however, single-cell cloning can be accelerated by limiting dilution and microscopically picking single colonies, as described in Fig. 4 and discussed in this section.

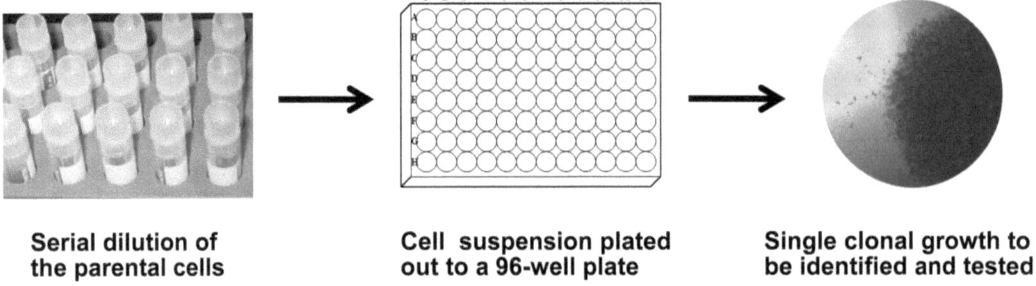


Fig. 4. Hybridoma subcloning by limiting dilution followed by microscopic selection of single cell colony. Parental hybridoma cells are diluted in culture medium by serial dilution to a final concentration of 10 cells/mL and 200 μL of the cell suspension plated into each well of a 96-well plate (2 cells/well). After incubation for 12–14 days, single clonal growths in the subcloning well are microscopically identified and tested for production of a specific antibody using hybridoma-screening protocols.

1. For subcloning, hybridoma cells are cultured either in hybridoma culture medium or HT medium, depending on the previously selected medium (see Note 7).
2. With a pipette, gently suspend hybridoma cells in culture. Transfer approximately 100 μL of cell suspension to a sterile vial labeled with the hybridoma clone name.
3. Count cells using a cell counter, and determine the initial concentration of cells.
4. Make serial dilutions of each hybridoma clone to a final concentration of 10 cells/mL in culture medium.
5. Using a multichannel pipette, plate out 200 μL of cell suspension (theoretically, 2 cells per well) into each well of a 96-well culture plate, which may have been pre-seeded with feeder cells as necessary.
6. Incubate plates in a 5% $CO_2$ incubator at 37°C, and microscopically examine the plates regularly for colony growth after the first week.
7. Examine and record the wells containing a single colony.
8. Sample supernatant from the single colony culture for antibody testing when the culture medium has turned an orange color.
9. Screen for specific antibodies from the subclone supernatant as described in Subheadings 3.4–3.6.
10. Based on antibody screening results, the desired subclones are selected, expanded for antibody production, and/or frozen for further studies.

### 3.8. Hybridoma Cryopreservation

1. Harvest hybridoma cells from culture plates or flasks. Transfer cell suspension to a centrifuge tube and spin for 5 min at $300 \times g$.
2. Remove supernatant and suspend cell pellets in a prechilled freezing medium at a density of $0.5–1 \times 10^7$ cells/mL.

3. Transfer 1-mL aliquots of cell suspension to a cryogenic vial.
4. Store cells in liquid nitrogen (see Note 8).
5. Record identity and location of cells in the liquid nitrogen freezer.

### 3.9. Antibody Isotyping

Identification of the antibody isotype not only provides information about the basic structure of an antibody and the isotype-related functions but also aids in selecting effective methods for antibody purification. The isotype of murine mAbs was traditionally determined by solid-phase ELISA or by immunodiffusion on agar plates, but both assays are less efficient and at times yield inconsistent results. In contrast, characterization of the antibody isotype with recently developed isotyping strips has made the process much easier, and as a result, the mAb isotype can be determined in minutes, especially for rat or murine antibodies. Since the isotyping strip bears immobilized bands of anti-rodent antibodies corresponding to each of the common antibody classes or subclasses and the κ or λ light chain, the strip reacts with any rodent antibody regardless of its isotype or purity. The detailed procedure to characterize the antibody isotype using isotyping strips is available in the manufacturer's instruction manual.

### 3.10. Thawing and Growth of Hybridoma Cells

Once the desired hybridoma clones have been identified and selected, the cells should be tested to ensure the absence of mycoplasma contamination in culture, and then frozen in several vials for long-term storage in a liquid nitrogen freezer. For production of mAbs from hybridoma cells, a vial of frozen hybridomas is thawed and grown in hybridoma culture medium to collect supernatant for antibody purification.

1. Locate and retrieve the cryovial of cells from a liquid nitrogen freezer.
2. Thaw cells immediately by placing the cryovial in a clean water-bath at 37°C. Agitate the cryovial in the water-bath gently until the frozen medium is completely thawed (see Note 9).
3. Submerge vial in 70% ethanol in a small beaker for 1–2 min and leave it to air-dry within the biosafety cabinet prior to opening.
4. Transfer thawed cell suspension from the cryovial into a 15-mL conical tube.
5. Add 10 mL of hybridoma culture medium gradually to the tube.
6. Centrifuge at 300 × *g* for 5 min and aspirate supernatant from the tube.
7. Suspend the cell pellet in hybridoma culture medium and transfer the cell suspension to a culture flask.

8. Add more medium to the culture as necessary (usually 8 mL of medium for a T-25 flask or 30 mL of medium for a T-75 flask).
9. Incubate the cell culture in a 5% $CO_2$ incubator at 37°C.
10. Examine growth of hybridomas regularly and expand the cells for mAb production (see Notes 10 and 11).

## 4. Notes

1. Normal lymphocytes and other cells from the mouse spleen die naturally after a few days in culture. Only hybridoma cells are able to survive in HAT medium and grow indefinitely because they are supplied from both the parental B-lymphocytes, from which the X-chromosome encodes the enzyme hypoxanthine-guanine phosphoribosyl transferase (HGPRT), and from the parental myeloma cells which have the ability to grow immortally in vitro. With the exception of hybridomas, almost all of the cells undergo death in selective HAT medium in the first couple of weeks after fusion. The HAT medium is gradually replaced by hypoxanthine-thymidine (HT) medium, followed by a routine hybridoma culture medium without either HAT or HT supplement. For fusion plates, when the hybridoma cells have grown to be half-confluent in the culture wells and the color of the medium has changed to an orange color (usually 10–15 days post-fusion), the culture supernatant is sampled for antibody screening by various immunoassays.
2. To enhance the cell fusion efficiency, different fusion partners or other fusion methods should be considered besides the PEG-mediated fusion. For example, electrofusion-based protocols have reportedly been established and optimized for generating hybridoma clones (40, 41). However, the PEG-mediated fusion is a conventional and convenient technique for hybridoma generation, and has remained one of the best approaches for cell fusion.
3. To promote hybridoma growth, mouse peritoneal exudate cells or fibroblasts are often seeded on the fusion plate as a feeder layer, if necessary (42).
4. To maintain good culture conditions, such as having a stable $CO_2$ concentration and constant temperature, do not open the incubator for the first 2 days post-fusion if possible.
5. The choice of which hybridoma screening assay to use depends largely on the nature of the antigen that is available and the prospective application of the mAbs that is being generated. However, it should be noted that the outcome of the antibody

reactivity usually varies depending on multiple factors, such as the binding antigen used to coat the plastic plates, the direct reactivity with the targeting antigen in cells, or the inhibition of binding of a ligand to its receptor. Moreover, the conformation of peptides and even proteins bound to plastic can be affected by charges present on the plastic surface.

6. Some antibodies from unfused B-lymphocytes in the early culture may yield a misleading positive reactivity in the initial screening of hybridomas from fusion plates. The false positives can be diminished by changing the culture medium in fusion plates twice with fresh medium.
7. In order to promote the growth of a single hybridoma cell during the subcloning stage, the culture plate may be pre-seeded with mouse peritoneal exudate cells or fibroblast lines as a feeder layer, or enhanced with commercially available hybridoma cloning supplements.
8. During the hybridoma freezing stage, cells in a cryovial can be directly placed into a liquid nitrogen freezer. This may appear contrary to the general recommendation to gradually lower the temperature by placing cells in a –80°C freezer or in the freezing chamber of liquid nitrogen before transferring the cells to a liquid nitrogen freezer; however, cells that have been frozen by the direct-freezing method routinely show no difference in the loss of cell viability on recovery.
9. It is critical that frozen hybridomas are thawed as quickly as possible when the cells are removed from the liquid nitrogen freezer. It is also important to assess the viability of the recovered cells upon thawing.
10. Most hybridoma cells in a conventional culture media, such as complete RPMI-1640, should steadily be adapted to either a medium with low-IgG serum or a serum-free medium by lowering the serum level in the culture medium gradually.
11. Traditional cell culture medium supplemented with serum contains a considerable level of immunoglobulins of animal origin, which are difficult to separate from the murine mAbs during purification. Therefore, a medium containing low-IgG serum or serum-free medium must be used to grow hybridoma cells for in vitro production of mAbs. The culture conditions in the absence of animal immunoglobulins and the low level of other proteins present make the purification of mAbs from the hybridoma supernatant much more effective and expedient. In order to maximize the yield of mAbs in the culture supernatant, hybridoma cells are allowed to grow until the medium is depleted of nutrients. When the cells reach saturated density and the medium has turned a yellow color, the culture supernatant is collected for mAb purification.

## Acknowledgments

The author gratefully acknowledges Lena Kikuchi and Nancy Chan for their expertise in hybridoma generation and the technical assistance for validating the protocols described here. The author is especially thankful to Dr. Peter LeMotte, Dr. Thomas Pietzonka and Dr. John Hastewell for helpful advice and support, and to Yuxiang Zhang for his assistance in editing the illustrations in this manuscript.

### References

1. Köhler G, Milstein C (1975) Continuous cultures of fused cells secreting antibody of predefined specificity. Nature 256:495–497
2. Little M, Kipriyanov SM, Gall FL, Moldenhauer G (2000) Of mice and men: hybridoma and recombinant antibodies. Immunol Today 21: 364–370
3. An Z (2010) Monoclonal antibodies—a proven and rapidly expanding therapeutic modality for human diseases. Protein Cell 1:319–330
4. Weiner LM (2007) Building better magic bullets—improving unconjugated monoclonal antibody therapy for cancer. Nat Rev Cancer 7: 701–706
5. Schlossman SF et al (1995) Leucocyte typing V: white cell differentiation antigens. Oxford University Press, Oxford
6. Matesanz-Isabel J, Sintes J, Llinàs L et al (2011) New B-cell CD molecules. Immunol Lett 134:104–112
7. Kung P, Goldstein G, Reinherz EL, Schlossman SF (1979) Monoclonal antibodies defining distinctive human T cell surface antigens. Science 206:347–349
8. Reinherz EL, Kung PC, Goldstein G, Schlossman SF (1979) Separation of functional subsets of human T cells by a monoclonal antibody. Proc Natl Acad Sci U S A 76:4061–4065
9. Meuer SC, Hussey RE, Hodgdon JC et al (1982) Surface structures involved in target recognition by human cytotoxic T lymphocytes. Science 218:471–473
10. Zhang C, Ao Z, Seth A, Schlossman SF (1996) A mitochondrial membrane protein defined by a novel monoclonal antibody is preferentially detected in apoptotic cells. J Immunol 157: 3980–3987
11. Zhang C (1998) Monoclonal antibody as a probe for characterization and separation of apoptotic cells. In: Zhu L, Chun J (eds) Apoptosis detection and assay methods. BioTechniques series on molecular laboratory methods. BioTechniques Books, Eaton Publishing, Natick, MA, pp 63–73
12. Bok RA, Small EJ (2002) Bloodborne biomolecular markers in prostate cancer development and progression. Nat Rev Cancer 2:918–926
13. Wagner PD, Maruvada P, Srivastava S (2004) Molecular diagnostics: a new frontier in cancer prevention. Exp Rev Mol Diagn 4:503–511
14. Jones PT, Dear PH, Foote J, Neuberger MS, Winter G (1986) Replacing the complementarity-determining regions in a human antibody with those from a mouse. Nature 321:522–525
15. Riechmann L, Clark M, Waldmann H, Winter G (1988) Reshaping human antibodies for therapy. Nature 332:323–327
16. Smith SL (1996) Ten years of Orthoclone OKT3 (muromonab-CD3): a review. J Transpl Coord 6:109–119
17. Lupo L, Panzera P, Tandoi F et al (2008) Basiliximab versus steroids in double therapy immunosuppression in liver transplantation a prospective randomized clinical trial. Transplantation 86:925–931
18. Van den Brande JM, Braat H, van den Brink GR et al (2003) Infliximab but not etanercept induces apoptosis in lamina propria T-lymphocytes from patients with Crohn's disease. Gastroenterology 124:1774–1785
19. Chan AC, Carter PJ (2010) Therapeutic antibodies for autoimmunity and inflammation. Nat Rev Immunol 10:301–316
20. Maloney DG, Grillo-López AJ, White CA et al (1997) IDEC-C2B8 (Rituximab) anti-CD20 monoclonal antibody therapy in patients with relapsed low-grade non-Hodgkin's lymphoma. Blood 90:2188–2195
21. Meissner HC, Welliver RC, Chartrand SA et al (1999) Immunoprophylaxis with palivizumab, a humanized respiratory syncytial virus monoclonal antibody, for prevention of respiratory syncytial virus infection in high risk infants: a consensus opinion. Pediatr Infect Dis J 18:223–231

22. Blattman JN, Greenberg PD (2004) Cancer immunotherapy: a treatment for the masses. Science 305:200–205
23. Reichert JM (2011) Antibody-based therapeutics to watch in 2011. mAbs 3:76–99
24. McCafferty J, Griffiths AD, Winter G, Chiswell DJ (1990) Phage antibodies: filamentous phage displaying antibody variable domains. Nature 348:552–554
25. Hoogenboom HR (2005) Selecting and screening recombinant antibody libraries. Nat Biotechnol 23:1105–1116
26. Traggiai E, Becker S, Subbarao K et al (2004) An efficient method to make human monoclonal antibodies from memory B cells: potent neutralization of SARS coronavirus. Nat Med 10:871–875
27. Lanzavecchia A, Bernasconi N, Traggiai E et al (2006) Understanding and making use of human memory B cells. Immunol Rev 211: 303–309
28. Nossal GJV (1992) The molecular and cellular basis of affinity maturation in the antibody response. Cell 68:1–2
29. Jakobovits A, Amado RG, Yang X, Roskos L, Schwab G (2007) From XenoMouse technology to panitumumab, the first fully human antibody product from transgenic mice. Nat Biotechnol 25:1134–1143
30. Brüggemann M, Neuberger MS (1996) Strategies for expressing human antibody repertoires in transgenic mice. Immunol Today 17: 391–397
31. Green LL (1999) Antibody engineering via genetic engineering of the mouse: XenoMouse strains are a vehicle for the facile generation of therapeutic human monoclonal antibodies. J Immunol Methods 231:11–23
32. Lonberg N (2005) Human antibodies from transgenic animals. Nat Biotechnol 23: 1117–1125
33. Davis CG, Gallo ML, Corvalan JRF (1999) Transgenic mice as a source of fully human antibodies for the treatment of cancer. Cancer Metastasis Rev 18:421–425
34. Zhang C, Xu Y, Gu J, Schlossman SF (1998) A cell surface receptor defined by a mAb mediates a unique type of cell death similar to oncosis. Proc Natl Acad Sci U S A 95:6290–6295
35. Yonehara S, Ishii A, Yonehara M (1989) A cell-killing monoclonal antibody (anti-Fas) to a cell surface antigen co-downregulated with the receptor of tumor necrosis factor. J Exp Med 169:1747–1756
36. Trauth BC, Klas C, Peters AMJ et al (1989) Monoclonal antibody-mediated tumor regression by induction of apoptosis. Science 245:301–305
37. Kearney JF, Radbruch A, Liesegang B, Rajewsky K (1979) A new mouse myeloma cell line that has lost immunoglobulin expression but permits the construction of antibody-secreting hybrid cell lines. J Immunol 123:1548–1550
38. Shi S-R, Shi Y, Taylor CR (2011) Antigen retrieval immunohistochemistry: review and future prospects in research and diagnosis over two decades. J Histochem Cytochem 59:13–32
39. D'Amico F, Skarmoutsou E, Stivala F (2009) State of the art in antigen retrieval for immunohistochemistry. J Immunol Methods 341:1–18
40. Glassy M (1988) Creating hybridomas by electrofusion. Nature 333:579–580
41. Ohnishi K, Chiba J, Goto Y, Tokunaga T (1987) Improvement in the basic technology of electrofusion for generation of antibody-producing hybridomas. J Immunol Methods 100:181–189
42. Long WL, McGuire W, Palombo A, Emini EA (1986) Enhancing the establishment efficiency of hybridoma cells: use of irradiated human diploid fibroblast feeder layers. J Immunol Methods 86:89–93

# Chapter 8

# The Application of Transgenic Mice for Therapeutic Antibody Discovery

E-Chiang Lee and Michael Owen

## Abstract

In 2006, panitumumab, the first fully human antibody generated from transgenic mice, was approved for clinical use by the US Food and Drug Administration (FDA). Since then, a further seven such antibodies have been approved. In this chapter, we discuss how transgenic mice technologies can provide a powerful platform for creating human therapeutic antibodies.

**Key words:** ES cells, Homologous recombination, Human antibody, Humanized mice, Ig locus, Immunoglobulin, Isotype, Phage display, Transgenic mice, Therapeutic antibody

## 1. Introduction

The B cell arm of the immune system has evolved to produce high affinity, antigen-specific antibodies in response to antigenic challenge. Antibodies are generated in B lymphocytes by a process of gene rearrangement in which variable (V), diversity (D; for the IgH locus), and joining (J) gene segments are recombined, transcribed, and spliced to a Cμ (for IgH) or a Cκ or Cλ (for Igκ or Igλ) constant region gene segment to form an IgM antibody. Depending on the stage of B cell development, IgM is either located on the cell surface or secreted. The recombination process generates a primary antibody repertoire with sufficient germ line diversity (~$10^{11}$) to bind a wide range of antigens. However, it is usually not large enough to provide the high affinity antibodies that are required for an effective immune response to an antigen such as an infectious agent. The primary response is limited further by the number of B cells circulating in the lymphoid organs and tissues at any particular time. This number ($10^{8}$–$10^{10}$ depending on the organism) is orders of magnitude less than the encoded

Gabriele Proetzel and Hilmar Ebersbach (eds.), *Antibody Methods and Protocols*, Methods in Molecular Biology, vol. 901,
DOI 10.1007/978-1-61779-931-0_8, © Springer Science+Business Media, LLC 2012

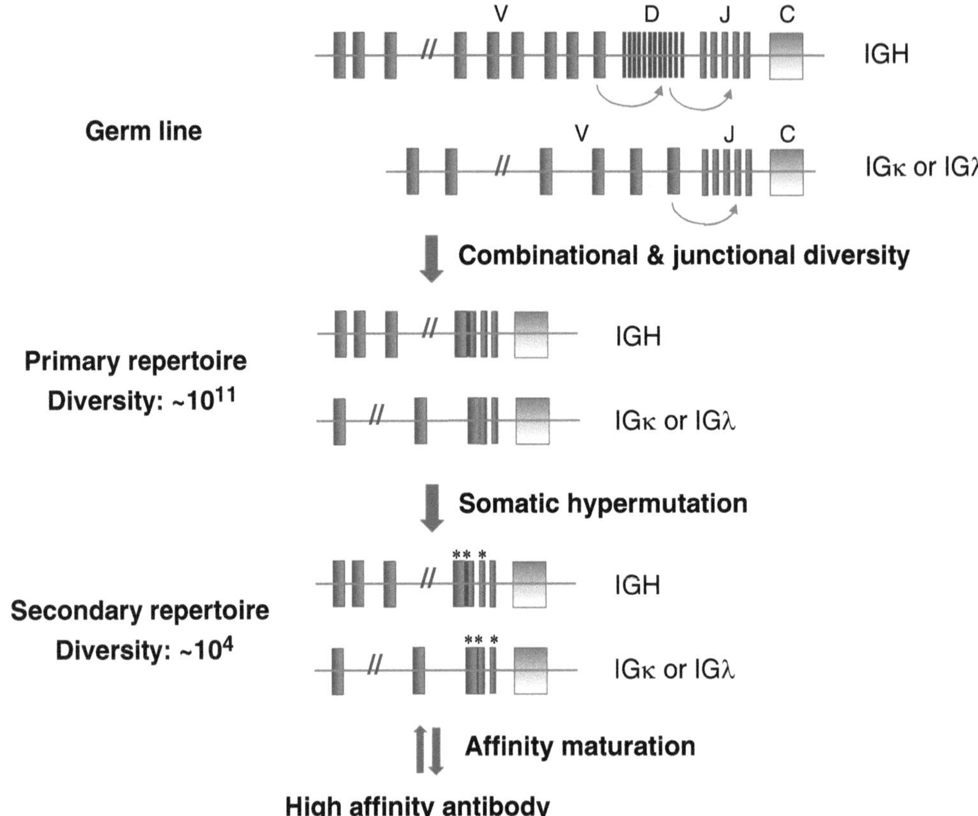


Fig. 1. Antibody diversification. The primary repertoire is formed by combination of germ line V, D, J segments for the heavy chain (IgH) and V, J segments for the light chains (Igκ or Igλ). During recombination, diversity is further increased by random insertions and deletions at the junctions between segments. Upon antigen challenge, engaged low-affinity antibodies are leads to somatic hypermutation to form the secondary repertoire. With intense competition for antigens, high-affinity antibodies are eventually selected out from the secondary repertoire. *Asterisks* indicate point mutations resulted from somatic hypermutation.

germ line diversity. Therefore, the immune system adopts a two-stage diversification process to increase diversity further (1) (Fig. 1). When challenged with antigens, B cells undergo selection and maturation by a process called somatic mutation. B cells expressing antibodies which bind to antigen undergo multiple rounds of diversification, clonal expansion, and antigen selection in the germinal centers (GCs) of the secondary lymphoid organs. During this process, the rearranged variable regions of the immunoglobulin genes acquire somatic hypermutation through nucleotide substitution. This stepwise process creates a secondary repertoire from the weak binders selected originally from the primary repertoire (2, 3) and combines rapid proliferation of antigen-reactive B cells with intense selection for quality of binding, eventually giving rise to high affinity antibodies with broad epitope coverage. During this process, antibodies undergo class switching in which the Cm constant region is replaced by Cγ, Cα, or Cε to produce IgG, A, or E classes of antibody with different effector functions.

The safety, specificity, and potency of antibodies have made them ideal candidates for pharmacological intervention in disease. Clearly, when used in a therapeutic setting, particularly during repeated administration, antibodies should contain no sequences that induce an immune response in patients which could produce an adverse reaction or alter the pharmacokinetic profile of the drug; ideally, they should be fully human. This requirement has resulted in a number of different strategies for "humanizing" monoclonal antibodies. Perhaps the most attractive of these approaches is the use of in vivo strategies such as transgenic mice that have harnessed the natural beauty of the two-stage diversification process and antigen-mediated selection for obtaining high affinity antibodies. The availability of these humanized mice has resulted in the development of powerful therapeutic agents against a number of human diseases.

## 2. Development of Human Immunoglobulin Transgenic Mice

Since the early 1980s, the introduction of rearranged immunoglobulin genes into the mouse germ line has been successfully exploited to study the mechanisms of assembly, expression, allelic exclusion, and somatic hypermutation of immunoglobulin (Ig) genes (4, 5). In 1985, Alt et al. noted that the transgenic mouse approach could not only enhance basic studies of immunology but also evolve to have a practical value in generating human antibodies through in vivo rearrangement, $V_H$ and $V_L$ assembly, and somatic mutation processes (4). There were four major challenges to the generation of such transgenic mice. Firstly, human Ig transgenes would be required to function as well as endogenous mouse Ig genes, properly utilizing the mouse machinery of the immune system, including gene rearrangement, heavy chain–light chain assembly, expression, allelic exclusion, hypermutation, class switch, and affinity maturation. Secondly, endogenous Ig genes would need to be inactivated to avoid expression of hybrid mouse–human antibodies. Thirdly, human sequence encoding sufficiently large repertoires would need to be inserted into mouse germ line. A limited repertoire may reduce the diversity of antibodies and constrain the application of the system. For the full human repertoire, this would necessitate the insertion of around 1 Mb of human DNA into the mouse germ line for each of the three Ig loci (Fig. 3). Finally, physiological levels of human Ig transgene products, equivalent to those in wild type mice, would need to be expressed. All of these challenges would need to be overcome to generate an uncompromised and fully functional immune system.

Four years after Alt's prediction, Bruggemann and her colleagues reported the generation of transgenic mice by pronuclear injection with a limited human repertoire of unrearranged $V_H$

and $D_H$ segments, six human $J_H$ segments, and a chimeric human/mouse μ constant region gene (6). In this process, the transgene randomly integrates into the mouse genome. This was the first study to demonstrate that human immunoglobulin gene segments are able to be rearranged and expressed in mice, suggesting that human cis-elements including IgH promoters, the intronic enhancer (iEμ), and recombination signal sequences (RSS) have at least some activity in transgenic mice. In 1992, Lonberg's group further showed that transgenic mice carrying an IgH minilocus including one human $V_H$, ten $D_H$s, six $J_H$s, Cμ, and Cγ1 genes together with their respective switch regions had detectable serum human IgM and IgG1 antibodies at levels ranging from 0.1 to 1 μg/ml, indicating that proper class switching of the human IgH transgenes had occurred (7). In addition, allelic exclusion was unimpaired in these mice since human and mouse IgM were never expressed on the surface of the same B cell. Both allelic exclusion and class switching require functional signaling from the transmembrane (cell surface-associated) form of human IgM. Therefore, the demonstration of that these functions were intact implies that the hybrid B-cell receptor (BCR) consisting of human IgM, mouse Igα, Igβ (essential co-receptors for B cell signaling), and other mouse signaling molecules can induce signaling during B cell development and activation.

The transgenic mouse lines generated by Bruggemann's and Lonberg's groups had a background of endogenous mouse Ig genes, which may have caused of the observed low expression of human antibodies. To overcome this problem, two groups reported the generation of human Ig gene-transgenic mice in a mouse IgH and IgK knockout background (8, 9). Lonberg's group created transgenic mice with a human $V_H$ minilocus having two more human $V_H$ segments than in their previous version, and a human $V_\kappa$ minilocus with four $V_\kappa$, five $J_\kappa$ segments and Cκ. Sequence analysis showed that the IgH minilocus did not only undergo VDJ rearrangement but also underwent somatic hypermutation following antigen challenge. In the absence of endogenous IgH and Igκ products, the levels of serum human IgM (~100 μg/ml) and human IgG1 (~0.1 to 10 μg/ml) were significantly higher than in transgenic mice harboring endogenous Ig genes (7, 8). The majority of human heavy chains were shown to be associated with human κ chains. A small portion (~1 to 5%) was complexed with mouse λ chains because the endogenous Igλ locus was not inactivated in these transgenic mice. Green's group used yeast artificial chromosomes (YACs) with human IgH or Igκ genes to generate transgenic mice through yeast protoplast fusion to embryonic stem (ES) cells (9). These YACs carried a much bigger fragment of genomic DNA (220 kb for IgH; 170 kb for Igκ) than the minilocus vectors used by Lonberg (80 kb for IgH; 40 kb for Igκ). Since YACs are able to accommodate more than 1 Mb of genomic DNA, this technology can be used as a vehicle to introduce a larger human Ig repertoire than with other types of vector.

Initial studies on the B cell immune response to the CD4 antigen in Lonberg's transgenic mice generated only low affinity antibodies ($8–9 \times 10^7$/M) (8). It was thus difficult to determine whether these antibodies underwent affinity maturation. His group subsequently reported the generation of new YAC transgenic mice carrying the same IgH minilocus but with a much larger Igκ locus comprising nearly half of the germ line human Vκ region (10). High-affinity antibodies with $5 \times 10^9$ to $1 \times 10^{10}$/M affinity to the CD4 antigen, were generated in these mice. In 1997, Mendaz et al. generated YAC transgenic mice carrying approximately 66 human $V_H$s and 32 $V_\kappa$s using modified YACs with sizes of 1,020 kb and 800 kb, respectively (11). With such diverse repertoires, they also generated specific antibodies with high affinities around $1 \times 10^9$ to $1 \times 10^{10}$/M to a variety of antigens including IL-8, EGFR, and TNFα. With persuasive evidence to support effective in vivo affinity maturation for human Ig transgenes in their transgenic mice, both groups provided a vital breakthrough in the use of transgenic strategies for therapeutic antibody discovery.

In 1999, Bruggemann and her colleagues reported the generation of YAC transgenic mice carrying all three human Ig loci, IgH (240 kb), Igκ (1.3 Mb), and Igλ (410 kb), in a strain with inactivated endogenous IgH and Igκ (12). Human IgM was detected in serum at levels of 50–400 μg/ml and was elevated after immunization. These levels are similar to those observed in wild-type mice. However, it was impossible to determine whether the IgG response was normal since the IgH locus in these mice only contained Cμ and Cδ genes and did not include any Cγ gene segments.

In addition to transgenic technologies using pronuclear microinjection of minilocus vectors and protoplast fusion of YACs, microcell-mediated chromosome transfer (MMCT) has been used to transfer large chromosome fragments carrying the Ig genes into mice. This approach enables transfer of single human chromosome or chromosome fragments with a centromere and two telomeres into pluripotent mouse ES cells by fusion of human primary fibroblast-derived microcells with mouse ES cells (13, 14). Although this technology offers the advantage of transfer of the complete Ig repertoire, the unpredictable transmission rates due to chromosome instability and somatic mosaicism significantly limit its application.

## 3. Is the Full Human Primary Repertoire Necessary?

The successful isolation of high-affinity antibodies from transgenic mice with a limited repertoire raises the question of whether the full human repertoire is necessary to identify clinically relevant monoclonal antibodies (10, 11). Studies on antibody binding to antigen have revealed that the CDRH3 region (complementarity determining region 3 of the IgH chain; the region spanning the VDJ junction) is responsible for most of the diversity of the primary repertoire. The additional diversity derived from CDRH1 and CDRH2 encoded by the $V_H$ segments in the primary repertoire seems less important. It has been proposed that the highly diverse CDRH3 sequences are the primary determinants of specificity of antigen recognition (15). In this context, Davis and colleagues demonstrated that transgenic mice with one $V_H$ segment are able to generate high affinity antibodies to variety of antigens through affinity maturation (16). However, it is possible that these antibodies bind to only limited epitopes because they were derived from one $V_H$ segment. Unlike the primary repertoire, the diversity of the secondary repertoire created by hypermutation involves all three CDRH regions. The limited diversity observed in germ line CDRH1 and CDRH2 $V_H$ sequences is thus amplified through second-phase diversification in GCs. From an antibody drug discovery perspective, broad epitope coverage is crucial for identifying clinical candidates. Therefore, the full primary repertoire may be required.

## 4. Compromised Immune Response from Transgenic Mice

Although the transgenic mouse approaches described above result in fully human antibodies, the level of antibody expression is lower than that found in wild-type mice. While the levels of serum human IgM in transgenic mice are usually around 10–400 μg/ml (8, 9, 12, 14) which are close to the serum IgM levels of wild-type mice (~500 μg/ml), the serum IgG concentration, around 10–600 μg/ml in transgenic mice, is much lower than the normal range of IgG levels (~2,000 μg/ml) (8, 11, 14). In addition, splenic B cell populations in these human Ig transgenic mice are usually only 5–40% of the number found in wild-type mice (8, 9, 12). Taken together, these results suggest that the immune response in these mice may be compromised with the consequence that obtaining high-affinity neutralizing antibodies usually requires more transgenic mice, a more intensive immunization schedule and more hybridoma screening when compared to wild-type mice (17).

This compromised immune response may be due to suboptimal use of human cis-regulatory elements within the immunoglobulin loci. Two critical long-range regulatory elements, the iEμ and the enhancer downstream of constant gene segments (the "3′ IgH regulatory region"), have been described in the IgH locus (18, 19). In both YAC and mini-locus transgenic mice, the human IgH

```
                         EMPD    /         TMD            /          CYT

IgM_H.sapien                  GEVSADEEGFENL WATASTFIVLFLLSLFYSTTVTLF KVK
IgM_M.musculus                GEVNAEEEGFENL WTTASTFIVLFLLSLFYSTTVTLF KVK

IgG1_H.sapiens     LQLEESCAEAQDGELDGL WTTITIFITLFLLSVCYSATVTFF KVKWIFSSVVDLKQTIIPDYRNMIGQGA
IgG2_H.sapiens     LQLEESCAEAQDGELDGL WTTITIFITLFLLSVCYSATITFF KVKWIFSSVVDLKQTIVPDYRNMIRQGA
IgG3_H.sapiens     LQLEESCAEAQDGELDGL WTTITIFITLFLLSVCYSATVTFF KVKWIFSSVVDLKQTIIPDYRNMIGQGA
IgG4_H.sapiens     LQLEESCAEAQDGELDGL WTTITIFITLFLLSVCYSATVTFF KVKWIFSSVVDLKQTIVPDYRNMIRQGA
IgG1_M.musculus    LQLDETCAEAQDGELDGL WTTITIFISLFLLSVCYSAAVTLF KVKWIFSSVVELKQTLVPEYKNMIGQAP
IgG2a_M.musculus   LDLDDVCAEAQDGELDGL WTTITIFISLFLLSVCYSASVTLF KVKWIFSSVVELKQTISPDYRNMIGQGA
IgG2b_M.musculus   LDLDDICAEAKDGELDGL WTTITIFISLFLLSVCYSASVTLF KVKWIFSSVVELKQKISPDYRNMIGQGA
IgG3_M.musculus    LELNETCAEAQDGELDGL WTTITIFISLFLLSVCYSASVTLF KVKWIFSSVVQVKQTAIPDYRNMIGQGA
```

Fig. 2. Alignment of amino acid residues comprising the transmembrane forms of human and mouse Igs. *EMPD* extracellular membrane proximal domain, *TMD* transmembrane domain, *CYT* cytoplasmic tail (45). The divergent residues are *underlined.*

transgenes use human instead of mouse regulatory elements. In addition, the low level of antibody expression can be due to the inefficient signaling of a hybrid BCR composed of human immunoglobulin, mouse Iga, Igβ, and other mouse signaling molecules. The Ig transmembrane region and cytoplasmic tail are crucial for BCR-mediated signaling (20–22). The mouse and human IgM transmembrane region and cytoplasmic tail are more similar than the equivalent mouse and human IgG regions (Fig. 2). Human IgM may, therefore, interact better with mouse Igα and Igβ than human IgG does, which could result in a normal range of human IgM but much lower levels of human IgG in transgenic mice (8, 11, 14). In this context, Rajewsky and colleagues generated mice in which mouse κ and γ1 constant regions were replaced with the corresponding human regions. The whole mouse Cκ region was replaced with the human Cκ region, whereas only the secreted exons of the mouse Cγ1 region were replaced in order to minimize the danger of disturbing membrane expression and signaling of the humanized IgG1 in the mouse. Interestingly, the serum levels of humanized IgG1 in transgenic mice were similar to those of mouse IgG1 in wild-type mice of either naïve or immunized status (23). This result suggests that mouse components of the transmembrane region and cytoplasmic tail or cis-regulatory elements are important to maintain antibody expression levels, particularly for IgG isotypes.

## 5. Learning the Lessons from Previous Studies

The pioneering studies described above have pointed the way to the creation of the second generation of transgenic mice expressing human immunoglobulin diversity. They have revealed the importance of maintaining the myriad of control elements within the Ig

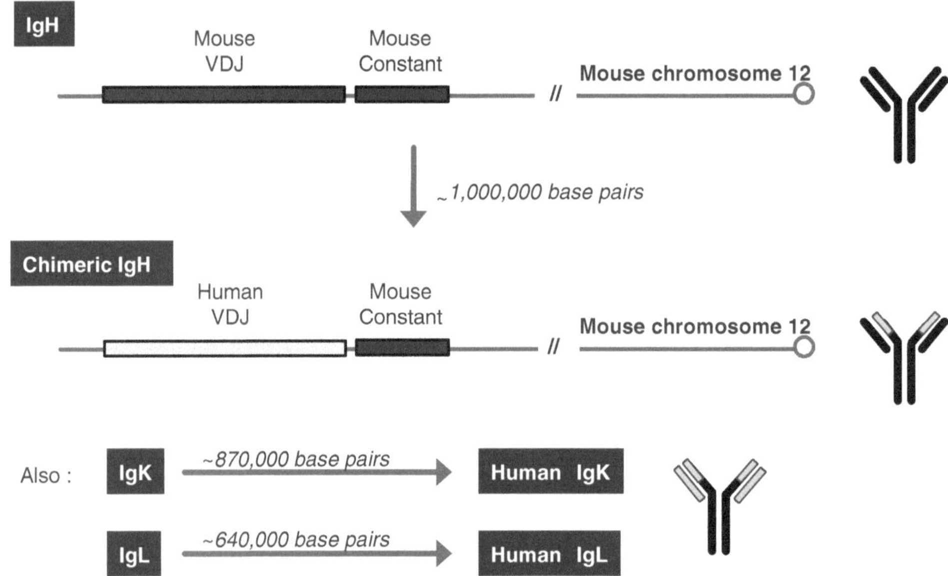


Fig. 3. Generation of a chimeric IgH locus with endogenous transcriptional control cis-elements and signaling machinery. The human variable region ($V_H$, $D_H$, and $J_H$) segments are inserted into the 5′ end of the endogenous mouse constant region to maintain the function of mouse cis-regulatory elements (Eμ and 3′ regulatory elements), and BCR signaling.

loci that regulate the processes of rearrangement, class switching, and somatic hypermutation and also the requirement of efficient signaling via the BCR for the optimal generation of the B cell compartment and the maturation of the B cell immune response. A new generation of transgenic mice has been constructed by precise replacement of mouse variable region genes with human counterparts in the Ig loci including the endogenous transcriptional control cis-elements and signaling machinery (17). These animals encode the mouse transmembrane domains and cytoplasmic tails and contain endogenous mouse iEμ and the 3′ regulatory elements (Fig. 3). The details of this transgenic mice technology have not been published, although it is likely that bacterial artificial chromosome (BAC) recombineering and homologous recombination of modified BACs in ES cells were applied to generate these transgenic mice (17, 24) and see also Chapter 9. Transgenic mice produced using this strategy generate chimeric antibodies with human variable regions and mouse constant regions and apparently possess normal serum levels of all isotype antibodies, and normal mature B cell numbers in blood, spleen, and lymph nodes (http://www.regeneron.com/velocimmune.html). Several antibodies produced from these transgenic lines are now in various stages of clinical development (25). The success of this new generation of transgenic mice in producing therapeutic grade human antibodies underpins the importance of the species-specific elements in the regulation of antibody signaling and expression.

## 6 Phage Display Technology: In Vitro Versus In Vivo

Phage display and other in vitro display technologies provide an alternative platform for generating human antibodies. In vitro technologies can be advantageous over transgenic approaches when applied to auto-antigens or when tailoring both affinities and cross-reactivities (26, 27) and see Chapters 3–5. However, antibodies against antigens that are similar between human and mouse can be generated in mice with a genetic knockout of the antigen-coding gene (28, 29). In addition, a wide range of adjuvants is available to modulate the immune response including breaking immune tolerance in mice (30, 31). These adjuvants, particularly agonists of Toll-like receptors (TLRs), will likely be useful in raising antibodies against auto-antigens.

Phage display technology is also amenable to high-throughput screening which relies critically on the quality of the libraries with sufficiently large effective diversity (26). One of the major drawbacks for phage display is that its diversity is generally limited to the range between $10^6$ and $10^{11}$ unique antibody molecules whether it is derived from naïve or synthetic repertoires (27). The diversity of phage display is constrained by the transformation efficiency practically achievable in *E. coli* (32). At its best, phage display captures only 0.01% of the potential diversity of in vivo antibody structures (i.e., $10^{15}$ B cell somatic diversity). A high affinity antibody usually cannot be directly isolated from such a library. Thus, for the phage display approach, the initially identified antibodies require further optimization or maturation, a manual step which takes time and can be tedious and problematic. While the phage display technology is limited by its overall efficiency, in vivo transgenic technologies can generate fully human antibodies that can be directly moved into clinical development without further optimization (33).

While transgenic technology generates fully human antibodies through in vivo affinity maturation in a normal physiological context, phage display technology usually requires optimization or in vitro affinity maturation. In vivo high affinity antibodies are generated by somatic hypermutation which is dependent on activation-induced cytosine deaminase (AID), an enzyme that induces mutation in DNA by error-prone repair of G:U lesions (34). Somatic hypermutation is not a random process that generates mutations distributed along the variable region (35, 36). Rather, the mutation spectrum of antibodies relies on the intrinsic substrate specificity of AID which exhibits a clear preference for certain major, strategically targeted hot spots within V regions (37–39). In contrast, the in vitro-introduced or synthetic sequences used during the library construction or affinity maturation for phage display may contain mutations not within the natural spectrum of AID, these less natural sequences potentially act as immunogenic human T-cell epitopes. Immunogenicity is an important issue for application of a therapeutic antibody. The development of an anti-therapeutic antibody response in antibody-treated patients can limit efficacy and reduce the safety of antibody treatments. Adalimumab, the first fully human antibody approved in the clinic, was developed from the phage display platform. It binds to TNFα with high affinity and effectively blocks TNFα activity. Clinical studies, however, revealed that up to 89% human anti-human antibody (HAHA) incidence in adalimumab-treated patients (40–42). Although it is not clear what causes the immunogenicity in adalimumab, golimumab, a human anti-TNFα antibody generated from a transgenic platform, did not show detectable neutralizing antibody in treated patients in clinical studies (43, 44). It is important to continuously monitor the immunogenicity of human antibodies derived from different platforms in clinical trials. The outcome may further change the trend of human antibody development.

## 7. Future Perspectives

In early 1990s, both phage display and transgenic mice technologies were developed to generate fully human monoclonal antibodies. By 2011, there were nine human antibodies approved by FDA for clinical uses. Two (adalimumab and belimumab) were generated from phage display platforms and seven (panitumumab, golimumob, canakinumab, ustekinumab, ofatumumab, denosumab, and ipilimumab) from transgenic platforms. The advantage of transgenic technology over phage display is clearly revealed by the numbers of approved therapeutic human antibodies generated from each technology. In particular, human antibodies generated from the transgenic technology have relatively higher phase II to III and Phase III approval transition rates than those from the phage display technology (25).

Although the utility of transgenic mice for human antibody development is already apparent, it is likely that we have only scratched the surface of its full potential. In our view, it is difficult for any in vitro technology to compete against the huge diversity that in vivo somatic mutation and selection provides. New technology development would further help us to explore this powerful in vivo system. Several new in vivo antibody formats including heavy-chain only and bispecifics are currently being explored. Advances in our understanding of what constitutes useful diversity should allow the generation of transgenic mice with increased levels of germ line diversity. With our ever increasing understanding of the basic mechanisms of immune regulation, we may be able to tune up the immune response by improving the cellular signaling and somatic hypermutation machinery, thus optimizing affinity maturation. The availability of these next-generation humanized mice will undoubtedly result in an ever increasing number of fully human therapeutic antibodies developed for diseases of unmet medical need.

## Acknowledgments

We thank Allan Bradley, Andrew Sandham, and Glenn Friedrich for critical comments, and all other colleagues at Kymab for helpful discussion.

### References

1. Ganesh K, Neuberger MS (2011) The relationship between hypothesis and experiment in unveiling the mechanisms of antibody gene diversification. FASEB J 25:1123–1132
2. Neuberger MS (2008) Antibody diversification by somatic mutation: from Burnet onwards. Immunol Cell Biol 86:124–132
3. Cyster JG (2010) Shining a light on germinal center B cells. Cell 143:503–505
4. Alt FW, Blackwell TK, Yancopoulos GD (1985) Immunoglobulin genes in transgenic mice. Trends Genet 1:231–236
5. Storb U, Peters A, Klotz E et al (1998) Immunoglobulin transgenes as targets for somatic hypermutation. Int J Dev Biol 42: 977–982
6. Bruggemann M, Caskey HM, Teale C et al (1989) A repertoire of monoclonal antibodies with human heavy chains from transgenic mice. Proc Natl Acad Sci U S A 86:6709–6713
7. Taylor LD, Carmack CE, Schramm SR et al (1992) A transgenic mouse that expresses a diversity of human sequence heavy and light chain immunoglobulins. Nucleic Acids Res 20: 6287–6295
8. Lonberg N, Taylor LD, Harding FA et al (1994) Antigen-specific human antibodies from mice comprising four distinct genetic modifications. Nature 368:856–859
9. Green LL, Hardy MC, Maynard-Currie CE et al (1994) Antigen-specific human monoclonal antibodies from mice engineered with human Ig heavy and light chain YACs. Nat Genet 7:13–21
10. Fishwild DM, O'Donnell SL, Bengoechea T et al (1996) High-avidity human IgG kappa monoclonal antibodies from a novel strain of minilocus transgenic mice. Nat Biotechnol 14: 845–851
11. Mendez MJ, Green LL, Corvalan JR et al (1997) Functional transplant of megabase human immunoglobulin loci recapitulates human antibody response in mice. Nat Genet 15:146–156
12. Nicholson IC, Zou X, Popov AV et al (1999) Antibody repertoires of four- and five-feature translocus mice carrying human immunoglobulin heavy chain and kappa and lambda light chain yeast artificial chromosomes. J Immunol 163:6898–6906
13. Tomizuka K, Yoshida H, Uejima H et al (1997) Functional expression and germline transmission of a human chromosome fragment in chimaeric mice. Nat Genet 16:133–143
14. Tomizuka K, Shinohara T, Yoshida H et al (2000) Double trans-chromosomic mice: maintenance of two individual human chromosome fragments containing Ig heavy and kappa loci and expression of fully human antibodies. Proc Natl Acad Sci U S A 97:722–727
15. Davis MM (2004) The evolutionary and structural 'logic' of antigen receptor diversity. Semin Immunol 16:239–243
16. Xu JL, Davis MM (2000) Diversity in the CDR3 region of V(H) is sufficient for most antibody specificities. Immunity 13:37–45
17. Scott CT (2007) Mice with a human touch. Nat Biotechnol 25:1075–1077
18. Khamlichi AA, Pinaud E, Decourt C et al (2000) The 3′ IgH regulatory region: a complex structure in a search for a function. Adv Immunol 75:317–345
19. Staudt LM, Lenardo MJ (1991) Immunoglobulin gene transcription. Annu Rev Immunol 9:373–398

20. Shaw AC, Mitchell RN, Weaver YK et al (1990) Mutations of immunoglobulin transmembrane and cytoplasmic domains: effects on intracellular signaling and antigen presentation. Cell 63: 381–392
21. Blum JH, Stevens TL, DeFranco AL (1993) Role of the mu immunoglobulin heavy chain transmembrane and cytoplasmic domains in B cell antigen receptor expression and signal transduction. J Biol Chem 268:27236–27245
22. DeFranco AL, Richards JD, Blum JH et al (1995) Signal transduction by the B-cell antigen receptor. Ann N Y Acad Sci 766:195–201
23. Zou YR, Muller W, Gu H et al (1994) Cre-loxP-mediated gene replacement: a mouse strain producing humanized antibodies. Curr Biol 4:1099–1103
24. Valenzuela DM, Murphy AJ, Frendewey D et al (2003) High-throughput engineering of the mouse genome coupled with high-resolution expression analysis. Nat Biotechnol 21: 652–659
25. Nelson AL, Dhimolea E, Reichert JM (2010) Development trends for human monoclonal antibody therapeutics. Nat Rev Drug Discov 9:767–774
26. Bradbury AR, Sidhu S, Dubel S et al (2011) Beyond natural antibodies: the power of in vitro display technologies. Nat Biotechnol 29: 245–254
27. Ponsel D, Neugebauer J, Ladetzki-Baehs K et al (2011) High affinity, developability and functional size: the holy grail of combinatorial antibody library generation. Molecules 16: 3675–3700
28. Prusiner SB, Groth D, Serban A et al (1993) Ablation of the prion protein (PrP) gene in mice prevents scrapie and facilitates production of anti-PrP antibodies. Proc Natl Acad Sci U S A 90:10608–10612
29. Williamson RA, Peretz D, Smorodinsky N et al (1996) Circumventing tolerance to generate autologous monoclonal antibodies to the prion protein. Proc Natl Acad Sci U S A 93: 7279–7282
30. Coffman RL, Sher A, Seder RA (2010) Vaccine adjuvants: putting innate immunity to work. Immunity 33:492–503
31. Verthelyi D, Wang V (2010) Trace levels of innate immune response modulating impurities (IIRMIs) synergize to break tolerance to therapeutic proteins. PLoS One 5:e15252
32. Roberts RW, Szostak JW (1997) RNA-peptide fusions for the in vitro selection of peptides and proteins. Proc Natl Acad Sci U S A 94: 12297–12302
33. Lonberg N (2008) Human monoclonal antibodies from transgenic mice. Handb Exp Pharmacol 181:69–97
34. Pavri R, Nussenzweig MC (2011) AID targeting in antibody diversity. Adv Immunol 110: 1–26
35. Rada C, Ehrenstein MR, Neuberger MS et al (1998) Hot spot focusing of somatic hypermutation in MSH2-deficient mice suggests two stages of mutational targeting. Immunity 9: 135–141
36. Ehrenstein MR, Neuberger MS (1999) Deficiency in Msh2 affects the efficiency and local sequence specificity of immunoglobulin class-switch recombination: parallels with somatic hypermutation. EMBO J 18: 3484–3490
37. Bransteitter R, Pham P, Scharff MD et al (2003) Activation-induced cytidine deaminase deaminates deoxycytidine on single-stranded DNA but requires the action of RNase. Proc Natl Acad Sci U S A 100:4102–4107
38. Kohli RM, Abrams SR, Gajula KS et al (2009) A portable hot spot recognition loop transfers sequence preferences from APOBEC family members to activation-induced cytidine deaminase. J Biol Chem 284:22898–22904
39. Wang M, Rada C, Neuberger MS (2010) Altering the spectrum of immunoglobulin V gene somatic hypermutation by modifying the active site of AID. J Exp Med 207:141–153
40. Bender NK, Heilig CE, Droll B et al (2007) Immunogenicity, efficacy and adverse events of adalimumab in RA patients. Rheumatol Int 27: 269–274
41. Coenen MJ, Toonen EJ, Scheffer H et al (2007) Pharmacogenetics of anti-TNF treatment in patients with rheumatoid arthritis. Pharmacogenomics 8:761–773
42. Getts DR, Getts MT, McCarthy DP et al (2010) Have we overestimated the benefit of human(ized) antibodies? MAbs 2:682–694
43. Shealy D, Cai A, Staquet K et al (2010) Characterization of golimumab, a human monoclonal antibody specific for human tumor necrosis factor alpha. MAbs 2:428–439
44. Kay J, Rahman MU (2010) Golimumab: a novel human anti-TNF-alpha monoclonal antibody for the treatment of rheumatoid arthritis, ankylosing spondylitis, and psoriatic arthritis. Core Evid 4:159–170
45. Varriale S, Merlino A, Coscia MR et al (2010) An evolutionary conserved motif is responsible for immunoglobulin heavy chain packing in the B cell membrane. Mol Phylogenet Evol 57: 1238–1244

# Chapter 9

# Production of Human or Humanized Antibodies in Mice

Brice Laffleur, Virginie Pascal, Christophe Sirac, and Michel Cogné

## Abstract

Mice are widely available laboratory animals that can easily be used for the production of antibodies against a broad range of antigens, using well-defined immunization protocols. Such an approach allows optimal in vivo affinity maturation of the humoral response. In addition, high-affinity antibodies arising in this context can readily be further characterized and produced as monoclonals after immortalizing and selecting specific antibody-producing cells through hybridoma derivation. Using such conventional strategies combined with mice that are either genetically engineered to carry humanized immunoglobulin (Ig) genes or engrafted with a human immune system, it is thus easy to obtain and immortalize clones that produce either fully human Ig or antibodies associating variable (V) domains with selected antigen specificities to customized human-like constant regions, with defined effector functions. In some instances, where there is a need for in vivo functional assays of a single antibody with a known specificity, it might be of interest to transiently express that gene in mice by in vivo gene transfer. This approach allows a rapid functional assay. More commonly, mice are used to obtain a diversified repertoire of antibody specificities after immunization by producing antibody molecules in the mouse B cell lineage from mouse strains with transgene Ig genes which are of human, humanized, or chimeric origin. After in vivo maturation of the immune response, this will lead to the secretion of antibodies with optimized antigen binding sites, associated to the desired human constant domains. This chapter focuses on two simple methods: (1) to obtain such humanized Ig mice and (2) to transiently express a human Ig gene in mice using hydrodynamics-based transfection.

**Key words:** B cells, ES cells, Genetic engineered mice, Homologous recombination, Humanized mice, Humanized antibodies, Hydrodynamics-based transfection, Immunoglobulin

## 1. Introduction

A major goal in the production of human and humanized antibodies is the initial identification of antibody molecules which combine high antigen specificity with defined effector functions. Well-defined methods now exist which allow production of recombinant modified animal antibodies which preserve the antigen binding sites while replacing the remainder of the molecule with human-like

Gabriele Proetzel and Hilmar Ebersbach (eds.), *Antibody Methods and Protocols*, Methods in Molecular Biology, vol. 901, DOI 10.1007/978-1-61779-931-0_9, © Springer Science+Business Media, LLC 2012

parts. However, such a "humanized antibody engineering" still carries the risk of affecting antigen recognition and/or retaining some level of immunogenicity. Further, it also obviously delays functional assays until the humanization of the molecule is achieved. This is also complicated by the fact that mouse antibodies have complex and rather unpredictable interactions with various activatory or inhibitory Fc receptors expressed on human effector cells. In short, mouse immunoglobulin (Ig) poorly mirrors the binding of human antibodies and this often makes it difficult to predict what will precisely be the efficacy of an antibody prior to its humanization. By contrast, mice in which the Ig constant genes have been modified provide an easy way for obtaining molecules with effector functions similar to human antibodies. This strategy also makes it possible to check early in the process that an antibody with the expected specificity also carries the expected efficacy in functional assays.

Antigen-specific monoclonal antibodies (mAbs) can be readily obtained after immortalization of rodent B cell clones as hybridomas (1). Since these techniques are easily mastered, the use of humanized mice thus constitutes a simple avenue for producing polyclonal as well as monoclonal humanized antibodies. However, a prerequisite to the humanization of antibodies in mouse is the removal of the endogenous mouse immunoglobulin sequences. Disruption of the IgH and Igκ loci is generally sufficient since Igλ represents only 5% of the total Ig light chains in mouse. Humanized mice have notably been generated by bringing human IgH and IgL large transgenes (HuMAb-Mouse®), YACs (XenoMouse®), or mini-chromosomes transfer (Transchromo mice), and have been successfully used for generating high-affinity antibodies against various targets (Fig. 1) (2–12). However, all these humanized mice are patented and are not readily available to academic laboratories. Further, such models remain hard to reproduce by conventional methodologies.

Several strains of mice have also been reported, which can allow direct production of chimeric antibodies with human constant regions. Zou et al. (9) first replaced the exons encoding the γ1 chain of murine IgG1 with the human γ1 gene, yielding mice with a normal endogenous VDJ repertoire, but with humanized IgG1 humoral responses after class switching, i.e., in a limited proportion of cells (Fig. 2). By contrast, insertion of the human gene at the most 5′ position of the mouse constant Ig gene cluster, either replacing or preceding the Cμ exons, allows it to be the first C gene expressed in naïve B cells. In this regard, an interesting strategy has been developed to make the insertion as a replacement of the switch μ (Sμ) target sequences that supports class switch recombination (CSR). The repetitive Sμ is a transcriptionally active region located immediately downstream of the heavy chain V–D–J variable region and upstream of the constant region Cμ. It is absolutely required for CSR so that Sμ replacement can block CSR to

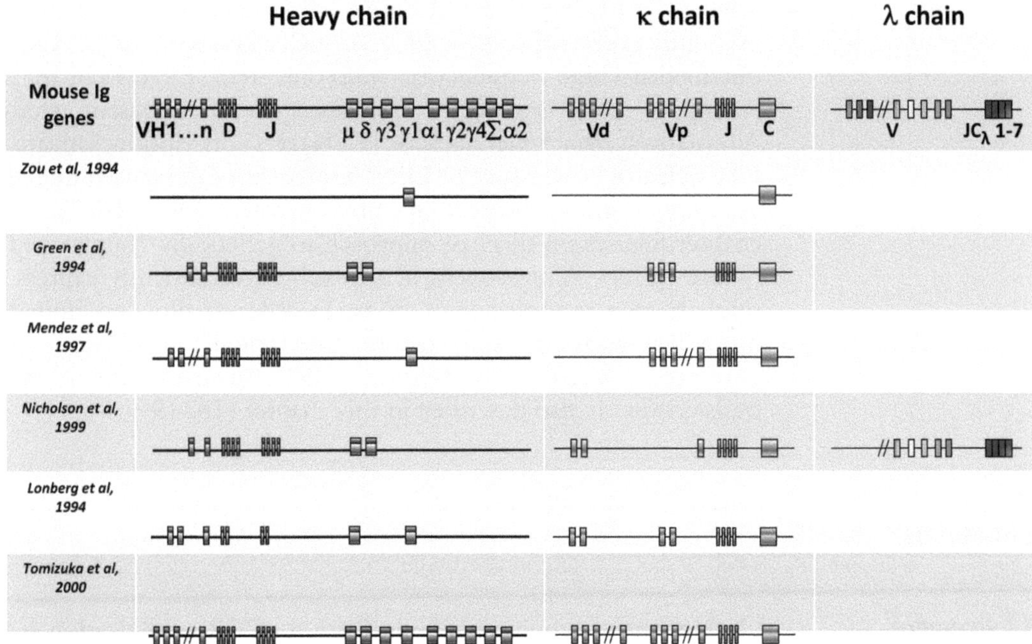


Fig. 1. The immunoglobulin (Ig) germline conformation for mouse at the *top* with the heavy- (μ, δ, γ, α, ε) and light-chain genes (κ and λ). Several strategies for humanization with randomly integrated human transgenes in the mouse genome are shown *below*.

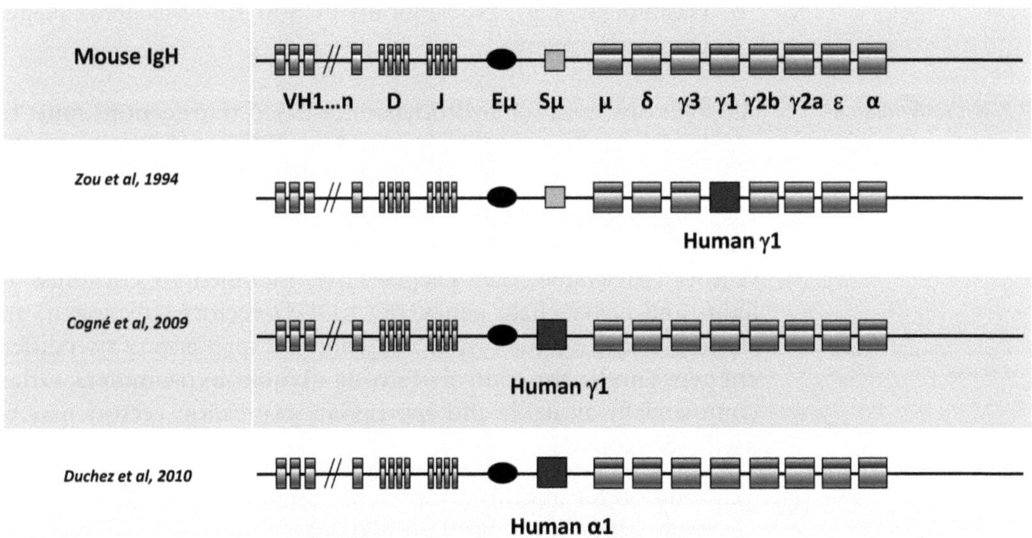


Fig. 2. The mouse IgH locus in germline conformation (*top*) with the μ, δ, γ, α, and ε genes, the intronic enhancer (Eμ), and the switch mu region (Sμ). Several strategies for humanization targeting the IgH locus are shown *below*.

downstream IgH genes and allows only the knock-in gene to be efficiently expressed (Fig. 2) (9, 13). Such a knock-in can be readily obtained at a high frequency in embryonic stem (ES) cells by transfecting a targeting vector described in the present study. Alternatively, zinc finger nuclease (ZFN) or Transcription Activator-Like Effector Nucleases (TALEN) approaches can be used directly in zygotes without the need of embryonic stem cells (14–17). This chapter focuses on this easy approach to genetically "humanized" mouse Ig loci. Alternatively, it is possible to transiently express a single human Ig molecule in mouse in order to allow preliminary functional assays in vivo before any tedious production and purification steps. This method called "hydrodynamics-based transfection" is also described in this chapter (18, 19).

## 2 Materials

### *2.1 Generation of a Targeting Vector for Homologous Recombination*

1. Human and mouse genomic DNA for PCR amplification (see Note 1).
2. Long-range high-fidelity taq polymerase (see Note 2) for amplification of genomic fragments from the mouse or human Ig loci.
3. Plasmid pBluescript II (SK+) (Agilent Technologies, Inc., Santa Clara, CA).
4. Bacterial strain *E. coli* TG1 (Agilent Technologies).
5. Plasmid kit, e.g., Nucleobond PC500 EF (Macherey-Nagel, Düren, Germany).

### *2.2. Hydrodynamics-Based Transfection*

All solutions used for hydrodynamics-based transfections must be sterile. Concentrated DNA is stored at −20°C and dilution buffer at room temperature. As the liver is the primary target for gene transfer, plasmids used for expression of the Ig genes contain preferentially liver-specific or ubiquitous promoters. We use pCpG-free vectors (Invivogen, San Diego, CA), modified to coexpress Ig light- and heavy-chain genes, but pDUO vectors (Invivogen) are especially adapted for easy cloning and coexpression of two different genes under the control of strong ubiquitous promoters. Other commercially available and appropriate expression vectors may be used (see Note 3).

1. Solution for injection: Use sterile Ringer's solution or, alternatively, saline solution: 0.9% NaCl.
2. 50-mL sterile plastic tubes to mix concentrated DNA in Ringer's solution.
3. Mice, over 8 weeks old, with a weight of at least 20 g.

4. 2-mL latex-free sterile syringe and 27-G needle. For bigger mice, provide extra 1 mL/10 g of weight and use 24-G needle.
5. Water bath.
6. Mouse restrainer box (see Note 4).
7. Bracket to maintain restrainer box.
8. pDUO plasmid (see Note 3).

## 3. Methods

### *3.1. Homologous Recombination to Modify Mouse Ig Genes*

Insertion of non-murine constant sequences within transcription units that link their coding sequences with endogenous Ig variable regions of the mouse genome can potentially be done at various positions within the IgH locus. Whatever the site of the insertion, production of secreted antibodies will only be possible after there is expression of the chimeric immunoglobulin at the B lymphocyte stage. For this reason, any inserted constant transgene will need to include the coding sequences for both the secreted form and the membrane-bound form of the molecule. Further, the intronic and 3′ flanking sequences are required, which are able to support the alternate splicing that normally drives maturation of either the membrane-form Ig mRNA at the B lymphocyte stage or the secreted-form mRNA at the plasma cell stage.

First, a targeting vector for the replacement of mouse Sμ by human constant Ig genes needs to be constructed (Fig. 3) (13), which is then transfected into ES cells. ES cells are screened for the targeted event and positive ES cell clones are used to generate mice by injecting them into mouse blastocysts to produce chimeras. Chimeric animals are then mated and their progeny checked by Southern blot and/or PCR with primers specific for the targeted and original murine IgH locus. A more functional based assay is to check by ELISA for expression of the transgenic Ig molecule in the serum.

1. For the 3′ arm of the targeting vector, amplify the mouse Cμ fragment (about 5 kb of sequence initiating downstream of Sμ, just before the Cμ exons), corresponding to positions 140,101–145,032 of murine chromosome 12(Genbank/EMBL AC073553, clone RP23-270B12). This is best achieved by long-range PCR with the aid of appropriate specific primers which also contain XhoI adapters. Post-XhoI digestion of the PCR fragment, insert the resulting fragment at the XhoI site of the pSK vector.
2. For the 5′ arm of the targeting vector, amplify the mouse DQ 52/JH fragment (about 5 kb of genomic fragment

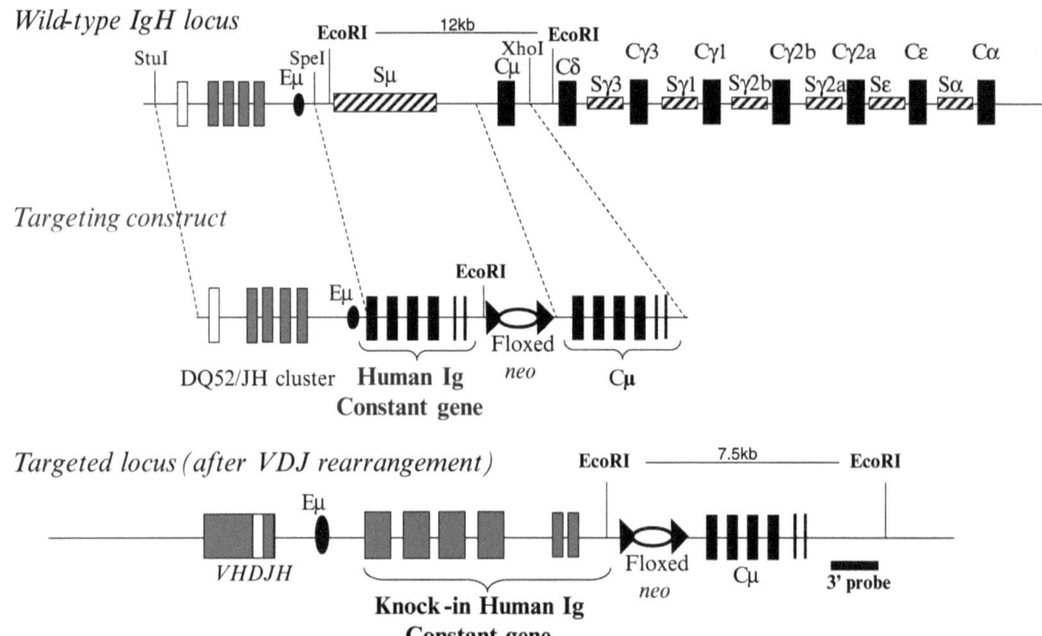


Fig. 3. A knock-in vector for humanized Ig production in mice. The targeting vector contains about 5-kb-long 5′ arm including the genomic JH region and located upstream of mouse S, a knock-in cassette including the human Ig constant gene to be expressed with all necessary splicing sites, a resistance (neoR) cassette ensuring resistance of transfected cells to the neomycin analog G418, and about 5-kb-long 3′ arm initiating downstream of Sμ. The EcoRI sites are used for the Southern blot and the lengths of the resulting fragments are indicated. The 3′ probe used for detection of the targeted event is represented as a *black box*. The locus and genes are not to scale.

located upstream of mouse Sμ of the IgH locus, encompassing DQ52, the JH cluster, and Eμ) corresponding to positions 131,281–136,441 of murine chromosome 12 (Genbank/EMBL AC073553, clone RP23-270B12) by PCR with the aid of appropriate specific primers containing EcoRV and ClaI adaptors (for forward and reverse primers, respectively). After EcoRV and ClaI digestion of the PCR fragment, insert the fragment between the EcoRV and ClaI sites of the pSK vector.

3. Insert the $neo^R$ cassette described in Pinaud (20) at the SalI site. Ensure that $neo^R$ gene is in the same orientation as the transcribed IgH locus, as the opposite orientation could influence human Ig gene expression (see Note 5).
4. Amplify the human Ig constant gene fragment, including all the exon and intron sequences necessary for complete Ig constant region expression and regulation (above-mentioned regulatory sites for expression of both membrane and secretory forms of Ig). Use appropriate specific primers containing ClaI adaptors and insert the resulting fragment at the ClaI site of the previous plasmid between the JH fragment (5′ arm) and the $neo^R$ cassette to get the final targeting vector. An example of primers used for amplification of the human γ1 gene is

**Table 1**
**Example of specific primers to amplify the human Cγ1 gene**

| | |
|---|---|
| Gam1CH1-5′F | 5′-CAA TCG ATG CCC GTG AGC CCA GAC-3′ |
| gam1 mbexon-3′R | 5′-AAA TCG ATG CTC CCA TCA CGA AGT ACA A-3′ |

presented in Table 1 (see Note 6). In addition, a negative selection marker can be included (see Note 7).

5. The final targeting vector is consequently grown using an endotoxin-free maxipreparation plasmid kit.
6. Verify the targeting vector by automated sequencing.
7. Linearize the vector for ES cells transfection using, for example, NotI enzyme. Store the DNA at –20°C until ready to use.

   Beyond targeted integration, further deletion of the neomycin resistance (neo$^R$) gene can be obtained either in ES cell clones or in mice, provided the resistance cassette was previously flanked with loxP sites, using a Cre recombinase (9). However, in the specific case of a gene insertion made as a replacement of Sμ into the IgH locus, it has been shown that the presence of a neo$^R$ gene downstream of the inserted Ig gene and in the same orientation does not compromise its expression so that deletion of the resistance marker can be omitted (13).
8. Electroporate ES cells with targeting vector.
9. Select ES cell clones with G418 for neomycin resistance.
10. Screen for the homologous recombination events by Southern blot and/or PCR. For Southern blots for example, the expected homologous recombination upstream of the mouse Cμ gene can be readily followed with EcoRI digests of the ES cell DNA which is then probed with a 3′ probe located downstream of the region homologous to Cμ used as the 3′ arm of the targeting vector (the 0.9 kb genomic XhoI–XbaI fragment located upstream of Cδ will serve as an adequate probe) (Fig. 3). This probe can be made by PCR amplification using primers corresponding to positions 145,032–145,945 of the murine chromosome 12 sequence (EMBL/Genbank AC073553). The presence of a recombinant allele is visualized with a fragment of about 7.5 kb (representing the murine μ fragment and the neo$^R$ cassette), whereas the wild-type allele corresponds to a fragment of 12 kb.
11. After this screening step, appropriately targeted ES cell clones can be microinjected in blastocysts to generate chimeras (21). Chimeric animals are mated with appropriate females and their progeny checked by the above-mentioned Southern blot and/or

PCR with primers specific for the mutated and non-mutated murine IgH locus. Alternatively, use ELISA for detection of the transgenic Ig molecule expression in the serum.

12. Using PCR, it is possible to check the presence of the non-mutated (wild-type) allele with the following primers: upstream SpeI Sμ primer (5′-GAG TAC CGT TGT CTG GGT CAC-3′) and SacI-3′ Imu primer (5′-GAG CTC TAT GAT TAT TGG TTA AC-3′). This PCR amplifies a 91 bp fragment delimiting the SpeI site specific for the non-mutated murine IgH locus. To check the presence of the mutated (human Ig gene insertion) allele, use the following primers: Neo1 primer (5′-GCA TGA TCT GGA CGA AGA GCA T-3′) and Neo2 primer (5′-TCC CCT CAG AAG AAC TCG TCA A-3′). This PCR amplifies a 120 bp fragment specific for the recombinant IgH locus carrying the human Ig genes and the $neo^R$. Both PCRs can be carried out using stranded conditions and an annealing temperature of 55°C for 30 cycles.

13. ELISA specific for the inserted gene product can be carried out on sera obtained by retro-orbital bleeding of the mice using a previously described method (13). ELISA can be used to discriminate either wild-type (negative ELISA) or targeted mice (positive ELISA). The ELISA can also be used to discriminate targeted heterozygous and homozygous mice as the former only reach few μg/ml of human Ig, compared to the hundreds of μg/ml obtained in the latter homozygous animals (13).

### 3.2. Hydrodynamics-Based Transfection

When seeking expression of a single Ig molecule in mice (for example to perform functional assays in vivo), an alternative method to transgenesis which also yields large amounts of recombinant proteins in mice (or rats) is the "hydrodynamics-based transfection" (18, 19). This method uses hydrostatic pressure induced by the rapid intravenous injection of a large volume of DNA in solution in order to mediate gene transfer into the cells of various organs. This is achieved by injecting DNA, at a ratio of 0.08–0.12 mL/g of body weight, very rapidly, e.g. in about 5 s for the complete injection. This process exceeds the cardiac output and results in the accumulation of injected DNA solution in the inferior vena cava. The higher pressure created within this venous section results in a reflux of the DNA solution into the liver and kidneys, making the liver the primary target for DNA entry into the cells and gene transfer. Transgene expression will reach a maximum level approximately 4–12 h post-injection and declines thereafter for over 1 month depending on the half-life of the encoded protein (22). After this time, a much lower but stable level of expression can persist for more than 6 months. Transfection efficiency depends upon DNA concentration and has to be optimized for each transgene. For proteins such as IgG, protein levels can reach grams per liter in serum at 24 h post-injection and can be maintained for several weeks above 100 μg/mL. This method thus provides an attractive tool for rapidly checking transgene expression in vivo, thus getting animals with long-term endogenous infusion of antibody for functional assays without any tedious protein production and purification.

1. cDNA coding for Ig heavy and light chains is cloned into a pDUO vector using standard molecular biology protocols.
2. Maxi preparations of plasmids are carried out with an endotoxin-free kit according to the manufacturer's protocol and the DNA resuspended in sterile ultrapure water at a final concentration of 1 μg/μL and frozen at −20°C until use.
3. Circular plasmid DNA concentrate is extemporaneously diluted in sterile Ringer's solution to a final concentration of 25 μg/mL, vortexed, and warmed at 37°C before injection. Use 50-mL plastic tubes for dilution. It is necessary to provide at least twice the required volume for the injections to anticipate losses during manipulation.
4. Warm the water bath to 45°C.
5. Prepare a syringe with its needle with appropriate volume of plasmid solution (1 mL/10 mg of weight). Carefully remove all bubbles in the syringe.
6. Introduce the mouse into the restrainer. If the restrainer is too big, add paper to the bottom but make sure that the mouse breathes normally. The animal must not move during the injection.
7. Warm animal tail into the water bath during at least 30 s in order to dilate the veins and immediately set restrainer on the bracket.
8. Locate one of the two lateral veins of the tail and align the needle exactly in line (bevel side up). Start at the tip of the tail and move closer to the body. This will allow injecting the animal more than once if necessary.
9. Inject the contents of the syringe at a constant but high speed. This should be done in 5 s for the complete injection. A shorter injection time may result in the breakage of the tail vein. A longer injection time may result in the absence of the required reflux of DNA-containing solution in the liver.
10. Carefully remove the mouse from the restrainer box and place it in a new cage. You should normally observe an immobilization of the mouse during a few minutes if the injection was successful. If the mouse does not stop moving this suggests that the injection was not successful.
11. 24 h after injection, collect a sample of blood using retro-orbital bleeding and proceed to ELISA or other protein quantification assay to check for the expression of the transgene.

## 4. Notes

1. The mouse genomic DNA should be obtained from the same mouse strain as the ES cells to be used to ensure a high frequency of the homologous recombination.
2. Examples of long-range polymerases: Takara LAtaq (Takara Bio, Shiga, Japan), Herculase II fusion DNA polymerase (Agilent Technologies), Phusion high-fidelity DNA polymerase (New England Biolabs, Ipswich, MA).
3. Examples of commercially available expression vectors: pLIVE (Mirus Bio Corporation, Madison, WI), pVIVO and pDUO (Invivogen, San Diego, CA) or, alternatively, pCMV-SPORT6 (Invitrogen, San Diego, CA), and pCI mammalian expression vector (Promega, Madison, WI).
4. Examples of restrainer box suppliers: Charles River (Wilmington, MA), Braintree Scientific, Inc. (Braintree, MA), Bel-Art products (Pequannock, NJ), Ellard Instrumentation Ltd. (Monroe, WA).
5. The $neo^R$ cassette can be purchased from GeneBridges GmbH (Heidelberg, Germany). The $neo^R$ cassette ensures resistance of transfected cells to G418, also known as Geneticin, which is used at 400 μg/mL for ES cells. Alternatively to neomycin, genes conferring resistance to hygromycin, puromycin, or zeocin can be used (23–25).
6. The primers to amplify the human Cγ1 gene in Table 1 amplify a genomic fragment of 6,860 bp. The ClaI adapters are underlined. A 200 bp intronic fragment is recommended before the first exon comprising the intronic polypyrimidine tract, the branch point, and an upstream acceptor site that will be joined with the JH donor site.
7. To enrich transfected clones with a targeted (rather than random) integration of the vector at the IgH locus, the thymidine kinase (tk) negative selection marker can be inserted in the vector at a position located outside of the homology arms. Random integration tends to preserve the tk gene and will result in cell death in the presence of ganciclovir (2 μM). Alternatively, the DT-A cassette encoding the diphtheria toxin A-chain can be used to counter-select random integration without the need for any drug added in the culture medium (26, 27).

## References


1. Kohler G, Milstein C (1975) Continuous cultures of fused cells secreting antibody of predefined specificity. Nature 256:495–497
2. Green LL, Hardy MC, Maynard-Currie CE et al (1994) Antigen-specific human monoclonal antibodies from mice engineered with human Ig heavy and light chain YACs. Nat Genet 7:13–21
3. Green LL, Jakobovits A (1998) Regulation of B cell development by variable gene complexity in

mice reconstituted with human immunoglobulin yeast artificial chromosomes. J Exp Med 188: 483–495

4. Kuroiwa Y, Tomizuka K, Shinohara T et al (2000) Manipulation of human minichromosomes to carry greater than megabase-sized chromosome inserts. Nat Biotechnol 18: 1086–1090
5. Le Provost F, Lillico S, Passet B et al (2010) Zinc finger nuclease technology heralds a new era in mammalian transgenesis. Trends Biotechnol 28:134–141
6. Mendez MJ, Green LL, Corvalan JR et al (1997) Functional transplant of megabase human immunoglobulin loci recapitulates human antibody response in mice. Nat Genet 15:146–156
7. Popov AV, Zou X, Xian J et al (1999) A human immunoglobulin lambda locus is similarly well expressed in mice and humans. J Exp Med 189: 1611–1620
8. Tomizuka K, Shinohara T, Yoshida H et al (2000) Double trans-chromosomic mice: maintenance of two individual human chromosome fragments containing Ig heavy and kappa loci and expression of fully human antibodies. Proc Natl Acad Sci U S A 97:722–727
9. Zou YR, Muller W, Gu H et al (1994) Cre-loxP-mediated gene replacement: a mouse strain producing humanized antibodies. Curr Biol 4:1099–1103
10. Ishida I, Tomizuka K, Yoshida H et al (2002) Production of human monoclonal and polyclonal antibodies in TransChromo animals. Cloning Stem Cells 4:91–102
11. Lonberg N, Taylor LD, Harding FA et al (1994) Antigen-specific human antibodies from mice comprising four distinct genetic modifications. Nature 368:856–859
12. Jakobovits A, Amado RG, Yang X et al (2007) From XenoMouse technology to panitumumab, the first fully human antibody product from transgenic mice. Nat Biotechnol 25:1134–1143
13. Duchez S, Amin R, Cogne N et al (2010) Premature replacement of mu with alpha immunoglobulin chains impairs lymphopoiesis and mucosal homing but promotes plasma cell maturation. Proc Natl Acad Sci U S A 107:3064–3069
14. Kiefer JC (2011) Primer and interviews: advances in targeted gene modification. Dev Dyn 240:2688–2696
15. Menoret S, Iscache AL, Tesson L et al (2010) Characterization of immunoglobulin heavy chain knockout rats. Eur J Immunol 40: 2932–2941
16. Flisikowska T, Thorey IS, Offner S et al (2011) Efficient immunoglobulin gene disruption and targeted replacement in rabbit using zinc finger nucleases. PLoS One 6:e21045
17. Li H, Haurigot V, Doyon Y et al (2011) In vivo genome editing restores haemostasis in a mouse model of haemophilia. Nature 475:217–221
18. Liu F, Song Y, Liu D (1999) Hydrodynamics-based transfection in animals by systemic administration of plasmid DNA. Gene Ther 6:1258–1266
19. Song YK, Liu F, Zhang G et al (2002) Hydrodynamics-based transfection: simple and efficient method for introducing and expressing transgenes in animals by intravenous injection of DNA. Methods Enzymol 346:92–105
20. Pinaud E, Khamlichi AA, Le Morvan C et al (2001) Localization of the 3′ IgH locus elements that effect long-distance regulation of class switch recombination. Immunity 15:187–199
21. Nagy A, Gertsenstein M, Vintersten K et al (2004) In: Cuddihy J (ed) Manipulating the mouse embryo, 3rd edn. Cold Spring Harbor Laboratory Press, Cold Spring Harbor, New York
22. Zuckier LS, Chang CJ, Scharff MD et al (1998) Chimeric human-mouse IgG antibodies with shuffled constant region exons demonstrate that multiple domains contribute to in vivo half-life. Cancer Res 58:3905–3908
23. Wilber A, Linehan JL, Tian X et al (2007) Efficient and stable transgene expression in human embryonic stem cells using transposon-mediated gene transfer. Stem Cells 25:2919–2927
24. Mortensen RM, Zubiaur M, Neer EJ et al (1991) Embryonic stem cells lacking a functional inhibitory G-protein subunit (alpha i2) produced by gene targeting of both alleles. Proc Natl Acad Sci U S A 88:7036–7040
25. Taniguchi M, Sanbo M, Watanabe S et al (1998) Efficient production of Cre-mediated site-directed recombinants through the utilization of the puromycin resistance gene, pac: a transient gene-integration marker for ES cells. Nucleic Acids Res 26:679–680
26. McCarrick JW 3rd, Parnes JR, Seong RH et al (1993) Positive-negative selection gene targeting with the diphtheria toxin A-chain gene in mouse embryonic stem cells. Transgenic Res 2:183–190
27. Yagi T, Nada S, Watanabe N et al (1993) A novel negative selection for homologous recombinants using diphtheria toxin A fragment gene. Anal Biochem 214:77–86

# Chapter 10

# Immortalization of Human B Cells: Analysis of B Cell Repertoire and Production of Human Monoclonal Antibodies

Elisabetta Traggiai

## Abstract

One of the major challenges in human B cell immunology field has been the objective to establish stable monoclonal cells lines that express the B cell receptor (BCR) on their cell surface and secrete antibodies. Such a system is extremely attractive not only for studying various aspect of BCR signaling but also for the generation of human monoclonal antibody and the analysis of the human B cell repertoire. This chapter describes an efficient method to immortalize and clone human B cells by Epstein–Barr Virus (EBV) transformation.

**Key words:** B cells, Cloning, Epstein–Barr Virus, Human B cell subsets, Human monoclonal antibodies, Immortalization, Polyclonal stimulation

## 1. Introduction

In recent years, it has become evident that there is a great need to develop in vitro methods allowing to analyze human B cell responses in order to understand their regulation in normal as well as pathological situation such as autoimmune disorders, immunodeficiency, and infection diseases (1). One of the main limitations is that mature B cells, naïve as well as memory, cannot be maintained efficiently in vitro. When B cells are cultured in vitro in the presence of CD40 ligand (CD40L), cytokines, BCR triggering and Toll-like receptor (TLR) agonists they do respond. However, as soon as the B cells respond they differentiate into terminal plasma cells (2). This process is accompanied by cell cycle arrest precluding the generation of long-term B cell lines. Recently, transduction of peripheral memory B cells with the transcriptional factors involved in the control of B cell proliferation and differentiation, B cell lymphoma-extra large (BCL-xl) and BCL-6, respectively, has allowed

Gabriele Proetzel and Hilmar Ebersbach (eds.), *Antibody Methods and Protocols*, Methods in Molecular Biology, vol. 901, DOI 10.1007/978-1-61779-931-0_10, © Springer Science+Business Media, LLC 2012

to immortalize and generate stable cell lines expressing BCR and are able to synthesize and secrete immunoglobulins (3).

Several approaches have been developed to dissect and investigate the molecular regulation of the human B cell repertoire. One successful method has been to combine immunoglobulin (Ig) gene repertoire analysis and Ig reactivity at the single cell level (4). This strategy has been successfully applied for autoimmunity and immunodeficiency questions, and for the first time in human for central and peripheral B cell tolerance (5).

Among the oldest techniques to generate stable human B cell lines is the immortalization with EBV (6). In the past, one of the major limitations was the very low efficiency of B cell infection and subsequent cloning (7). Thus, alternative methods to produce human monoclonal antibodies have been developed, such as immunization of transgenic mice expressing human Ig loci, phage display library, and humanization of mouse antibodies via genetic engineering (8–10).

We recently described an improved method to infect and immortalize human B cells with EBV, in the presence of the TLR9 agonist, CpG 2006, during viral transformation and cloning (11). We have used this method to isolate neutralizing as well as non-neutralizing antibodies against severe acute respiratory syndrome coronavirus (SARS-CoV) (11). These antibodies have been generated from one individual, who recovered from SARS infection. The obtained antibodies display a high in vitro potency to neutralize viral replication. This approach is not only applicable to the area of infectious diseases but also other clinical conditions, such as autoimmune diseases and cancer, and allows exploiting the breadth and the avidity of the human B cell repertoire (12, 13). The method consists of four sequential steps: (a) human B cell subset isolation, (b) EBV infection, (c) B cell cloning, and (d) screening (Fig. 1).

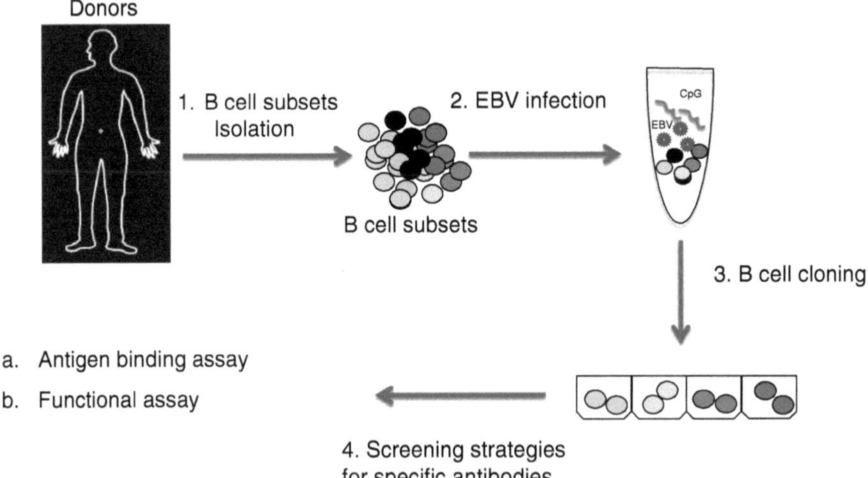


Fig. 1. Screening strategy for isolating antibodies from human B cells. Scheme of the different steps required for human B cell immortalization.

## 2. Materials

***2.1. Isolation of Human B Cells Subsets from PBMC***

1. Human peripheral blood mononuclear cells (PBMCs) or peripheral blood or cryopreserved mononuclear cells.
2. Phosphate-buffered saline (PBS) containing 2% fetal calf serum (FCS).
3. Ficoll-Hypaque density gradient.
4. CD22 or CD20 MicroBeads (Miltenyi Biotec, Bergisch Gladbach, Germany).
5. MACS buffer: PBS, 0.5% bovine serum albumin (BSA), 2 mM EDTA, prepare fresh and keep on ice.
6. SuperMACS separator (Miltenyi Biotec).
7. Complete culture medium: RPMI 1640 (Gibco, Life Technologies, Carlsbad, CA, USA), sodium pyruvate (1 mM, Gibco), penicillin (100 U/mL, Gibco), streptomycin (100 μg/mL, Gibco), kanamycin (100 μg/mL, Gibco), L-glutamine (2 mM, Gibco), nonessential amino acids (10 μM, Gibco), 2-beta-mercaptoethanol ($5 \times 10^{-2}$ μM), 10% FCS (Hyclone, ThermoScientific, Waltham, MA, USA).
8. LS column and LS column adaptor (Miltenyi Biotec.).
9. 5, 15, and 50 mL propylene conical tubes (Falcon, BD Biosciences, Franklin Lakes, NJ, USA).
10. Monoclonal antibodies for surface antigens to sort B cell subsets.
11. Refrigerated centrifuge.
12. Cell strainer, 40 μm (Falcon cat. no. 352340, BD Biosciences).
13. BD FACSAria Cell Sorter (BD Biosciences).

***2.2. B95.8 Cell Expansion Epstein–Barr Virus B Cell Infection***

1. EBV Virus, produced from B95.8 cell line (Sigma Aldrich, St. Louis, MO, USA).
2. Complete culture medium: RPMI 1640, sodium pyruvate (1 mM), penicillin (100 U/mL), streptomycin (100 μg/mL), kanamycin (100 μg/mL), L-glutamine (2 mM), nonessential amino acids (10 μM), 2-beta-mercaptoethanol ($5 \times 10^{-2}$ μM), 10% FCS.
3. 70% Ethanol.
4. 5, 15, and 50 mL propylene conical tubes (Falcon, BD Biosciences).
5. 6-Well tissue culture plates.

#### 2.3. Epstein–Barr Virus B Cell Infection

1. Complete culture medium (see Subheading 2.1).
2. Sorted B cells (see Subheading 2.1).
3. CpG 2006, TLR9 agonist (CpG 2006, 5′ TCg TCg TTT TgT CgT TTT gTC gTT 3′ (phosphotio bonds)) (Invivogen, San Diego, CA, USA).
4. EBV virus (see Subheading 2.2).

#### 2.4. EBV-B Cell Cloning Protocols

1. Cell irradiator.
2. Ficoll-Hypaque density gradient.
3. Complete culture medium (see Subheading 2.1).
4. CpG 2006, TLR9 agonist (CpG 2006, 5′ TCg TCg TTT TgT CgT TTT gTC gTT 3′ (phosphotio bonds)).
5. Irradiated allogeneic PBMCs isolated from peripheral blood from normal donors.
6. EBV virus (see Subheading 2.2).
7. 384-Well plates (Corning-Costar, Corning Incorporated Life Sciences, Lowell, MA, USA).
8. Multichannel for 384 plates.
9. 5, 15, and 50 mL propylene conical tubes (Falcon).
10. Freezing media: 90% FCS, 10% DMSO.
11. Cryovials.

#### 2.5. ELISA Screening

1. ELISA plates, medium binding (Greiner Bio-One, Frickenhausen, Germany).
2. Coating buffer: $Na_2HPO_4$ 0.1 M pH 9.6 or PBS.
3. Blocking solution: PBS 10% FCS.
4. Tween 20.
5. Developing buffer: 1.59 g $Na_2CO_3$, 2.93 g $NaHCO_3$, and 0.2 g $NaN_3$ in 1 L, pH 9.6.
6. ELISA substrate 104, conc. 1 mg/mL in developing buffer (cat. no. N2765, Sigma-Aldrich).
7. Goat anti-human IgG alkaline phosphatase (cat. no. 2040-04, Southern Biotech, Birmingham, AL, USA).

## 3. Methods

#### 3.1. Isolation of Human B Cells Subsets from PBMC

The human peripheral B cell pool is composed of cells at different stage of development, characterized by different signal requirements to differentiate into immunoglobulin secreting cells and carrying different Ig isotypes on the cell surface: (a) immature transitional

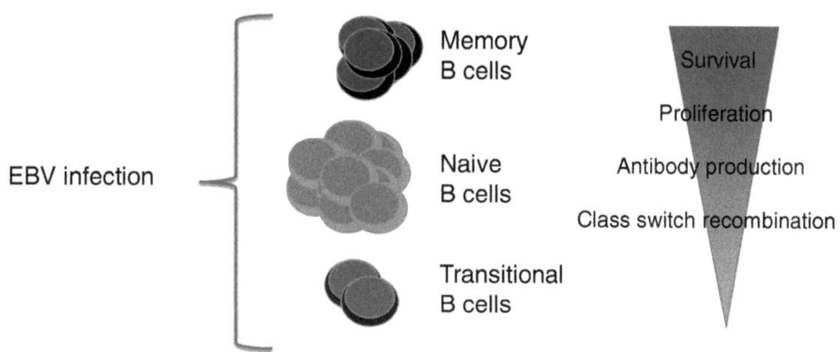


Fig. 2. Representation of the human peripheral B cell pool, which can be transformed by EBV. As soon as B Cell mature from the transtional stage to the haire and then the memory stage some of the functional properties as survival, proliferation, antibody production and class switch recombination increase.

**Table 1**
**Summarization of antibody combinations**

| B cell subtype | Antibodies | Gating strategy |
|---|---|---|
| Transitional immature B cells | CD3, CD14, CD16 in PE-Cy5; CD20 in PE-Cy7; CD24 in PE; CD38 in FITC; IgG, IgA in APC | IgG/A$^-$, CD3/14/16$^-$, CD20$^+$, CD24$^{high}$, CD38$^{high}$ |
| Naïve B cells | CD3, CD14, CD16 in PE-Cy5; CD20 in PE-Cy7; CD27 in FITC; IgG/A in APC | IgG/A$^-$, CD3/14/16$^-$, CD20$^+$, CD27$^-$ |
| IgM memory B cells | CD3, CD14, CD16 in PE-Cy5; CD20 in PE-Cy7; CD27 in FITC; IgG/A in APC | IgG/A$^-$, CD3/14/16$^-$, CD20$^+$, CD27$^+$ |
| IgG switch memory B cells | CD3, CD14, CD16 in PE-Cy5; CD20 in PE-Cy7; CD27 in FITC; IgM/A in APC; IgD in PE | IgA/M/D$^-$, CD3/14/16$^-$, CD20$^+$, CD27$^+$ |
| Switch memory IgA B cells | CD3, CD14, CD16 in PE-Cy5; CD20 in PE-Cy7; CD27 in FITC; IgM/G in APC; IgD in PE | IgG/M/D$^-$, CD3/14/16$^-$, CD20$^+$, CD27$^+$ |

B cells, (b) naïve B cells, (c) IgM memory B cells, and (d) switch memory B cells (Fig. 2). EBV can transform all peripheral resting B cell subsets. To immortalize the desired human B cell subset immunomagnetic beads enrichment followed by cell sorting are sequentially applied for purification. Enriched B cells can be labeled with different combinations of monoclonal antibodies specific for surface antigens to identify and sort the B cell subpopulation of interest. A wide number of antibody combinations can be used and is summarized in Table 1.

1. Prepare mononuclear cells by Ficoll-Hypaque density gradient centrifugation from peripheral blood or thaw cryopreserved mononuclear cells (see Note 1).
2. Count cells and adjust cell concentration to $10^7$ cells per 265 μL MACS buffer.
3. Add 65 μL of CD22 (or CD20) microbeads per $10^8$ cells and incubate 30 min in the dark at 4°C.
4. Add 10 mL of cold MACS buffer and centrifuge at 330×*g* for 10 min, 4°C. Carefully remove the supernatants by aspiration. Make sure not to disturb the pellet.
5. Resuspend cells in 4 mL of cold MACS buffer at a concentration of $2 \times 10^8$ cells/mL.
6. Insert the LS column adaptor in the magnetic field of the SuperMACS separator. Place the LS column into the adaptor and a 15 mL conical tube (see Note 2).
7. Prepare columns by rinsing with 4 mL cold MACS buffer. Discard the effluent and change the collection tube. Make sure that the LS columns does not run dry.
8. Transfer the cell suspension to the column and let flow through.
9. Wash three times by adding 3 mL of MACS buffer, add new buffer when the column is empty. Collect the effluent containing the B cell negative fraction.
10. Remove columns from the separator and place each on top of 15 mL propylene conical tubes.
11. Pipette 4 mL of cold MACS buffer onto columns. Flush the magnetically labeled cells by pushing the plunger into the column. Bring the volume of the cells to 10 mL with cold MACS buffer.
12. Centrifuge at 330×*g* for 10 min at 4°C and carefully remove the supernatants by aspiration.
13. Resuspend the pellet in 2 mL of PBS 2% FCS in 5 mL propylene conical tubes.
14. After this step, cells are sorted according to B cell subset populations.
15. Dilute mAbs in 400 mL of PBS 2% FCS to stain the cells (see Table 2 for the dilution factor).
16. Centrifuge the 5 mL tube with the cells recovered from the enrichment, at 330×*g* per 10 min, 4°C. Remove supernatants carefully.
17. Add mAbs solution to the pellet, and dissociate into single cell suspension by pipetting.
18. Incubate for 20 min in the dark, at 4°C.

**Table 2**
**Dilution factors**

| mAb | Provider | Code/clone | Dilution |
|---|---|---|---|
| CD3 Cy5 | Beckman Coulter | A07749/UCHT1 | 1:100 |
| CD14 Cy5 | Beckman Coulter | A07765/RMO52 | 1:100 |
| CD16 Cy5 | Beckman Coulter | A07767/3G8 | 1:100 |
| CD20 PECy7 | Beckman Coulter | IM/3629/B9E9 | 1:50 |
| CD24 PE | BD, Pharmingen | 555428/ML5 | 1:50 |
| CD38 FITC | Beckman Coulter | A07778/T16 | 1:100 |
| CD27 FITC | BD Pharmingen | 555440/M-T271 | 1:50 |
| IgG APC | Jackson ImmunoResearch | 109 496 098 | 1:400 |
| IgM APC | Jackson ImmunoResearch | 109 496 129 | 1:400 |
| IgA APC | Jackson ImmunoResearch | 109 496 011 | 1:400 |
| IgD PE | BD Pharmingen | 555779/IA6-2 | 1:100 |

19. Add 4 mL PBS, 2% FCS and centrifuge at 330×*g* per 10 min. Repeat this once.
20. Resuspend cells in 0.5 mL PBS, 2% FCS and filter the cell suspension with a cell strainer (40 μm nylon) into a fresh 5 mL tube in order to eliminate cellular aggregates that could interfere with the sorting procedure.
21. Prepare 15 mL collection tubes with 2 mL complete culture medium.
22. Sort with a BD FACSAria according to the desired phenotype (see Note 3).

### 3.2. B95.8 Cell Expansion

1. Prewarm complete culture medium at 37°C.
2. Thaw the cryo-preserved B95.8 cells by gently agitating the cryovial in a 37°C water bath.
3. In a sterile tissue culture hood spray the vial with 70% ethanol.
4. Very gently transfer the content of the vial in a 15 mL tube and add drop by drop up to 10 mL of warm complete medium.
5. Centrifuge at 330×*g* per 10 min at room temperature (RT).
6. Carefully aspirate the supernatants. Do not disturb the pellet.
7. Resuspend the cells in warm complete culture medium and transfer them in a 6-well plates at $1\times10^6$ cell/mL. Monitor cells for growth (see Note 4).

8. After 10 days, remove all cells by centrifugation at 350×*g* for 10 min.
9. Filter the supernatants with 0.8 μm filters.
10. Aliquot the supernatants in polypropylene tube, 5 mL per tube, and store at –80°C until used for EBV infection.

### *3.3. Epstein–Barr Virus B Cell Infection*

1. Add prewarmed complete medium up to 10 mL to sorted B cells, centrifuge at 330×*g* for 10 min at RT. Remove the supernatant carefully and add 1 mL of complete culture medium with CpG 2006 at 2.5 μg/mL.
2. Add 1 mL of EBV virus (from Subheading 3.2), mix gently, and incubate for 5 h at 37°C, 5% $CO_2$ (tube cap open).

### *3.4. EBV-B Cell Cloning Protocols*

1. Prepare mononuclear cells by Ficoll-Hypaque density gradient of the allogeneic buffy coat. Resuspend cells in complete culture medium and irradiate at 6,000 rad. These cells will be used as feeder.
2. B cells infected with EBV are diluted in prewarmed complete culture medium containing: CpG 2006 2.5 μg/mL, 1% EBV, irradiated PBMCs at $2.5 \times 10^5$ cells/mL. Dispense 50 μL of the cloning mixture with a multichannel pipette in 384-well plates. Different concentrations of B cells are plated at 25, 5, and 1 cells/well.
3. Complete medium with CpG 2006 2.5 μg/mL, 1% EBV, irradiated PBMCs at $2.5 \times 10^5$ cells/mL without sorted B cells are dispensed in two 384-well plates. These plates are the negative control plates to check for potential overgrowth of irradiated feeder cells.
4. Plates are transferred into the incubator at 37°C, 5% $CO_2$.
5. After 7 days, check cells with a microscope for growth.
6. Supernatant of the growing clones is tested for the presence of the specific antibody by a binding or functional assay.
7. Specific clones are expanded in complete culture medium, without CpG 2006 and EBV.
8. As soon as the clones are growing, they can be frozen in 90% FCS, 10% DMSO. The minimum amount of EBV-B cells to be frozen is $5 \times 10^6$ per vial.

### *3.5. ELISA Screening*

The screening strategy to select the "good" antibodies is a crucial part of the human antibody development. Humoral responses to vaccination or infection can be quantitatively but also qualitatively different. This reflects various level of protection in vivo, related to the differences in antibody function, which can be measured in vitro. All antibodies, which bind to a given antigen can be measured by enzyme-linked immunoabsorbent assay (ELISA).

Alternatively, if the specific antigen can be expressed in the plasma membrane of a given cell line upon transfection of the relevant gene the binding of the antibody to the cell surface can be evaluated in flow cytometry. The ability to neutralize the specific pathogen in vitro is another possible measurement of antibody function.

1. Add 70 μL antigen resuspended in coating buffer per well (final concentration 10 μg/mL) in ELISA plates and incubate overnight at 4°C or 4 h at RT.
2. Wash 3× with PBS, 0.05% Tween 20.
3. Add 200 μL of blocking solution PBS 10% FCS, 2 h RT.
4. Wash 3× with PBS, 0.05% Tween 20.
5. Add 50 μL of B cell supernatant, incubate overnight at 4°C.
6. Wash 3× with PBS, 0.05% Tween 20.
7. Add 50 μL of anti-Ig-alkaline phosphatase 1/500 in PBS 10% FCS, 2 h at RT.
8. Wash 3× with PBS, 0.05% Tween 20.
9. Add 100 μL of ELISA substrate 104.
10. Read at absorbance of 405 nm in ELISA reader.

## 4. Notes

1. The number of B cells obtained from peripheral blood varies greatly between different donors. Percentage of peripheral B lymphocytes can range from 5 to 12% and this is age dependent. Usually elder people have fewer B cells. In order to minimize the loss of B cells, it is better to process the blood as soon as possible. Anti-coagulant such as heparin must be used. It is crucial to keep B cells on ice during all the different steps. Depletion of platelets form peripheral blood (800 rpm × 8 min), avoid the formation of clumps and aggregates. Also see Current Protocols in Immunology, Unit 7.1, April 2009.
2. These columns separate $1 \times 10^8$ magnetically labeled cells from up to $10^9$. Smaller or larger column are also available. Alternatively an automated column separator (e.g., autoMACS, Miltenyi) can be used.
3. In order to obtain a pure B cell population, it is necessary to use a positive selection method with immunomagnetic beads, followed by cell sorting. The positive selection method has the advantage that B cells are isolated with high degree of purity. However, unless Fab antibodies are used there is also the theoretical disadvantage that cells bearing high affinity Fc receptors (monocytes), may bind to the antibodies. In addition, the

antibodies utilized to select B cells, such as anti-surface Ig could provide a signal to the B cell that can influence the EBV infection. Indeed in all the antibodies combinations mentioned in Table 1 the surface Ig is used to negatively select the B cell population. Moreover, it is crucial to use anti-CD22 or CD20 microbeads to enrich B cells, instead of anti-CD19 microbeads. The latter induces the internalization of CD19 surface and consequently also of CD21, which is responsible for EBV entry into B cells (14).

4. Make sure that B95.8 do not grow in big clusters, some cells adhere to the plastic, and are intolerant to acid conditions. It is crucial to split them every 2 days with a 1/2 or 1/3 dilution factor. The goal is to gradually expand these cells to obtain the needed amount, which depends on the size of the infection you plan to perform. When the desired volume is reached, all cells maintenance procedures (including medium change) are stopped.

## References


1. DiLillo DJ, Horikawa M, Tedder TF (2011) B-lymphocytes effector functions in health and disease. Immunol Res 49:281–292
2. Jourdan M, Caraux A, Caron G, et al (2011) Characterization of a transitional preplasmablast population in the process of human B cell to plasma cell differentiation. J Immunol 87:3931–3941
3. Kwakkenbos MJ, Diehl SA, Yasuda E, Bakker AQ, van Geelen CMM, Lukens MV, van Bleek GM, Widjojoatmodjo MN, Bogers WMJ, Mei H, Radbruch A, Scheeren FA, Spits H, Beaumont T (2010) Generation of stable monoclonal antibody-producing B cell receptor-positive human memory B cells by genetic programming. Nat Med 16:123–129
4. Tiller T, Meffre E, Yurasov S, Tsuiji M, Nussenzweig MC, Wardemann H (2008) Efficient generation of monoclonal antibodies from single human B cells by single cell RT-PCR and expression vector cloning. J Immunol Methods 329(1–2):112–124
5. Meffre E, Wardemann H (2008) B-cell tolerance checkpoints in health and autoimmunity. Curr Opin Immunol 20:632–638
6. Steinitz M, Klein G, Koskimies S, Makel O (1977) EB virus-induced B lymphocyte cell lines producing specific antibody. Nature 269: 420–422
7. Kozbor D, Roder JC (1981) Requirements for the establishment of high-titered human monoclonal antibodies against tetanus toxoid using the Epstein-Barr virus technique. J Immunol 127:1275–1280
8. McCafferty J, Griffiths AD, Winter G, Chiswell DJ (1990) Phage antibodies: filamentous phage displaying antibody variable domains. Nature 348:552–554
9. Burton DR, Barbas CF III (1994) Human antibodies from combinatorial libraries. Adv Immunol 57:191–280
10. Jones PT, Dear PH, Foote J, Neuberger MS, Winter G (1986) Replacing the complementarity-determining regions in a human antibody with those from a mouse. Nature 321: 522–525
11. Traggiai E, Becker S, Subbarao K, Kolesnikova L, Uematsu Y, Gismondo MR, Murphy BR, Rappuoli R, Lanzavecchia A (2004) An efficient method to make human monoclonal antibodies from memory B cells: potent neutralization of SARS coronavirus. Nat Med 10:871–875
12. Traggiai E, Lunardi C, Bason C, Dolcino M, Tinazzi E, Corrocher R, Puccetti A (2010) Generation of anti-NAG-2 mAb from patients' memory B cells: implications for a novel therapeutic strategy in systemic sclerosis. Int Immunol 22(5):367–374
13. Lanzavecchia A, Bernasconi N, Traggiai E, Ruprecht CR, Corti D, Sallusto F (2006) Understanding and making use of human memory B cells. Immunol Rev 211:303–309
14. Fingeroth JD, Weis JJ, Tedder TF, Strominger JL, Biro PA et al (1984) Epstein-Barr virus receptor of human B lymphocytes is the C3d receptor CR2. Proc Natl Acad Sci U S A 81: 4510–4514

# Chapter 11

# Kinetic Screening in the Antibody Development Process

Michael Schräml and Matthias Biehl

## Abstract

Kinetic screening is of paramount importance when it is to select custom-made antibodies, tailored for their respective scientific, diagnostic, or pharmaceutical application. Here a kinetic screening protocol is described, using a Biacore A100 surface plasmon resonance biosensor instrument. The assay is based on an Fc-specific antibody capture system. Antibodies from complex mixtures, like from mouse hybridoma supernatants are captured on the sensor surface in an oriented manner. The method uses a single injection of one antigen concentration for the determination of six relevant screening parameters, which comprehensively describe the antibody's kinetic rate profile and its valence mode. The method enables the scientist to rank and finally select rare and outstanding antibodies according to their kinetic signatures.

**Key words:** Kinetic screening, Molar Ratio, Valence, Dissociation half-life ($t_{1/2\ \mathrm{diss}}$), Binding Late, Stability Late, Antibody Capture Level, $k_\mathrm{d}$, Surface plasmon resonance

## 1. Introduction

The term kinetic antibody screening (1–4) means to select antibodies according to their antigen binding kinetic rate properties, rather than to their sole equilibrium dissociation constant $K_\mathrm{D}$ (M). Typically, kinetic screening is integrated in a workflow, where it refines the hit selection of a preceding ELISA-based screening, from which the outcome is initial information about an antigen binding event from sometimes hundreds of potentially suitable binders (see Note 1).

Based on an automated surface plasmon resonance (SPR) instrument, a method is described, which uses six easy-to-access parameters and two simple graphical depictions to quickly select best in class antibodies, even from large sample sets. The screening parameters are: the amount of antibody captured on the sensor surface (Capture Level, CL); the antigen-binding signal at the end

Gabriele Proetzel and Hilmar Ebersbach (eds.), *Antibody Methods and Protocols*, Methods in Molecular Biology, vol. 901, DOI 10.1007/978-1-61779-931-0_11, 

of the antigen association phase (Binding Late, BL) and the antigen binding signal at the end of the antigen dissociation phase (Stability Late, SL). The Molar Ratio (MR) describing the antibody–antigen binding valence mode. The dissociation rate constant $k_d$, also called the "off rate" describes how fast the antigen dissociates from the antibody–antigen complex. Another way, to describe this is to calculate the antibody–antigen complex half-life $t_{1/2 \text{ diss}}$ in minutes. A high $t_{1/2 \text{ diss}}$ value indicates an antibody as binder with high antigen complex stability. The parameters are relevant for all binding molecules, no matter whether they will be used for a pharmaceutical, diagnostic, or research application. An example demonstrates how kinetic screening facilitates how to adapt the antibody selection process according to the latter antibody application specifications.

An antibody for its use in an in vitro diagnostic instrument, which is characterized by a short sample incubation at 37°C, followed by stringent washing steps prior to analysis is to be produced. The antibody is kinetically screened according to the following selection scheme: first, to adapt the instruments physical parameters, the screening takes place at 37°C. Second, an antibody is selected for rapid antigen complex formation (high BL value), so that enough binding signal can be generated in the limited period of the instrument's incubation time. Third, an antibody with sufficiently high antigen complex stability (BL=SL) is to be selected to withstand the stringent washing steps (small $k_d$ means high $t_{1/2 \text{ diss}}$ value). The antibody's binding valence should indicate a functional antigen-binding mode. The Molar Ratio should be between MR=1 and MR=2. The exploration of these kinetic screening parameters facilitates the production of fit for purpose antibodies, kinetically tailored for their respective application. The method supports the scientist with a high degree of information, already at early project states, and is suitable for diagnostic as well as therapeutic antibodies.

## 2. Materials

### 2.1. Biacore Sensor Preparation

1. Biacore A100 (GE Healthcare, Piscataway, NJ, USA).
2. A100 antibody extension package software (GE Healthcare).
3. CM5 series S sensor (GE Healthcare).
4. 96-Well microtiter plates and deep well reagent plates (GE Healthcare).
5. At least 50 μl of hybridoma supernatant.
6. 0.2 μm Filtrated and degassed Bidest. water.
7. Biadesorb solution 1 (GE Healthcare).
8. Biadesorb solution 2 (GE Healthcare).
9. Bianormalization solution (GE Healthcare).

10. HBS-N buffer: 10 mM HEPES pH 7.4, 150 mM NaCl.
11. Activation buffer: 10 mM Sodium acetate, 150 mM NaCl pH 4.5, 0.05% Tween 20.
12. Polyclonal rabbit anti-mouse RAMFcy antibody (GE Healthcare).
13. EDC: 400 mM 3-(*N*,*N*,-dimethylamino)propyl-*N*-ethylcarbodiimide.
14. NHS: 100 mM *N*-hydroxysuccinimide.
15. 10 mM Sodium acetate pH 5 buffer (immobilization buffer).
16. 1 M Ethanolamine pH 8.

### 2.2. Kinetic Screening

1. Biacore A100 (GE Healthcare).
2. A100 antibody extension package software (GE Healthcare).
3. A100 Biaevaluation Software 1.1 (GE Healthcare).
4. CM5 series S sensor (GE Healthcare).
5. RAMFcy sensor.
6. 96-Well microtiter plates and deep well reagent plates (GE Healthcare).
7. At least 50 μl of hybridoma supernatant.
8. 1 mg/ml Antigen solution.
9. 0.2 μm Filtrated and degassed Bidest. water.
10. HBS-ET+CMD buffer: 10 mM HEPES pH 7.4, 150 mM NaCl, 1 mM EDTA, 1 mg/ml CMD, 0.005% Tween 20.
11. HBS-ET buffer: 10 mM HEPES pH 7.4, 150 mM NaCl, 1 mM EDTA, 0.05% Tween 20.
12. Carboxymethyl Dextran (CMD) 100 mg/ml stock solution in water.
13. 10 mM Glycine buffer pH 1.7 (regeneration buffer).

### 2.3. Data Processing

1. A100 antibody extension package software (GE Healthcare).
2. A100 Biaevaluation Software 1.1 (GE Healthcare).

## 3. Methods

### 3.1. Sensor Preparation

1. A Biacore CM5 sensor series S is mounted into a Biacore A100 system and is hydrodynamically addressed and normalized according to the manufacturer's instructions (see Note 2).
2. HBS-N buffer, activation buffer, immobilization buffer, and the Biadesorb solution 1 and 2 are used as buffers during the immobilization.
3. An antibody species specific Fc capture system (1) is prepared. In each flow cell, a polyclonal rabbit anti-mouse RAMFCy

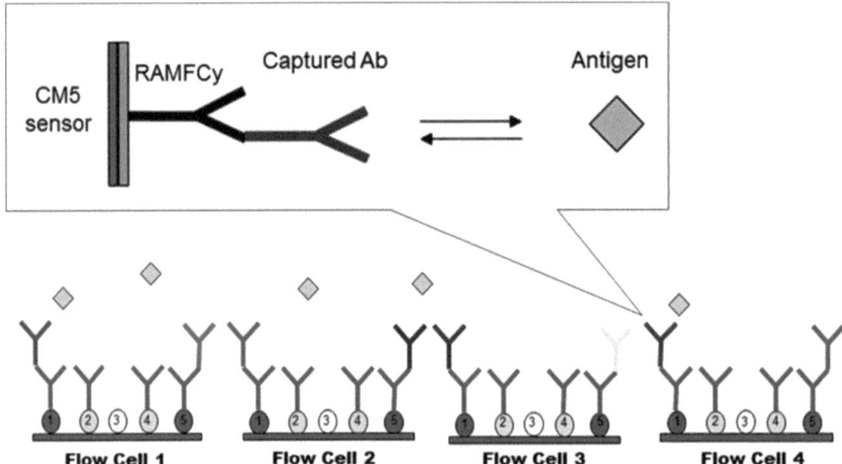


Fig. 1. Biacore A100 biosensor setup. A mouse Fc-specific antibody is covalently immobilized. In each flow cell, spot 1 and spot 5 are used to capture antibodies. Referenced binding signals are calculated from spot 1 minus 2 and spot 5 minus 4. Spot 3 is a blank spot, which serves as a control spot for unspecific binding to the blank sensor surface. Four flow cells can handle eight different antibodies in a single analyte injection. Acidic regeneration of the sensor elutes all complexes from the capture system.

antibody is immobilized on the spots 1, 2, 4, and 5 (Fig. 1). RAMFcy antibody is covalently immobilized using EDC/NHS coupling via primary amines (5).

4. After EDC/NHS activation of all spots on the sensor by a 10 min injection of EDC/NHS at 25°C, 30 µg/ml RAMFcy in 10 mM sodium acetate pH 5 buffer are injected for 10 min at 10 µl/min at 25°C. 10,000 Relative response units (RU) are immobilized on spots 1, 2 and 4, and 5.
5. The sensor's chemical binding capacity is saturated by a 2 min injection of 1 M ethanolamine at pH 8. The assay setup of the sensor references unspecific binding and corrects drifting baselines (spot 3).
6. For more details on the sensor preparation, immobilization procedure and instrument handling, please refer to the Biacore Methodology Handbook.

### 3.2. Kinetic Screening

At least 50 µl of hybridoma supernatant should be available for each antigen to be measured by kinetic screening. The hybridoma supernatants are diluted at least 1:2 with HBS-ET + CMD buffer (see Note 3). HBS-ET buffer is used as system running buffer during the kinetic screening. The screening temperature should be adjusted to the temperature of the antibody's latter field of application (see Note 4), like described in the introductory example.

Prior to each analysis run, the sensor is conditioned by 5 cycles capturing 25 nM of an arbitrary monoclonal mouse antibody.

Every 25th cycle, this antibody is repeatedly injected to control the stable antibody capture level performance of the surface.

Roughly calculated, one cycle takes 30 min to analyze eight antibodies. Depending on the regeneration stability of the sensor, a kinetic screening cycle can be repeated several hundred times. In this way, within 15 h, 120 hybridoma primary cultures can be analyzed for their kinetic properties, including double referencing (see Note 5).

One assay cycle comprises four steps:

(a) Antibody capturing.

(b) Antigen association phase monitoring.

(c) Antigen dissociation phase monitoring.

(d) Regeneration of the sensor.

1. Before the antibody is injected the baseline is defined by the setting of the Baseline Start (BS [RU]) report point (Fig. 5 and see Note 6).
2. The antibody capturing step is done at 10 μl/min for 2 min injection time on the measurement spots 1 and 5 (Fig. 1).
3. The amount of captured antibody is monitored as Capture Level (CL [RU]) at the end of the antibody association phase (see Note 7).
4. The antigen is injected at 150 nM for 2 min at 30 μl/min (see Notes 8 and 9) over all four flow cells.
5. At the end of the antigen's association phase, the Binding Late (BL [RU]) report point is taken. When the antigen injection is stopped, system buffer is floating over the sensor again and only the dissociation of the antigen from the captured antibody is monitored.
6. Dissociation is monitored for 3 min at 30 μl/min. At the end of the dissociation phase, the Stability Late (SL [RU]) report point is set.
7. The RAMFcy sensor is regenerated by a 1 min injection of 10 mM glycine buffer pH 1.7 at 30 μl/min over all flow cells (see Note 6).
8. After the regeneration procedure the Baseline End (BE [RU]) report point is set.

### 3.3. Data Processing and Visualization for Binding Late/Stability Late Report Points

Kinetic screening data can be quickly evaluated by plotting the Stability Late (SL) report points over the Binding Late (BL) report points (Fig. 2), which dramatically simplifies the visualization of the complex kinetic behavior of the molecular interactions. Antibodies populating on the BL = SL trendline show no measurable antigen complex dissociation within the monitored time frame and thus form tight antigen complexes.

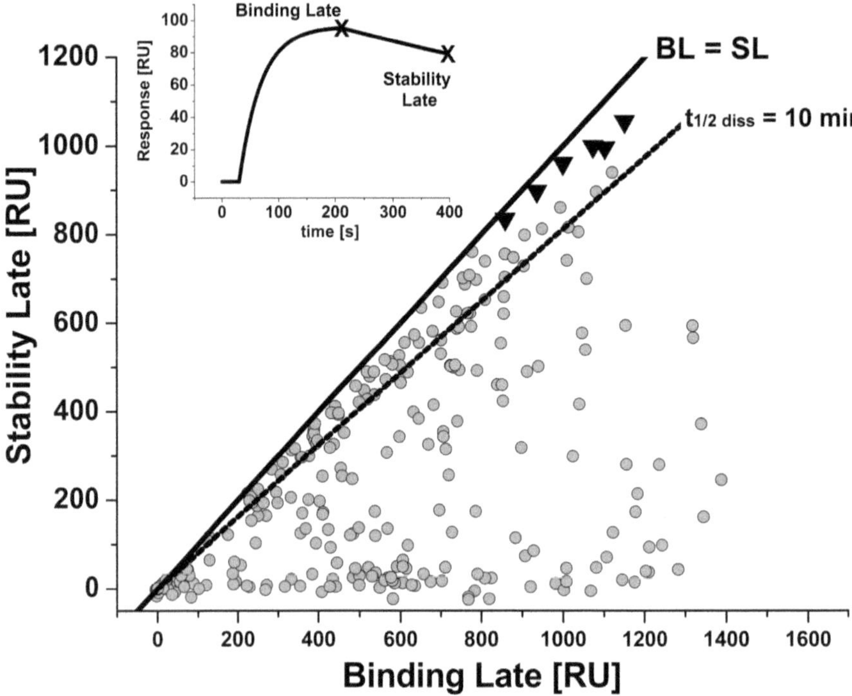


Fig. 2. 37°C kinetic screening of 296 mouse hybridoma clone culture supernatants versus a 72-kDa protein receptor analyte. Each data spot in the Stability Late (SL)/Binding Late (BL) plot represents an antigen–antibody interaction. The origin of the report points is shown in the enframed Biacore sensorgram (Response Units RU over time in seconds). The *black line* indicates values, where BL = SL. *Black triangles* mark antigen-antibody interactions of hybridoma supernatants, which are selected for further processing.

Best in class antibodies show highest BL values and at the same time populate as close as possible to the BL = SL trendline (see Note 10).

Figure 2 outlines the value of kinetic screening. From 225 ELISA preselected binders six antibodies were selected for being further developed into clone cultures. Kinetic screening is the ultimate filter for the selection of rarely occurring antibodies.

### *3.4. Data Processing and Visualization*

The detection of an antibody forming a tight complex with its respective antigen is not sufficient to classify an antibody as a positive hit. The functionality and specificity of the interaction is to be proven, because e.g. unspecific binding hydrophobic artifacts can also produce highly stable complexes.

An important tool is the calculation of the Molar Ratio of the antibody–antigen interactions.

The Molar Ratio is calculated from the Binding Late value, the antibody Capture Level and the Molecular Weights (MW) of the interacting molecules:

MR = (BindingLate(RU)/CaptureLevel(RU)) × (MW(antibody)/MW (antigen)).

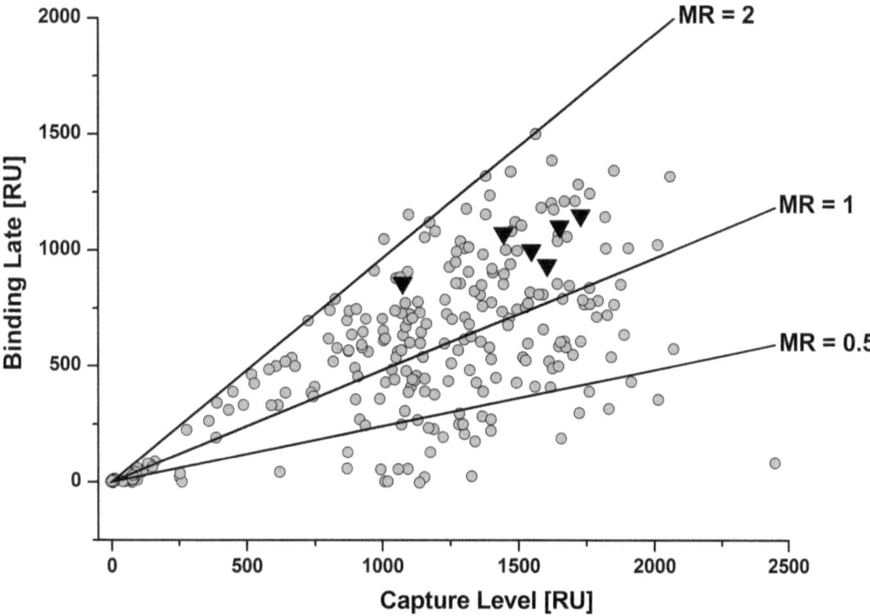


Fig. 3. Exemplary valence analysis of the data set from Fig. 2. Binding Late (RU) is plotted over the antibody Capture Level (RU). Corridors are formed by *lines*, indicating areas of the same Molar Ratios. The *lines* help to quickly classify antibodies according to their valences. The antibodies populate all corridors and therefore bind to their 72-kDa antigen with different valences. *Black triangles* indicate the selected clone cultures from Fig. 2.

To graphically visualize the valence analysis, Binding Late is plotted over the antibody Capture Level. Valence corridors, calculated using the MR formula, allocate the antibodies according to their virtual Binding Late values (Fig. 3), e.g., for the plotting of the MR=2 trendline use the formula: BL at MR(2)=(MW(antigen)×2×Capture Level (RU)/MW (antibody)). Just replace the Molar Ratio values to calculate different trendlines.

When the antibody shows a MR=1, it binds to an antigen with single valence. Obviously, there is some steric hindrance, which avoids full bivalent antibody binding.

When the antibody shows MR=2, it is able to simultaneously bind to two antigens.

Here antibodies in the range of MR=1 and MR=2 were selected, when they showed a suitable BL/SL ratio (Fig. 3) at the same time. For further details about the valence analysis see Notes 9 and 11.

### 3.5. Data Analysis for $k_d$ Ranking

If possible, calculate the "off rate", which means the antigen dissociation rate constant $k_d$ (1/s) (6). The dissociation rate constant $k_d$ describes the decay of complexes per second. $k_d$ is calculated from a linear regression fitting of the antigen dissociation phase, which is a function of the Biaevaluation software. Using the dissociation rate constant, the complex half life $t_{1/2\ diss}$ in minutes

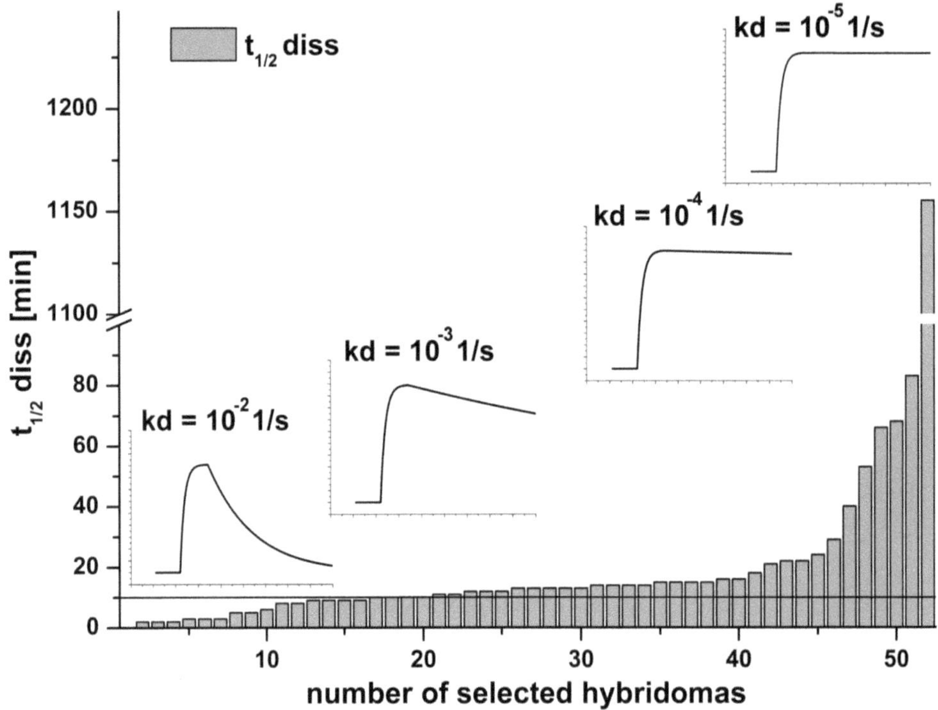


Fig. 4. From a set of 529 ELISA positive mouse hybridoma primary cultures, 51 cultures were selected at 37°C and ranked according to their $t_{1/2\ \mathrm{diss}}$ values (*filled bars*) versus a 6 kDa antigen. The sensorgrams reflect the $t_{1/2\ \mathrm{diss}}$ values. The *line* indicates the $t_{1/2\ \mathrm{diss}} = 10$ min value.

is calculated according to the first order kinetics half life law: $t_{1/2\ \mathrm{diss}} = \ln(2)/(60 \times k_{\mathrm{d}})$ (7). Finally the antibodies are ranked according to their antigen complex half-lives (Fig. 4).

In Fig. 4, a single antibody labeled as rare event and showing outstanding kinetic properties was identified among 529 ELISA hits. Antibodies with an antigen complex stability of $t_{1/2\ \mathrm{diss}} > 10$ min at 37°C are suitable binders for the use in an in vitro diagnostic assay as described in Subheading 1 (see Notes 11 and 12).

## 4. Notes

1. Kinetic screening succeeding after high throughput ELISA assays is a recommendable workflow. Most ELISA formats coat the antigen unspecific in microtiter plates, which denatures the antigen and blocks epitopes. The bivalent antibody recognizes the antigen in an avidity mode, which deteriorates the affinity information. The antibody concentration in primary hybridoma supernatants is mostly unknown in early process steps. A strong ELISA binding signal could originate from a high antibody

concentration, binding with low avidity. The protocol described here delivers kinetically resolved affinity information, as long as the analyte in solution is monomeric and efficiently selects binders from a pool of just potentially suitable ELISA-preselected antibodies.

2. The A100 performs hydrodynamic addressing, which separates four sensor flow cells each into five sensitive measurement spots, which then can be triggered singly or in certain combinations. 20 signals are simultaneously monitored. Applying Figs. 2 and 3 and the Subheading 3, the protocol can be effectively transferred to other Biacore instruments, such as 2000, 3000, T100/200, 4000, or any other commercially available biosensor-based kinetic systems.
3. 1 mg/ml CMD minimizes unspecific binding to the dextran layer on the CM5 sensor surface.
4. When enough antibody and antigen is available, try to screen at different temperatures, e.g., at 13, 25, and 37°C. This allows you to select antibodies according to their optimal temperature-dependent kinetic binding rate signatures.
5. Whenever possible, sample buffer is injected (0 nM antigen) to double reference. The antibody/antigen binding signals are referenced versus their control spots and additionally versus a 0 nM antigen injection to avoid baseline drifts or positively drifting signals during the dissociation phase. When a higher throughput is necessary you can omit the double referencing or reduce the association and dissociation time. But keep in mind that data quality is the top priority. When the throughput allows it, perform double referencing or add more antigen analytes, e.g., for off-target or cross-reactivity tests.
6. It is important that the captured antibodies are tightly captured without dissociation, but finally are completely regenerated from the surface. An important control is the setting of two additional report points before the antibody capturing (Baseline Start, BS) and after the regeneration step (Baseline End, BE). Both report points shouldn't deviate much. Sometimes, it is necessary to perform a regeneration buffer scouting to figure out suitable regeneration conditions, which do not harm the capture system and guarantee constant capture performance (Fig. 5).
7. Since SPR is a mass-sensitive system, the antibody capture level impacts the latter assay sensitivity. This is especially an issue when one needs to screen primary hybridoma supernatants with low antibody concentrations or antigens with low molecular weight. The smaller the analytes' molecular weight, the higher the antibody capture level is needed. For an antigen range of about 10 kDa, at least 500 RU antibody capture level

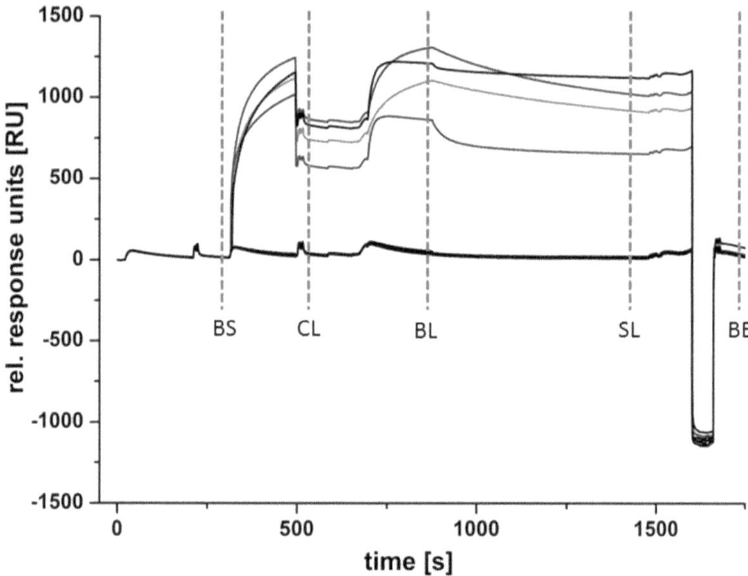


Fig. 5. A sensorgram (relative response units over time in seconds) overlay plot of four unreferenced screening cycles. *Dashed lines* indicate the time points of the report point settings. BS: Baseline Start defines the baseline signal prior to the antibody capturing. *CL* Antibody Capture Level is determined after the injection of the antibody containing solutions. *BL* Binding Late determined at the end of the antigen injection. *SL* Stability Late is determined at the end of the antigen dissociation phase. Clearly, different antigen association and dissociation phase signatures can be identified. *BE* Baseline End is determined after the regeneration of the capture system.

is recommended. To increase the antibody capture level increase the injection time, but do not use a more concentrated hybridoma supernatant due to the risk of unspecific binding and instrument clogging.

8. When the antigen is not available at sufficiently high concentration or generally slowly associates, increase the association time to up to 10 min. However, keep in mind that this increases the antigen consumption and the instrument's runtime.
9. The oriented presentation of the captured antibodies allows the selection of antibodies according to their valence by calculating their Molar Ratio. The correct calculation of the Molar Ratio requires saturating the antibody during the antigen association phase. In order to get information of low affinity antibodies it is useful to inject the antigen at higher concentration of at least 150 nM.
10. A high Binding Late (BL) value resembles a fast association rate constant $k_a$ (1/Ms), even when $k_a$ is not quantified. To select an antibody with highest $k_a$ value is the most important screening parameter when it is to select diagnostic and pharmaceutical antibodies.

11. Primary hybridoma cultures mostly show low Molar Ratio values. In contrast, clone culture hybridoma supernatants should show reasonable Molar Ratios (Fig. 3). Usually, the whole data set is characterized by small MR values, when high molecular weight antigens (MW > 50 kDa) are used, because neighboring antibodies presented on the sensor surface are sterically blocked simply by the antigens' size. When the MR values statistically distribute, cultures with too low Molar Ratio (MR = 0.01) or overstoichiometric binding (MR > 2.5) should be deselected. If the complete run is characterized by generally understoichiometric or overstoichiometric Molar Ratio values, check the antigen's stability, buffer formulation, p*I*, molecular weight, and oligomeric status. In the worst case, the Molar Ratio indicates that the data obtained by the run is not meaningful. Always visually check the sensorgrams and do not just rely on $k_d$ and $t_{1/2\ diss}$ values. A $k_d = 1.0\text{E}{-05}$ 1/s resulting in $t_{1/2\ diss} = 1{,}155$ min and a binding late signal of BL = 0.5 RU is an artifact, identifiable by low Molar Ratio values. Therefore, carefully consider all six parameters in a comprehensive way. It is not relevant to focus only on antibody–antigen complex stability. Fast association rates, reflected by considerable Binding Late values, are equally important. For an application in an equilibrium system (= without washing), a fast antibody–antigen association rate (= high BL value) is even of more of importance than just a high complex stability.
12. A comprehensive kinetic screening is shown in a table with Binding Late (BL), Stability Late (SL), $k_d$ (1/s), $t_{1/2\ diss}$ (min), antibody Capture Level (CL) and the Molar Ratio (MR) at a specific temperature.

## References


1. Canziani GA, Klakamp S, Myszka DG (2004) Kinetic screening of antibodies from crude hybridoma samples using biacore. Anal Biochem 325(2):301–307
2. Rich RL, Myszka DG (2007) Higher-throughput, label-free, real-time molecular interaction analysis. Anal Biochem 361(1):1–6
3. Wassaf D, Kuang G, Kopacz K et al (2006) High-throughput affinity ranking of antibodies using surface plasmon resonance microarrays. Anal Biochem 351(2):241–253
4. Safsten P, Klakamp SL, Drake AW et al (2006) Screening antibody–antigen interactions in parallel using biacore a100. Anal Biochem 353(2): 181–190
5. Johnsson B, Lofas S, Lindquist G (1991) Immobilization of proteins to a carboxymethyldextran-modified gold surface for biospecific interaction analysis in surface plasmon resonance sensors. Anal Biochem 198(2): 268–277
6. Leonard P, Safsten P, Hearty S et al (2007) High throughput ranking of recombinant avian scfv antibody fragments from crude lysates using the biacore a100. J Immunol Methods 323(2): 172–179
7. Pasqualucci L, Guglielmino R, Houldsworth J et al (2004) Expression of the aid protein in normal and neoplastic B cells. Blood 104(10): 3318–3325

# Chapter 12

# Temperature-Dependent Antibody Kinetics as a Tool in Antibody Lead Selection

Michael Schräml and Leopold von Proff

## Abstract

Antibody–antigen interactions can principally be classified into three different temperature-dependent kinetic rate profiles. The affinity $K_D$ can persist, decrease, or increase in the temperature gradient. Today, the impact of temperature-dependent antibody kinetics is recognized, especially as part of the development of best in class monoclonal antibodies. Here, a robust surface plasmon resonance-based protocol is presented, which describes a sensitive temperature-dependent kinetic measurement and evaluation method.

**Key words:** Surface plasmon resonance, SPR, Kinetics, $k_a$, $k_d$, $K_D$, Temperature, Thermodynamics

## 1. Introduction

The measurement of the temperature-dependence of antibody binding kinetics generates a unique thermodynamic fingerprint of each antibody–antigen interaction (1, 2). The dissociation constant $K_D$ is a temperature-dependent variable, which becomes clear by the Gibbs equation $\Delta G° = -RT\ln K_D$, which relates the free standard binding enthalpy $\Delta G°$ to the dissociation constant $K_D$. A large negative value of $\Delta G°$ characterizes a high affinity interaction by summing up all its energy contributions in the antibody–antigen interface. Since $K_D$ is the quotient from $k_d$ and $k_a$, the equation can be rearranged into $\Delta G° = -RT\ln(k_d/k_a)$. Therefore, the temperature-dependency of the rate constants reflects the quantity and quality of the noncovalent interactions. Here, a higher resolution kinetic analysis is described, which is applied at advanced project states, where a lead candidate with optimized temperature-dependent kinetic rate properties is finalized from a pool of antibodies.

Gabriele Proetzel and Hilmar Ebersbach (eds.), *Antibody Methods and Protocols*, Methods in Molecular Biology, vol. 901, DOI 10.1007/978-1-61779-931-0_12, 

For example, an antibody–antigen interaction, which is dominated by short ranged hydrophobic forces (3) or which is sterically hindered in its epitope accessibility, usually generates slow association rate constants $k_a$. This is especially observable in the kinetic signature below 25°C (4). When temperature catalyzes the Brownian motion of the molecules $k_a$ can accelerate by orders of magnitudes and finally the antibody pretends being an unobtrusive binder at 37°C (5). Here, the analysis of the temperature-dependency of the rate constants helps us to unmask a suboptimal interface amino acid composition.

Another example is an antibody–antigen interaction, which is dominated by long ranged, electrostatic forces (6). Charged residues, which can generate an optimal antibody–antigen surface complementarity (7) contribute to antigen specificity and are known to induce fast association rate constants $k_a$ (8, 9). This is observable also at temperatures far below 25°C. When such an interface is lacking any hydrophobic moment (7) or when the interface is simply too small, an insufficient antigen complex stability at elevated temperature will dominate kinetics resulting in a too low affinity. Therefore, the goal is to use temperature-dependent kinetics as a method to investigate and select antibodies with optimal rate properties reflecting an optimal antibody–antigen binding site size and amino acid composition.

Of course, this method supports antibody engineering and antibody quality control efforts well. It can be analyzed whether an exchange of the Fc compartment (10), a point mutation in the CDR or frame region, a posttranslational modification, a chemical labeling moiety, or a humanization approach lead to an inferior, persisting, or improved temperature-dependent kinetic performance.

## 2. Materials

1. Biacore T100 (GE Healthcare, Piscataway, NJ, USA).
2. T100 Biaevaluation Software 1.1 (GE Healthcare).
3. CM5 series S sensor (GE Healthcare).
4. Polyclonal rabbit anti-mouse antibody (RAMIgG) (GE Healthcare).
5. 0.1% SDS in 50 mM NaOH, 10 mM HCl.
6. 100 mM $H_3PO_4$.
7. 100 mM *N*-hydroxysuccinimide (NHS).
8. 400 mM 3-(*N*,*N*,-dimethylamino) propyl-*N*-ethylcarbodiimide (EDC).
9. 1 M Ethanolamine pH 8.

10. Biadesorb solution 1 (GE Healthcare).
11. Biadesorb solution 2 (GE Healthcare).
12. Bianormalization solution (GE Healthcare).
13. HBS-N buffer: 10 mM HEPES pH 7.4, 150 mM NaCl.
14. Immobilization buffer: 10 mM NaAc pH 4.5.
15. System Buffer (HBS-ET buffer): 10 mM HEPES pH 7.4, 150 mM NaCl, 1 mM EDTA, 0.05% Tween 20.
16. Stock solution 100 mg/mL Carboxymethyl Dextran (CMD).
17. System Buffer with CMD: 10 mM HEPES pH 7.4, 150 mM NaCl, 1 mM EDTA, 1 mg/mL Carboxymethyl Dextran (CMD), 0.005% Tween 20.
18. Regeneration Buffer: 10 mM glycine–HCl buffer pH 1.7.
19. 100 μg of each monoclonal mouse antibody.
20. 1 mg Antigen solution at 1 mg/mL.
21. 0.2 μm Filtrated and degassed Bidest. water.

## 3. Methods

### *3.1. Sensor Preparation*

A Biacore CM5 sensor series S is mounted into a Biacore T100/200 system driven by Biacore control software V1.1.1 and is preconditioned by 1 min injections at 100 μL/min of 0.1% SDS in 50 mM NaOH, 10 mM HCl, and 100 mM $H_3PO_4$. HBS-ET is used as System Buffer.

In case of screening antibodies of murine origin, a polyclonal rabbit anti-mouse antibody (RAMIgG) (see Note 1) at 20 μg/mL is immobilized at 6,000 response units (RU) on flow cells 1, 2, 3, 4 with EDC/NHS chemistry according to the manufacturers' instruction's using 10 mM sodium acetate buffer at pH 4.5 as preconcentration buffer. Finally the sensor is blocked with 1 M ethanolamine pH 8. The sensor surface is used as an Fc-specific capture system for murine antibodies. The antibodies can be captured from crude mixtures.

### *3.2. Homogenous Adjustment of Antibody Capture Levels at Varying Temperatures*

The antibody's capturing kinetics are strongly influenced by temperature. A prerun is recommended to optimize the antibody capture concentrations at different temperatures. In Table 1, a monoclonal mouse antibody is temperature-dependently titrated at different concentrations on the capture system to determine the RAMIgG capture capability at different temperatures.

1. Murine antibody (see Note 1) is injected for 1 min at 10 μL/min at different concentrations: 25, 50, 75, and 100 nM (Table 1). Each concentration series is measured at different

**Table 1**
**This table shows a typical matrix for temperature-dependent antibody capturing to optimize constant antibody capture levels on the sensor surface**

| Anti-thyrotropin (TSH) antibody (nM) | RU at °C | | | | | |
|---|---|---|---|---|---|---|
| | 17°C | 21°C | 25°C | 29°C | 33°C | 37°C |
| 25 | 91 | 106 | 122 | 137 | 153 | 170 |
| 50 | 187 | 206 | 226 | 248 | 273 | 295 |
| 75 | 225 | 248 | 270 | 293 | 318 | 340 |
| 100 | 270 | 292 | 315 | 342 | 369 | 394 |

temperatures from 17 to 37°C. The sensor is regenerated by 3-min injection of 10 mM glycine buffer pH 1.7 at 10 μL/min (Regeneration Buffer).

2. A matrix is established (Table 1) with the obtained data. To produce constant antibody capture levels at different temperatures, determine the optimal antibody concentration according to the matrix. Extrapolate or interpolate between concentrations, if necessary (see Note 2).

### 3.3. Temperature-Dependent Kinetic Measurements

After the antibody capture system has been established according to Subheading 3.2 you can start to analyze monoclonal antibodies of interest (see Note 3).

1. The antibody capture solution is prepared in System Buffer supplemented with 1 mg/mL CMD to suppress unspecific binding. Antibody (Figs. 1 and 3) is injected at 100 nM at 17°C, 80 nM at 21°C, 60 nM at 25°C, 50 nM at 29°C, 40 nM at 33 and 37°C. Antibody capturing is done for 1 min at 10 μL/min. Flow cell 1 is used as reference. Any murine monoclonal antibody can be used as control antibody on flow cell 1, as long as it does not bind to the antigen. For calculation of the Molar Ratio, the amount of captured antibody is monitored in response units (RU) at the end of each antibody capturing phase.
2. The antigen is injected over all flow cells at concentration steps of 0 nM (see Note 3), 1.2, 4, 2× 11, 33, 100, and 300 nM for 3 min at 100 μL/min. The antigen in solution must be monomeric, temperature-stable in the gradient and should not tend to aggregate. Finally, the interaction should follow a binary interaction model, which is fitted according to a Langmuir model. Complex kinetics are more difficult to evaluate and should be handled with care. The dissociation is monitored for

10–15 min at 100 μL/min. The sensor is fully regenerated by a 3 min injection of 10 mM glycine buffer pH 1.7 (Regeneration Buffer) at 10 μL/min.

3. In this way, concentration-dependent kinetics are measured at (13°C) (see Note 4), 17, 21, 25, 29, 33, and 37°C (see Note 5). A Langmuir 1:1 model (see Note 6) is fitted to the data using the Biacore evaluation software 1.1. The kinetic parameters $k_a$ (1/Ms), $k_d$ (1/s), $K_D$ (M), and $R_{MAX}$ (RU) are calculated (see Note 7). The Molar Ratio (see Note 8) is calculated using the $R_{MAX}$ values:

MR = (antigen $R_{MAX}$ (RU)/antibody Capture Level (RU)) × (MW (antibody)/MW (antigen)). The complex half-life $t_{1/2\ diss}$ in minutes is calculated according to the first-order kinetics half-life law: $t_{1/2\ diss} = \ln(2)/(60 \times k_d)$ (11).

### 3.4. Graphical Depictions, Data Processing and Evaluation

Start to evaluate the sensorgrams by a visual inspection at the respective temperatures (Figs. 1 and 3).

1. Common temperature-dependent binding kinetics
The shape of the sensorgrams in Fig. 1 indicate, that the association rate constant $k_a$ and the dissociation rate constant $k_d$ both accelerate in the temperature gradient (see Note 9). Compare the 17°C with the 37°C sensorgrams (see Note 10) and learn how the kinetic rates are changing. The mAb in Fig. 1 is a typical representative for an antibody with reduced antigen complex stability at increasing temperature. The kinetic rates are depicted in Fig. 1. Antibodies with a massive affinity-decrease due to a lacking temperature-dependent antigen complex stability frequently occur. This could be due to a smaller antibody–antigen interface, or an interface with less hydrophobic residues, but more polar amino acids (see Note 11) (Fig. 2).

2. Rare temperature-dependent binding kinetics
Another example of an antibody–antigen interaction is depicted in Fig. 3. Here, a rare event is shown, where the kinetic rates seem nearly not to change in the temperature gradient. This is my personally desired outcome of a temperature-driven selection process. The monoclonal antibody depicted is on market in the Roche Elecsys PTH Immunoassay. The association rate constant $k_a$ increases and the dissociation rate constant $k_d$ persists. Compare the 17 and 37°C data points and think about the sensorgram kinetic rate properties. These are very different from the sensorgrams in Fig. 1. The rates determined from the sensorgrams in Fig. 3 are depicted in Fig. 4.

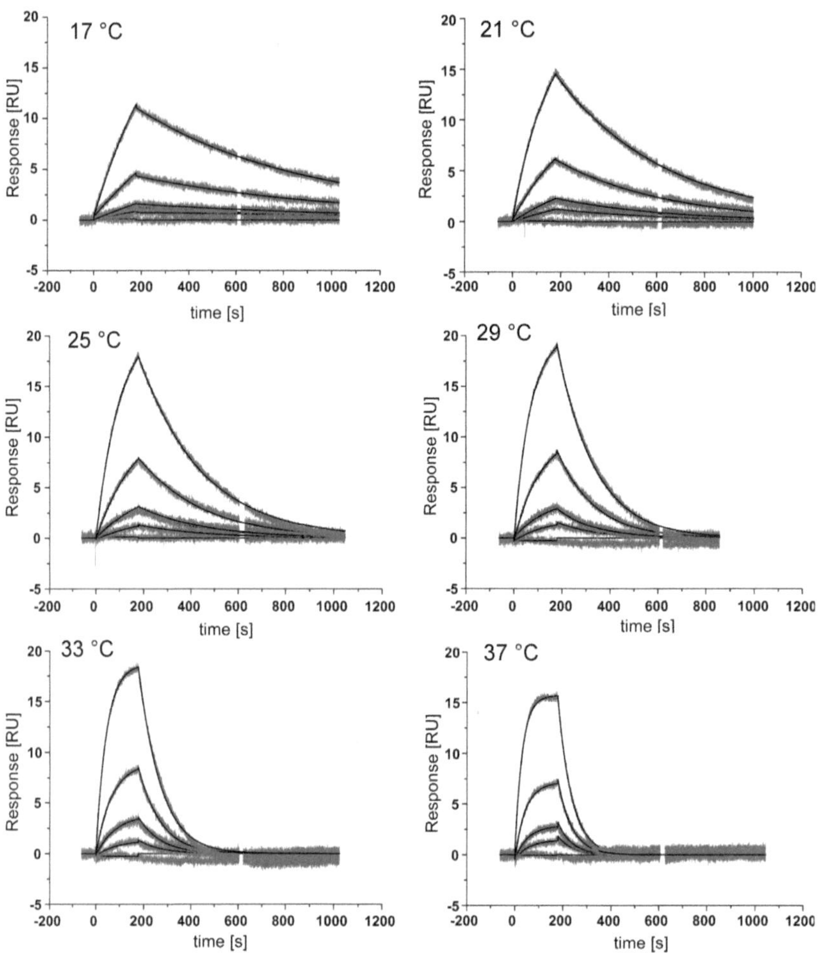


Fig. 1. Biacore sensorgrams, showing concentration-dependent kinetics of a murine monoclonal antibody binding to a 25-kDa protein analyte at different temperatures. The Langmuir fitting model is superposed on the kinetic data.

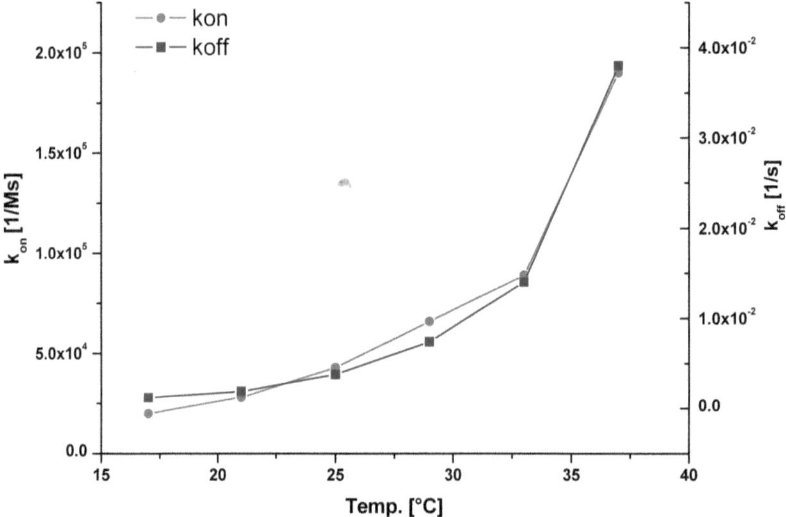


Fig. 2. Rate map of the temperature-dependent kinetic rates of Fig. 1. $k_a$ ($k_{on}$) and $k_d$ ($k_{off}$) increases in the temperature gradient. The affinity $K_D$ decreases with increasing temperature.

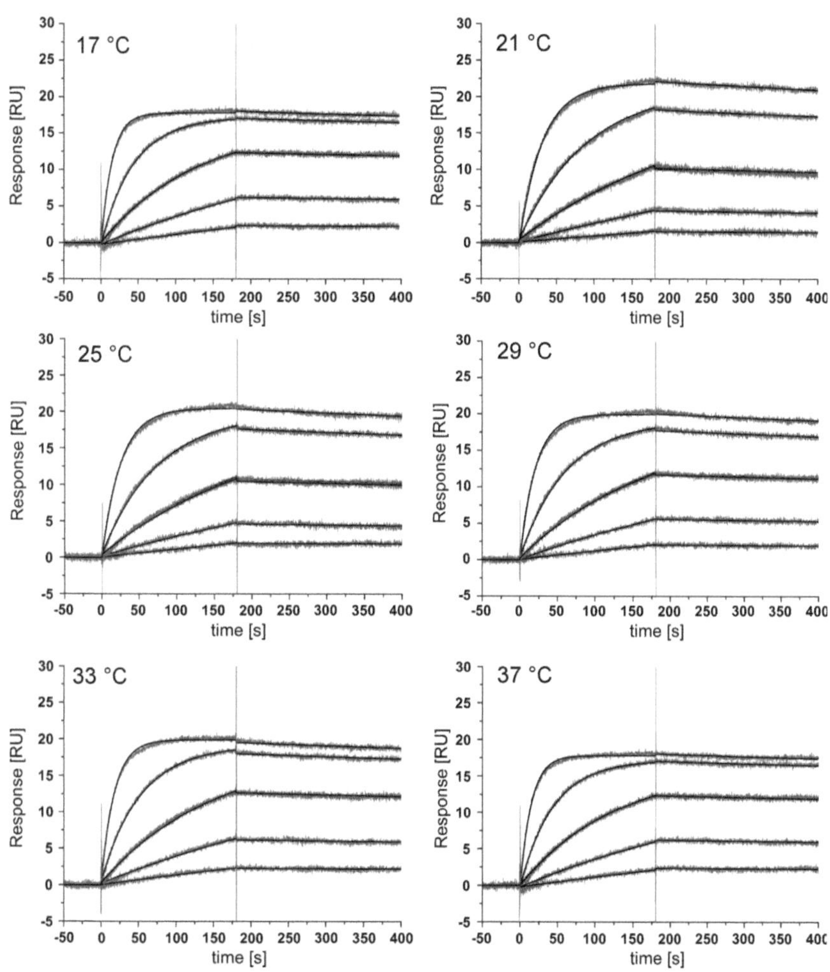


Fig. 3. Biacore sensorgrams, showing concentration-dependent kinetics of a murine monoclonal antibody binding to a 7.5-kDa antigen analyte at different temperatures. The Langmuir fitting model is superposed on the kinetic data.

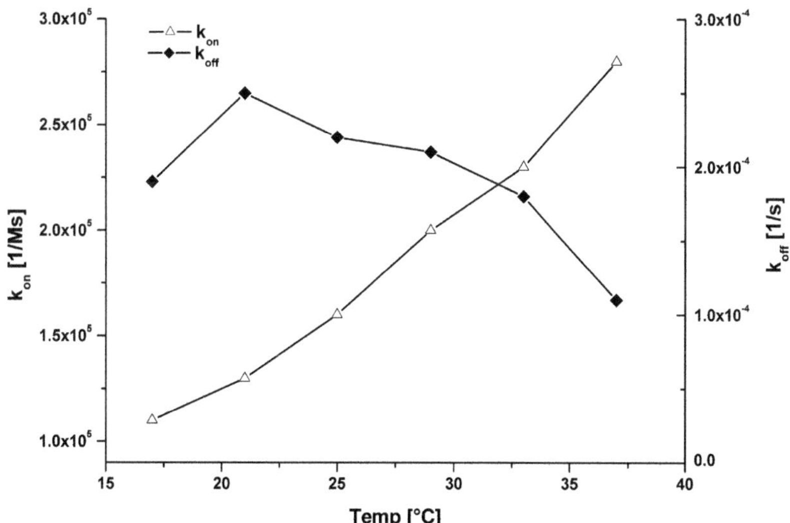


Fig. 4. Rate map of the temperature-dependent kinetic rates quantified from the sensorgrams in Fig. 3. *Triangles* indicate a regularly increasing association rate constant $k_a$ ($k_{on}$). *Filled rectangles* indicate, that the dissociation rate constant $k_d$ ($k_{off}$) remains constant and even decelerates at 37°C. This antibody increases its affinity with increasing temperature.

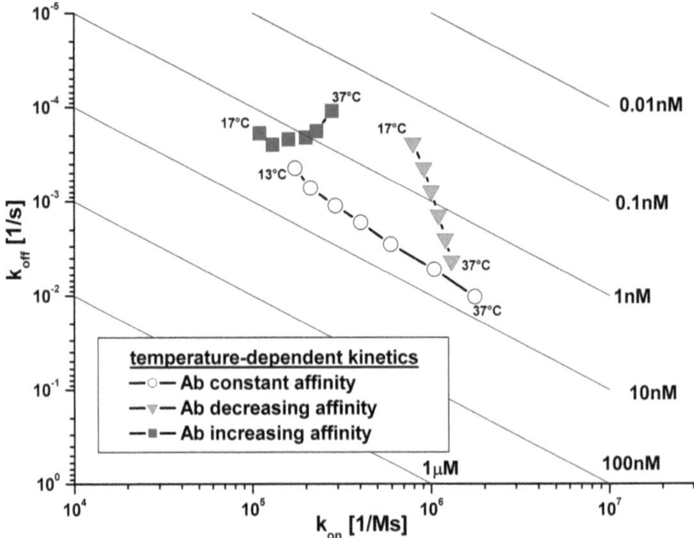


Fig. 5. Rate map, where the dissociation rate constant $k_d$ ($k_{off}$) is double logarithmically plotted over the association rate constant $k_a$ ($k_{on}$). *Isometric lines* indicate areas of the same affinity $K_D$. Three typical temperature-dependent antibody–antigen kinetic profiles are depicted and indicated in the *enframed box*.

### 3.5. Three Typical Temperature-Dependent Kinetic Signatures

The goal of the method becomes obvious in Fig. 5. In general, antibodies can be classified into three groups, according to their temperature-dependent rate properties. Select your antibody lead candidate according to your latter preferred or intended use.

Usually, the association rate constant $k_a$ increases in the temperature gradient. The dissociation rate constant $k_d$ then classifies the antibody into three possible categories:

First, the antibody loses affinity, because the antigen complex stability dramatically decreases in the temperature gradient (Figs. 1 and 2, and see Note 11).

Second, $k_a$ and $k_d$ compensate each other (see Note 12). The antibody shows a constant dissociation rate constant $K_D$ (Fig. 5, open circles). Nevertheless, the antibody loses antigen complex stability.

Third, but rare, the antibody gains in affinity, because $k_d$ decelerates or persists despite an increasing temperature. Such rare antibodies, which perform like the antibody in Fig. 5 (filled rectangle), are immunity reagents for applications, where key parameters are optimal kinetic rates also at elevated or low temperatures, e.g., in diagnostic applications.

### 3.6. Production of Humanized Lead Candidates

The method described is also suitable for the selection of humanized lead antibodies in a pharmaceutical antibody development process. Optimally, a successful humanization process leaves

**Table 2**
**Temperature-dependent kinetics vs. a 7-kDa antigen monitoring the humanization process from the murine to chimeric into a fully humanized mAb**

| $T$ (°C) | CL (RU) | $k_a$ (1/Ms) | $k_d$ (1/s) | $t_{1/2\ diss}$ | $K_D$ (nM) | $R_{MAX}$ (RU) | MR |
|---|---|---|---|---|---|---|---|
| *Murine mAb RAMIgG* | | | | | | | |
| 17 | 513 | 6.50E+05 | 1.20E−04 | 81 | 0.19 | 38 | 1.1 |
| 21 | 486 | 8.10E+05 | 2.00E−04 | 49 | 0.25 | 40 | 1.2 |
| 25 | 525 | 1.10E+05 | 3.00E−04 | 33 | 0.29 | 46 | 1.3 |
| 29 | 468 | 1.20E+05 | 4.70E−04 | 22 | 0.39 | 45 | 1.4 |
| 33 | 490 | 1.50E+05 | 7.70E−04 | 13 | 0.52 | 50 | 1.5 |
| 37 | 430 | 1.70E+05 | 1.10E−03 | 9 | 0.65 | 44 | 1.5 |
| *Chimeric mAb GaHu* | | | | | | | |
| 17 | 503 | 5.60E+05 | 3.60E−05 | 276 | 0.07 | 38 | 1.1 |
| 21 | 509 | 6.50E+05 | 6.90E−05 | 145 | 0.11 | 39 | 1.2 |
| 25 | 467 | 7.10E+05 | 9.50E−05 | 106 | 0.13 | 45 | 1.3 |
| 29 | 465 | 8.00E+05 | 1.70E−04 | 59 | 0.21 | 45 | 1.4 |
| 33 | 451 | 8.60E+05 | 2.40E−04 | 41 | 0.28 | 50 | 1.5 |
| 37 | 401 | 9.40E+01 | 4.00E−04 | 25 | 0.43 | 45 | 1.5 |
| *Humanized mAb GaHu* | | | | | | | |
| 17 | 340 | 7.60E+05 | 7.70E−06 | o.o.s. | o.o.s. | 33 | 1.4 |
| 21 | 349 | 9.30E+05 | 2.20E−05 | 454 | 0.02 | 35 | 1.5 |
| 25 | 362 | 1.10E+06 | 6.00E−05 | 167 | 0.05 | 39 | 1.6 |
| 29 | 373 | 1.30E+06 | 8.80E−05 | 114 | 0.07 | 42 | 1.7 |
| 33 | 361 | 1.50E+06 | 1.50E−04 | 68 | 0.10 | 42 | 1.7 |
| 37 | 326 | 1.80E+06 | 2.40E−04 | 42 | 0.13 | 38 | 1.7 |

*CL* antibody capture level, *GAHu* polyclonal goat anti-human antibody capture system, *O.o.s.* out of specifications of the Biacore instrument $t_{1/2\ diss}$ in minutes.

the kinetic rate contribution unaffected or it even improves $k_a$ and $k_d$, whereby the valence mode (Molar Ratio) should persist. A one-sided decrease of $k_a$, could indicate issues in the epitope accessibility after humanization (6). As mentioned in Subheading 1, this effect can especially be identified at temperatures below 25°C (see Note 13). A one-sided slow down of $k_d$ at elevated temperature could indicate stickiness of the humanized antibody. Stickiness or instabilities due to a suboptimal CDR graft complementarity on the human frame can be avoided by carefully selecting antibodies by temperature-dependent kinetics. In Table 2, the kinetic signatures of a parental murine antibody, the chimerized antibody, and the successfully humanized antibody are shown (12).

Finally, you can understand temperature-dependent kinetics as a chance to further improve the kinetic performance of the antibody by its humanization. In Table 2, the rate properties, complex half-life ($t_{1/2\ \mathrm{diss}}$), and affinity $K_D$ of the humanized antibody were all improved when compared to the murine parental antibody.

## 4. Notes

1. For the analysis of other species than mouse or antibody fragments use appropriate capture antibodies, e.g., goat anti-human pAbs. Before introducing a new capture system evaluate, whether the captured antibodies or fragments thereof are tightly bound and generate stable instrument baselines, also at 37°C. The capture system must be capable to be regenerated without loss of performance over many measurement cycles! Perform a temperature-dependent regeneration buffer scouting to figure out suitable regeneration conditions, which do not harm the capture system and guarantee constant capture performance. A capturing by anti-kappa or anti-lambda light chain antibodies is not optimal, because it might interfere with kinetics. Since SPR is a mass sensitive analysis method, the antibody capture level governs the latter assay sensitivity. Optimally, an antibody capture level is adjusted so that 10–20 RU are obtained at antigen saturation ($R_{MAX}$).
2. If necessary, implement additional antibody capture concentrations. The data are established for a species specific capture system and can be used as a template for other antibodies from the same species. When you need to test other antibody species or antibody fragments the matrix layout is useful to optimize the new assay in the same format.
3. Always use the 0 nM antigen injection and double reference the data, especially for the analysis of antibody–antigen interactions with high complex stabilities ($k_d$ = 1E−5 1/s and $t_{1/2\ \mathrm{diss}}$ = 1,155 min). Like in Fig. 4, one needs to avoid positively drifting dissociation rates. The dissociation rate fitting quality can be improved by increasing the dissociation times. However, consider that such will extend the assay run time.
4. The temperature interval between 17 and 37°C in steps of +4°C is optimal. Below 13°C, the antibody capture association rates are getting extremely slow and would require prolonged injection time or much higher antibody concentrations. This is valid for the antibody to be captured, as well as for the antigen later on. Of course, it is possible to measure at 4°C and at 40°C. For technical reasons, the run time increases, when one needs to

cool down the instrument to 4°C. At temperatures around 40°C, antibody or antigen stability issues can occur.

5. The overall run time usually takes about 72 h for the testing of three antibodies.
6. The method works well with a Langmuir 1:1 kinetic model fitted with a local or global $R_{MAX}$ calculation. If you cannot fit the sensorgrams to a 1:1 model, use the shape of the sensorgrams to discuss the kinetic profiles.
7. Sometimes, the interactions change with increasing temperature from Langmuir kinetics into complex kinetics. This could be due to instable or heterogeneous analytes, e.g., temperature-induced oligomerization. Always calculate the Molar Ratio to identify issues with aggregates or oligomers. Molar Ratios MR > 2.5 (oligomers) or MR < 0.1 (loss of functionality) indicate issues with the analytes.
8. Always try to produce sensorgrams with antigen saturation at $R_{MAX}$. Therefore use up to 300 nM antigen concentration. Try to keep the $R_{MAX}$ values constant over the whole temperature gradient. This is relevant for the correct calculation of the Molar Ratios, which indicate the influence of the temperature on the valence mode of binding.
9. For a fast-track analysis use a two spot measurement at 17 and 37°C. A hypothermic measurement below 25°C and a hyperthermic measurement at 37°C guarantee the classification of the antibodies into one of the three thermodynamic signatures in Fig. 5. This can also be performed in a high throughput mode.
10. It is worthwhile analyzing temperature-dependent antibody kinetics. You can select antibodies with outstanding kinetic properties adapted to their exact field of application.
11. Antibodies with a massive temperature-dependent affinity-decrease due to a lacking temperature-dependent antigen complex stability frequently occur. To investigate to which extent electrostatic forces are driving the interaction you can check the salt-dependency of the interaction. Increase the salt concentration from 150 mM NaCl to up to 1 M NaCl and check whether $k_a$ slows down. A negative salt effect can decrease $k_a$ by a factor of 4–5 (11).
12. "I tested my antibody at 25 and 37°C and it had the same affinity" does not contain any information unless the kinetic rates are dissolved. An antibody with a rate signature like depicted in Fig. 5 (open circles) shows low complex stability at 37°C, despite constant affinity $K_D$.
13. It is recommended to deselect antibodies, which show a two or more orders of magnitude acceleration of $k_a$ in the temperature gradient 17–37°C. Such a temperature signature is a clear evidence for a highly entropy-burdened interaction (5, 8, 10).

## References

1. Leonard P, Hayes CJ, O'Kennedy R (2011) Rapid temperature-dependent antibody ranking using Biacore A100. Anal Biochem 409: 290–292
2. Roos H, Karlsson R, Nilshans H et al (1998) Thermodynamic analysis of protein interactions with biosensor technology. J Mol Recognit 11: 204–210
3. Young L, Jernigan RL, Covell DG (1994) A role for surface hydrophobicity in protein–protein recognition. Protein Sci 3:717–729
4. Willcox BE, Gao GF, Wyer JR et al (1999) TCR binding to peptide-MHC stabilizes a flexible recognition interface. Immunity 10:357–365
5. Gabdoulline RR, Wade RC (2001) Protein-protein association: investigation of factors influencing association rates by brownian dynamics simulations. J Mol Biol 306:1139–1155
6. Wang Y, Shen BJ, Sebald W (1997) A mixed-charge pair in human interleukin 4 dominates high-affinity interaction with the receptor alpha chain. Proc Natl Acad Sci U S A 94:1657–1662
7. Stites WE (1997) Proteinminus signProtein interactions: interface structure, binding thermodynamics, and mutational analysis. Chem Rev 97:1233–1250
8. Selzer T, Schreiber G (1999) Predicting the rate enhancement of protein complex formation from the electrostatic energy of interaction. J Mol Biol 287:409–419
9. Sinha N, Smith-Gill SJ (2002) Electrostatics in protein binding and function. Curr Protein Pept Sci 3:601–614
10. Zeder-Lutz G, Zuber E, Witz J et al (1997) Thermodynamic analysis of antigen–antibody binding using biosensor measurements at different temperatures. Anal Biochem 246: 123–132
11. Pasqualucci L, Guglielmino R, Houldsworth J et al (2004) Expression of the AID protein in normal and neoplastic B cells. Blood 104: 3318–3325
12. Torres M, Fernandez-Fuentes N, Fiser A et al (2007) Exchanging murine and human immunoglobulin constant chains affects the kinetics and thermodynamics of antigen binding and chimeric antibody autoreactivity. PLoS One 2:e1310

# Chapter 13

# Determination of Antibody Glycosylation by Mass Spectrometry

**Christiane Jäger, Claudia Ferrara, Pablo Umaña, Anne Zeck, Jörg Thomas Regula, and Hans Koll**

## Abstract

Immunoglobulin (Ig) G is formed by two antigen-binding moieties termed Fabs and a conserved Fc portion, which interacts with components of the immune systems. Within the Fc, N-linked carbohydrates are attached to each conserved asparagine residue at position 297 within the CH2 domain. These oligosaccharide moieties introduce a higher degree of heterogeneity within the molecule, by influencing stability of the antibody and its mediated effector functions, such as antibody-dependent cellular cytotoxicity and complement-dependent cytotoxicity (CDC).

The carbohydrate moieties can vary strongly depending on the production host and can be manipulated by different fermentation conditions, thereby influencing the function of the antibody. Therefore it is necessary to carefully monitor changes in the carbohydrate composition during cell line development and production processes. This chapter describes two different mass spectrometry based methods used for analyses of the carbohydrate moieties attached to the Fc-part of human IgG1. In the first approach, the glycans are released from the antibody by endoglycosidase (Peptide N Glycosidase F) digestion and monitored by matrix-assisted laser desorption ionization-time-of-flight mass spectrometry (MS), whereas in the second method the carbohydrate structures, still attached to an enzymatically produced Fc-fragment, are analyzed by electrospray ionization mass spectrometry.

**Key words:** N-linked glycosylation, MALDI-TOF, LC-MS, ESI-MS, IdeS, IgG, PNGase F, Endoglycosidase

## 1. Introduction

Carbohydrate structures attached to the conserved N-glycosylation site at asparagine 297 (Asn297) within the CH2-domain of the heavy chain of an immunoglobulin are influencing structure, stability, and biological activity of recombinant monoclonal antibodies (1–4).

These oligosaccharides are generally heterogeneous. The natural compositions are predominantly biantennary (biant) complex-type

Gabriele Proetzel and Hilmar Ebersbach (eds.), *Antibody Methods and Protocols*, Methods in Molecular Biology, vol. 901, DOI 10.1007/978-1-61779-931-0_13, © Springer Science+Business Media, LLC 2012

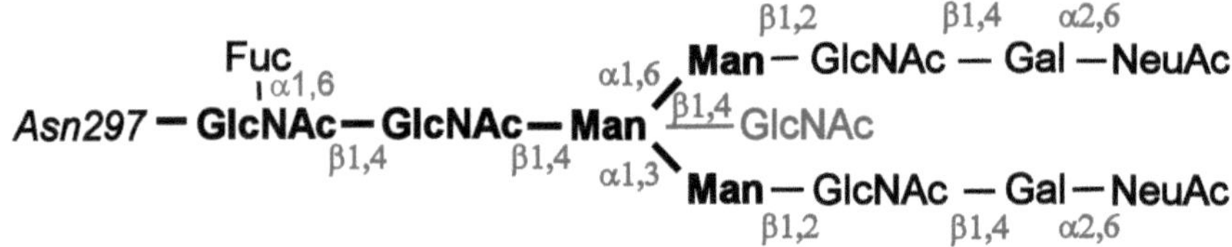


Fig. 1. Carbohydrate moiety attached to Asn-297 of human IgG1-Fc. The sugars in *bold* define the pentasaccharide core; the addition of the other sugar residues is variable. *GlcNAc N*-acetylglucosamine, *Fuc* fucose, *Man* mannose, *Gal* galactose, *NeuAc N*-acetylneuraminic acid.

structures varying in the content of bisecting *N*-acetylglucosamine (GlcNAc), terminal galactoses, core fucose, and sialic acids. The major heterogeneity is introduced by incomplete processing of the terminal galactose residues resulting in structures carrying two (G2), one (G1), or no (G0) galactose residues (Fig. 1) (5). Additionally, the presence of oligomannose and hybrid-type glycoforms is described in some cases (6).

Various studies have shown that the composition of carbohydrates strongly affects the antibody-mediated immune effector functions (3, 4, 7). Low level of galactosylation positively affects complement activation, whereas the lack of core fucose results in higher affinity to Fc gamma receptor IIIa (FcγRIIIa) and thereby enhances antibody-dependent cellular cytotoxicity (ADCC) (7–9). Several approaches have been developed to manipulate the glycosylation profile to generate therapeutic antibodies with improved biological functions (10–12). Besides directly engineering the carbohydrate profile of an antibody, glycosylation can also vary depending on the production host cell line, during clone selection and is affected by different cultivation conditions (13–15). As the carbohydrate composition can be affected by all these factors, it is essential to monitor and characterize the glycan moieties of recombinant immunoglobulin in detail, thereby ensuring product consistency, as well as understand the relationship between glycan structure and function.

Several methods have been described for detailed characterization of the glycosylation profile of human IgGs, e.g., analysis of enzymatically released and fluorescence-labeled carbohydrates by capillary electrophoreses or HPLC, or oligosaccharide profiling by HPAEC/PAD (5, 16). Mass spectrometry based methods are also commonly used to characterize the glycan structures attached to human IgGs (5, 17–22).

Using matrix-assisted laser desorption ionization-time-of-flight mass spectrometry (MALDI-TOF MS) biomolecules such as proteins, peptides, and oligosaccharides embedded in a UV light-absorbing matrix are irradiated by a laser pulse. Since most of the laser energy is absorbed by the matrix, unwanted fragmentation of the sample is prevented. The ionized samples are accelerated in an electric field and enter the flight tube, where they are separated according to their mass-to-charge (*m/z*) ratio (23). MALDI-TOF MS can be used for in-depth characterization and relative quantitation of neutral oligosaccharides, to a concentration level of 50–80 fM, released by Peptide N Glycosidase F (PNGase F) from glycosylated IgG1 (19).

Electrospray ionization mass spectrometry (ESI-MS) is another type of mass spectrometry widely used to characterize proteins like IgGs and their glycosylation profiles (24–26). For desalting of samples prior analysis by ESI-MS, automated sample analysis or analytically separation of individual isoforms, the mass spectrometer is often coupled to reversed-phase liquid chromatography (LC). LC-coupled ESI-MS is also a fast and effective analytical tool for the evaluation of the glyco pattern, with the carbohydrates still attached to the polypeptide chain. Resolution of modern ESI-MS instruments [>10,000 full width half maximum (FWHM)] is well suited to separate individual glycan species even when linked to an intact protein like the heavy chain of an IgG or the Fc-fragment. An obstacle, however, is the presence of potential heterogeneities in the protein part, like oxidation, C-terminal lysine heterogeneity, or N-terminal pyroglutamic acid formation, which may interfere with the mass of individual glycan structures, thereby requiring complex data interpretation.

To reduce the heterogeneity related to the protein part in the analysis of Fc-associated glycans and to make optimal use of the MS instrument's resolution, enzymatic pretreatment is the method of choice. The immunoglobulin G degrading enzyme S (IdeS) of *S. pyogenes* cleaves an IgG highly specific, resulting in a defined Fc-fragment lacking the Fab moiety (27, 28). The heterogeneity of such glycosylated Fc-fragments is further reduced by combining IdeS digestion with carboxypeptidase B (CpB), an enzyme removing the C-terminal lysine. The LC-MS analysis of such prepared glycosylated Fc-fragments can be easily performed with a total of 20 pmol of antibody and even less.

## 2. Materials

### *2.1. Release of N-Linked Oligosaccharides*

1. Centrifugal filter units with 5,000 Da molecular weight cut off (MWCO) (Millipore, Billerica, MA, USA).
2. 2 mM Tris–Base solution in analytical-grade water, adjust pH to 7.0 using HCl (Sigma-Aldrich, St. Louis, MO, USA).
3. PNGase F, at a concentration of 5 U/mL (cat. no. E-PNG05, QA-Bio, Palm Desert, CA, USA).
4. Empty spin chromatography columns (Micro Bio-Spin, Bio-Rad Laboratories, Hercules, CA, USA).
5. Cation exchange resin (AG 50W-X8, Bio-Rad Laboratories).

### 2.2. MALDI-TOF Mass Spectrometry

1. DHB (2,5-dihydroxybenzoic acid) (Bruker, Billerica, MA, USA).
2. 10 mM NaCl solution in analytical-grade water (Sigma-Aldrich).
3. Ethanol, HPLC gradient grade (Carl Roth GmbH, Karlsruhe, Germany).
4. Microtiter MTP target plate ground steel TF (MTP) (Bruker).
5. Bruker autoFlex MALDI-TOF mass spectrometer (Bruker).

### 2.3. Fragmentation of Human IgG

1. Formic acid solution (1%v/v): Add 1 mL formic acid p.a. to 99 mL analytical-grade water.
2. Digestion buffer: 50 mM Tris–Base (e.g., Merck) in analytical-grade water, adjust pH to 8.0 using HCl p.a.
3. CpB stock solution: 5 mg/mL (cat. no. 10103233001, Roche, Penzberg, Germany).
4. CpB working solution (1 mg/mL): Add 4 volumes of digestion buffer to 1 volume of CpB stock solution.
5. IdeS stock solution: 66 U/μL (reconstituted FabRICATOR lyophilisate) (cat. no. A0-FR1-020, Genovis, Lund, Sweden).
6. IdeS working solution (22 U/μL): Add 2 volumes of digestion buffer to 1 volume of IdeS stock solution.
7. NanoSep centrifugal filter units with 10,000 Da MWCO (e.g., Pall Life Sciences, Port Washington, NY, USA).

### 2.4. LC-MS Analysis

1. Eppendorf bench top centrifuge.
2. Eluent A: 0.1%v/v formic acid in Type 2 analytical-grade water (LC-MS Chromasolv) (Fluka, Buchs, Switzerland or Sigma-Aldrich).
3. Eluent B: 0.1%v/v formic acid in acetonitrile (LC-MS Chromasolv) (Fluka).
4. HPLC sample vials: 300 μL (Chromacol, Welwyn Garden City, UK, or Thermo Fisher Scientific, Waltham, MA, USA).
5. RP column: ACE-213-0202, C4, 2.1 mm × 20 mm, 3 μm, 300 Å [Advanced Chromatography Technologies (ACT), Aberdeen, UK].
6. HPLC instrument capable of micro flow rates of about 200 μL/min.
7. Renin peptide: 10 pmol/μL [Applied Biosystems part no. 4405239, Life Technologies (ABI), Carlsbad, CA, USA].
8. MTP sample plate (cat. no. 1002611, Advion, Ithaca, NY, USA).
9. TriVersa NanoMate System (Advion).

10. Electrospray Ionization Quadrupole-Time-of-Flight (ESI-Q-ToF) mass spectrometer (e.g., Q-Star Elite) (Applied Biosystems, Life Technologies).
11. Data acquisition software: e.g., Analyst software in case of Q-Star Elite (Applied Biosystems, Life Technologies).

## 3. Methods

### 3.1. Release of N-Linked Oligosaccharides from Human IgG

1. 10–50 μg purified protein samples are prepared by buffer exchange at least two times into 2 mM Tris–HCl, pH 7.0 using a centrifugal filter unit with 5,000 Da MWCO. Concentrate samples to a final volume of 25 μL.
2. Oligosaccharides are enzymatically released by PNGase F digestion at 0.05 mU/mg protein in 2 mM Tris, pH 7.0 for at least 3 h at 37°C.
3. Acetic acid is added to final concentration of 150 mM followed by incubation for 1 h at room temperature (19).

#### 3.1.1. Optional: Desalting on Cation-Exchange Resin

High concentrations of salt might disturb the crystallization procedure. Therefore cleanup of carbohydrates after PNGase F treatment is recommended (see Note 2). Here carbohydrate cleanup using ion exchange chromatography is described (20).

1. 5 g Cation exchange resin is rinsed four times in eightfold excess analytical-grade water and finally suspended in 5 mL water.
2. 900 μL of the suspension is packed into a micro-bio-spin chromatography column and centrifuged twice for 30 s at 1,000 × *g*.
3. The digest is loaded onto the column and purified by centrifugation at 1,000 × *g* for 1 min.

### 3.2. Matrix-Assisted Laser Desorption Ionization-Time-of-Flight Mass Spectrometry

1. 80 mg DHB is dissolved in 2 mL ethanol (HPLC gradient grade).
2. Aliquots of 25 μL are prepared, dried under vacuum, and stored until usage at 20°C.
3. One aliquot of the vacuum-dried DHB is dissolved by adding 125 μL 10 mM NaCl solution, which is the matrix for positive ion mode.
4. 0.5 μL of the protein sample prepared in Subheading 3.1 is mixed with 0.5 μL matrix and applied on the MTP target plate (see Note 1).
5. Samples are air-dried.

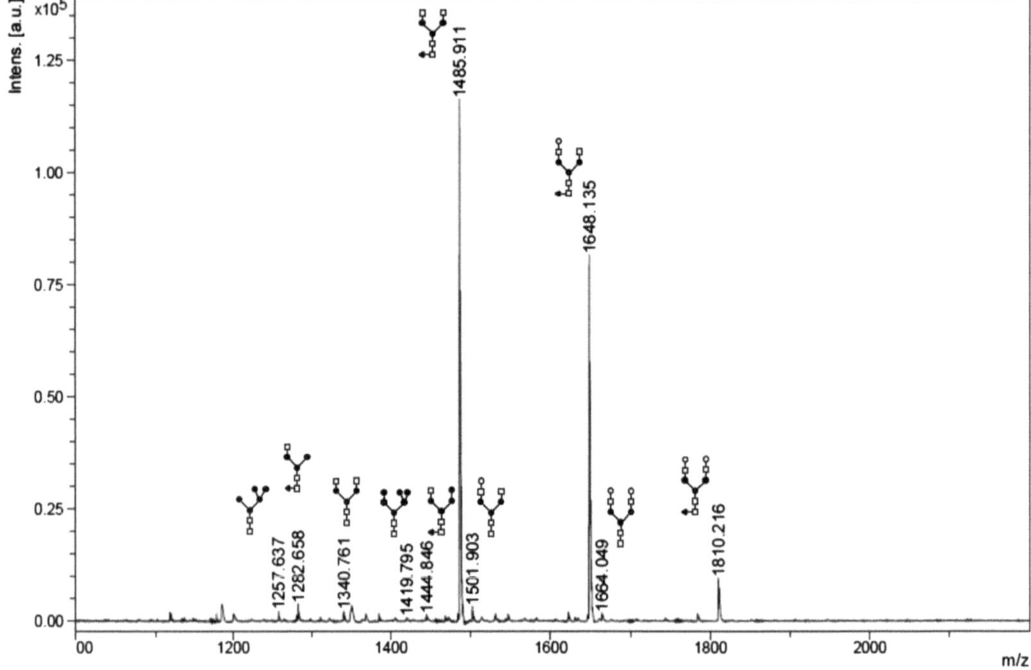


Fig. 2. Positive-ion MALDI-TOF mass spectra of the N-linked oligosaccharides released from recombinant IgG produced in CHO. Carbohydrate structures corresponding to the respective *m/z* peak are shown. *Square* GlcNAc, *filled circle* Man, *open circle* Gal, *filled left-pointing pointer* Fuc.

6. Mass spectra are acquired in positive ion mode. Ions are accelerated to 20 kV after an 80-ns delay. Spectra are acquired in a range between 1,000 and 2,220 *m/z* (see Note 3).
7. Spectra from 500 to 1,000 laser shots are summed to obtain the final spectrum.
8. For evaluation and quantification the relative percentage of the single peak height compared to the total sum of the intensity of each peak is determined (Fig. 2; Table 1, see Notes 4–6).

### 3.3. Fragmentation of Human IgG Using IdeS and Carboxypeptidase B

1. Dilute 25 µg purified IgG into 50 µL digestion buffer. Antibody solutions >1 mg/mL can be diluted directly into digestion buffer; antibody solutions <1 mg/mL need to be concentrated to >1 mg/mL using a NanoSep centrifugal filter unit of 10,000 Da MWCO.
2. Add 1.5 µL IdeS working solution and incubate for 2.5 h at 37°C.
3. Add 2 µL CpB working solution and incubate for another 30 min at 37°C.
4. Stop the enzymatic reactions by adding 50 µL 1%v/v formic acid.

**Table 1**
**Distribution of the neutral, Fc-associated oligosaccharides of human IgG1 determined by MALDI-TOF MS in positive ion mode**

| *m/z* | Symbol | Relative percentage (%) |
|---|---|---|
| 1,257 | 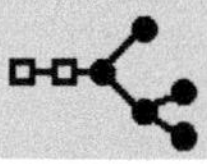 | 0.98 |
| 1,282 | 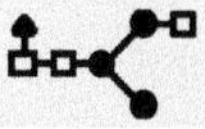 | 1.70 |
| 1,340 | 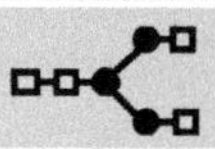 | 1.00 |
| 1,419 | 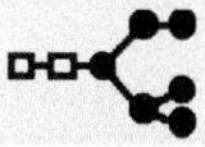 | 0.32 |
| 1,444 | 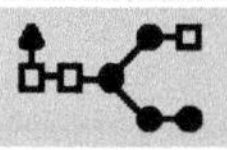 | 0.64 |
| 1,485 | 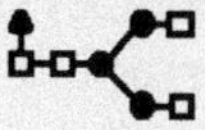 | 52.10 |
| 1,501 | 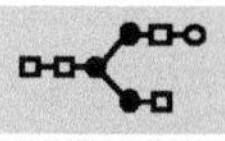 | 1.46 |
| 1,648 | 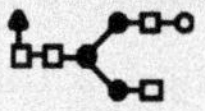 | 36.60 |
| 1,664 | 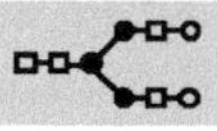 | 0.80 |
| 1,810 | 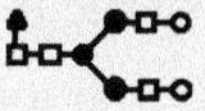 | 4.32 |

Carbohydrate structures corresponding to the respective *m/z* are shown. *Square* GlcNAc, *filled circle* Man, *open circle* Gal, *filled left-pointing pointer* Fuc

**3.4. LC-MS Analyses of the Fc-Fragment**

1. Centrifuge samples obtained in Subheading 3.3 for 5 min at 9,000 × *g* and transfer supernatant into HPLC sample vials.
2. Assemble the ACE-213-0202 column into the HPLC instrument, warm up the column to 75°C, and subsequently equilibrate with 5% eluent B at a flow rate of 200 μL/min until baseline and pressure value are constant.
3. Calibrate the MS instrument using the renin peptide according to manufacturer's instructions for accuracy, resolution, and sensitivity (see Notes 7 and 8).
4. Connect the outlet capillary of the HPLC to the TriVersa NanoMatc interface and induce a spray by applying 1.7 kV at the nozzle at a flow rate of 200 μL/min, splitting 500 nL/min into the mass spectrometer using a post-column splitter (T-fitting) (see Note 9).

**Table 2**
**Parameters of the MS instrument (here Q-Star ELITE) optimized for data acquisition**

| Parameter | Value |
|---|---|
| Polarity | Positive mode |
| Spray voltage | 1.7 kV |
| Declustering potential | ~50 |
| Focusing potential | ~200 |
| ToF *m/z* range | 800–2,000 |

5. For data acquisition run the mass spectrometer according to manufacturer's instructions with parameters optimized as listed in Table 2 (see Note 10).
6. Inject 10 μL of each sample onto the ACE-213-0202 column and separate into Fc- and $F(ab')_2$-fragments using an 11-min gradient as specified in Table 3. Run a blank sample (eluent A) at the beginning of the sequence and subsequent of each protein sample (see Note 11).
7. For the first 2 min of the gradient direct the eluate from the HPLC into the waste. Then direct ~500 nL/min into the ESI-ToF mass spectrometer using a post-column splitter (T-fitting) and record the ion current.
8. A typical total ion current chromatogram (TIC) representing the eluted antibody fragments from the RP column is shown in Fig. 3. Peak 1 consists of the glycosylated Fc-fragment. Upon IdeS digestion the interchain disulfide bridges within the hinge region of the IgG1 are not any longer connecting the Fc-part, thus the Fc-fragment elutes in the monomeric form under the conditions applied for RP-LC. Peak 2 represents the $F(ab')_2$-fragment held together by the hinge disulfide bridges. Due to the defined mass range of 600–2,000 *m/z*, peak 1 should be the highest peak in the TIC.
9. For data analysis of individual oligosaccharide species attached to the Fc-fragment, convert the MS raw data into a data format suited for further evaluation with an appropriate software tool. Here, an in-house developed software tool supporting peak assignment and relative quantitation from the *m/z* signal series instead of deconvoluted data is used (see Note 6).
10. Create a combined spectrum from TIC peak 1 representing the glycosylated Fc-fragment in order to generate the *m/z* peak series of individual Fc-fragments containing distinct glycan structures (Fig. 4). Figure 4 illustrates a single *m/z* charge

**Table 3**
**Gradient applied for LC separation of Fc-fragment and F(ab)′$_2$-fragment**

| Time (min) | Eluent A (%) | Eluent B (%) |
|---|---|---|
| 0 | 95 | 5 |
| 0.5 | 95 | 5 |
| 0.51 | 85 | 15 |
| 7 | 50 | 50 |
| 7.5 | 0 | 100 |
| 8 | 95 | 5 |
| 8.75 | 0 | 100 |
| 9.0 | 0 | 100 |
| 9.5 | 95 | 5 |
| 10.0 | 0 | 100 |
| 10.25 | 95 | 5 |
| 11 | 95 | 5 |

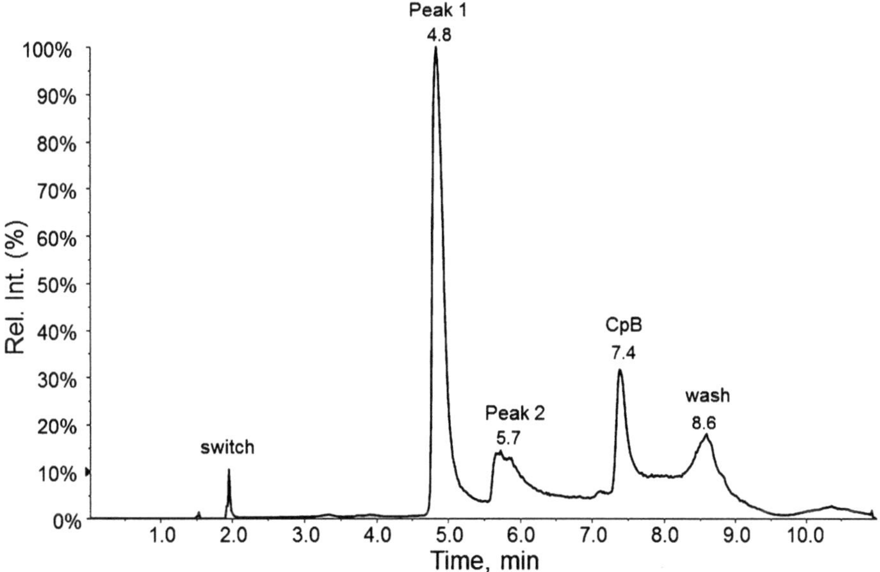


Fig. 3. Total ion chromatogram of the IdeS- and Carboxypeptidase B-treated IgG1 separated by RP-HPLC and detected by ESI-MS. *Peak 1* indicates the glycosylated Fc-fragment, *peak 2* is the F(ab)′$_2$-fragment. Additional peaks are marked: (1) switch, point where the eluate is directed into the waste by splitting 0.25% into the MS instrument; (2) CpB, its elution; and (3) wash, of the column.

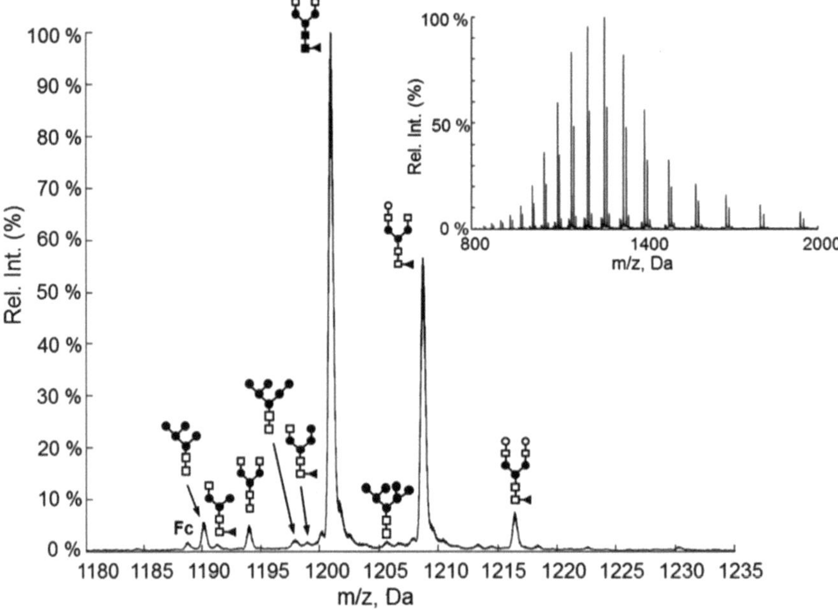


Fig. 4. Single *m/z* charge state of the glycosylated Fc-fragment detected by ESI-MS in the positive mode zoomed from the combined *m/z* spectrum (see *insert*). Each assigned peak represents an individual glycan species attached to the Fc-fragment. Carbohydrate structures corresponding to the respective *m/z* peaks are shown. The *insert* illustrates the combined spectrum representing the complete envelope of *m/z* peak series for all glycosylated Fc-fragments contained in *peak 1* of the TIC (see Fig. 3). *Square* GlcNAc, *filled circle* Man, *open circle* Gal, *filled left-pointing pointer* Fuc.

state of the glycosylated Fc-fragment. Each peak assigned represents an individual glycan species attached to the Fc-fragment.

11. Individual peak series are assigned to specific glycans attached by comparing the experimental $m/z$ peak series with theoretically calculated $m/z$ series expected for distinct glycan structures linked to the Fc-fragment.

12. Relative quantitation of the glycan structures at the Fc-fragments is also performed at the level of $m/z$ peak series (see Table 4). The relative ratios of peak areas of all $m/z$ peak series representing glycosylated Fc-fragments are calculated. The sum of all $m/z$ peak series representing glycosylated Fc-fragments is 100%.

## 4. Notes

1. Sample amount for MALDI-TOF MS analyses must be between 10 and 50 μg. Protein amount higher than 50 μg might disturb the crystallization process of the matrix with oligosaccharides.

**Table 4**
**Oligosaccharide distribution of the neutral Fc-associated glycans of human IgG1 determined by LC-ESI-MS**

| Fc-fragment plus | Symbol | Relative percentage (%) |
|---|---|---|
| Man5 w/oFuc | 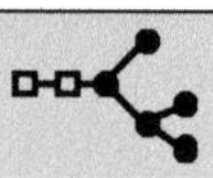 | 3.5 |
| Man3+ GlcNAc w/ Fuc | 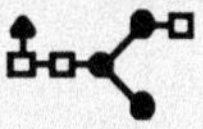 | <1 |
| Biant Gal0 w/oFuc | 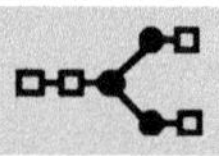 | 2.4 |
| Man6 w/oFuc | 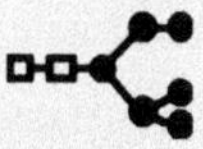 | ~1 |
| Man4+GlcNAc w/Fuc | 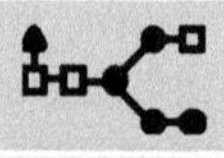 | <1 |
| Biant Gal0 w/Fuc | 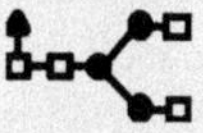 | 55 |
| Man7 w/oFuc | 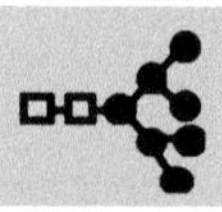 | <1 |
| Biant Gal1 w/Fuc | 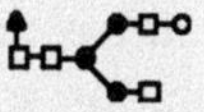 | 31.7 |
| Biant Gal2 w/Fuc | 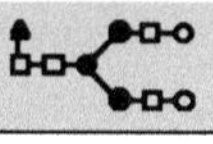 | 4.7 |

Carbohydrate structures corresponding to the respective *m/z* are shown. *Square* GlcNAc, *filled circle* Man, *open circle* Gal, *filled left-pointing pointer* Fuc, *Biant* biantennary

This can be prevented by varying the ratio between matrix and sample, but optimization is required.

2. High concentrations of salt (e.g., NaCl, CaCl2, KH2PO4), detergents (e.g., Tween, Triton, SDS), urea, guanidine, DMSO or glycerol disturb the crystallization process. It is necessary to clean up the samples by ion exchange, RP-HPLC, Zip-Tips, or dialyses prior to PNGase F digest.
3. Impurities like polyethylene glycol (PEG) appear in the MALDI-TOF spectra between 1,000 and 1,800 *m/z*. They might be removed by RP-HPLC treatment of the samples.
4. Recombinant antibody preparations typically contain only low amount of sialic acids (29, 30). Carbohydrate structures carrying sialic acids will not appear in the MALDI-TOF spectrum in positive ion mode. To remove sialic acids, treatment with sialidase following manufacturer's instructions prior to PNGase F treatment is recommended (10).

5. Analysis of sialic acid content in negative ion mode using MALDI-TOF is not described in this chapter (19).
6. Limitations to both approaches described in this chapter are isobaric structures of various glycans, like some hybrid- and complex-type structures. To assign the peaks to the respective structure, combinatory treatment using PNGase F and exoglycosidases or endoglycosidases such as Endo H is recommended (11). For the ESI-MS approach isobaric species resulting from a protein modification like oxidation could occur. For example, an Fc-fragment with a biantennary, complex G1 glycan lacking core fucose is isobaric to an oxidized Fc-fragment with a biantennary, complex G0 glycan with core fucose. In such cases an additional analysis of the PNGase F-treated Fc-fragment is recommended.
7. The mass spectrometer (here the Q-star Elite) is calibrated by off-line infusion using the TriVersa NanoMate for sample application according to manufacturer's instructions of theinstruments. For this, 40 μL of the renin peptide are pipetted in a well of the MTP sample plate and placed in the TriVersa NanoMate. Before calibration is started, spray conditions are defined and spray stability is controlled according to manufacturer's instructions. Solvent spray is accepted as stable when current deviations are within ±20 nA, and typical spray current value is >50 nA. Calibration is performed by spraying the calibration solution off-line at conditions inducing fragmentation of the peptide used. The average of ten scans with an intensity of $6e^4$–$5e^5$ counts is used for calibration. Calibration is successful, when predefined specifications for mass accuracy, resolution at FWHM, and intensity are met.
8. Resolution of ESI-MS-instrument should be at least above 10,000 FWHM. In order to resolve also minor differences like the presence of fucose vs. galactose/glucose ($\Delta m$ 16 Da) in a glycan attached to the protein, a resolution of 15,000 FWHM and above is recommended.
9. Stability of the spray is given, if the current (70–120 nA) is constant for about 1–2 min.
10. Parameters for data acquisition: The MS settings have to be specifically defined for the instrument used. In addition for measurement of intact proteins (e.g., Fc-fragment) special attention has to be turned on (1) a high signal intensity for intact proteins (>10 kDa); (2) good solvation conditions; and (3) avoidance of protein fragmentation by, e.g., source fragmentation.
11. The blank sample subsequent to each protein sample is introduced to ensure that no carryover effect occurs. For samples not prone to carryover, this can be omitted.

## References


1. Wright A, Morrison SL (1997) Effect of glycosylation on antibody function: implications for genetic engineering. Trends Biotechnol 15: 26–32
2. Krapp S et al (2003) Structural analysis of human IgG-Fc glycoforms reveals a correlation between glycosylation and structural integrity. J Mol Biol 325:979–989
3. Raju TS (2008) Terminal sugars of Fc glycans influence antibody effector functions of IgGs. Curr Opin Immunol 20:471–478
4. Jefferis R (2009) Recombinant antibody therapeutics: the impact of glycosylation on mechanisms of action. Trends Pharmacol Sci 30: 356–362
5. Huhn C et al (2009) IgG glycosylation analysis. Proteomics 9:882–913
6. Jefferis R (2007) Antibody therapeutics: isotype and glycoform selection. Expert Opin Biol Ther 9:1401–1413
7. Hodoniczky J, Zheng YZ, James DC (2005) Control of recombinant monoclonal antibody effector functions by Fc N-glycan remodeling in vitro. Biotechnol Prog 21:1644–1652
8. Malhotra R et al (1995) Glycosylation changes of IgG associated with rheumatoid arthritis can activate complement via the mannose-binding protein. Nat Med 3:237–243
9. Shields RL et al (2002) Lack of fucose on human IgG1 N-linked oligosaccharide improves binding to human Fcgamma RIII and antibody-dependent cellular toxicity. J Biol Chem 277:26733–26740
10. Umana P et al (1999) Engineered glycoforms of an antineuroblastoma IgG1 with optimized antibody-dependent cellular cytotoxic activity. Nat Biotechnol 17:176–180
11. Ferrara C et al (2006) Modulation of therapeutic antibody effector functions by glycosylation engineering: influence of Golgi enzyme localization domain and co-expression of heterologous beta1, 4-*N*-acetylglucosaminyltransferase III and Golgi alpha-mannosidase II. Biotechnol Bioeng 93:851–861
12. Kanda Y et al (2006) Comparison of biological activity among nonfucosylated therapeutic IgG1 antibodies with three different N-linked Fc oligosaccharides: the high-mannose, hybrid, and complex types. Glycobiology 17:104–118
13. Kunkel JP et al (1998) Dissolved oxygen concentration in serum-free continuous culture affects N-linked glycosylation of a monoclonal antibody. J Biotechnol 62:55–71
14. Baker KN et al (2001) Metabolic control of recombinant protein N-glycan processing in NS0 and CHO cells. Biotechnol Bioeng 73: 188–202
15. Hills A et al (2001) Metabolic control of recombinant monoclonal antibody N-glycosylation in GS-NS0 cells. Biotechnol Bioeng 75:239–251
16. Weithandler M et al (1994) Analysis of carbohydrates on IgG preparations. J Pharm Sci 83: 1670–1675
17. Mock KK, Davey M, Cottrell JS (1991) The analysis of underivatized oligosaccharides by matrix-assisted laser desorption mass spectrometry. Biochem Biophys Res Commun 177: 644–651
18. Huberty MC et al (1993) Site-specific carbohydrate identification in recombinant proteins using MALD-TOF MS. Anal Chem 65: 2791–2800
19. Papac DI, Wong A, Jones AJ (1996) Analysis of acidic oligosaccharides and glycopeptides by matrix-assisted laser desorption/ionization time-of-flight mass spectrometry. Anal Chem 68:3215–3223
20. Papac DI et al (1998) A high-throughput microscale method to release N-linked oligosaccharides from glycoproteins for matrix-assisted laser desorption/ionization time-of-flight mass spectrometric analysis. Glycobiology 8:445–454
21. Sinha S et al (2008) Comparison of LC and LC/MS methods for quantifying N-glycosylation in recombinant IgGs. J Am Soc Mass Spectrom 19:1643–1654
22. Karg SR et al (2009) A small-scale method for the preparation of plant N-linked glycans from soluble proteins for analysis by MALDI-TOF mass spectrometry. Plant Physiol Biochem 47: 160–166
23. Schiller J et al (2004) Matrix-assisted laser desorption and ionization time-of-flight (MALDI-TOF) mass spectrometry in lipid and phospholipid research. Prog Lipid Res 43:449–488
24. Dillon TM et al (2004) Development of an analytical reversed-phase high-performance liquid chromatography-electrospray ionization mass spectrometry method for characterization of recombinant antibodies. J Chromatogr A 1053:299–305
25. Yan B et al (2007) Analysis of post-translational modifications in recombinant monoclonal antibody IgG1 by reversed-phase liquid chromatography/mass spectrometry. J Chromatogr A 1164:153–161
26. Lim A et al (2008) Glycosylation profiling of a therapeutic recombinant monoclonal antibody

with two N-linked glycosylation sites using liquid chromatography coupled to a hybrid quadrupole time-of-flight mass spectrometer. Anal Biochem 375:163–172

27. Von Pawel-Rammingen U et al (2002) IdeS, a novel streptococcal cysteine proteinase with unique specificity for immunoglobulin G. EMBO J 21:1607–1615
28. Chevreux G et al (2011) Fast analysis of recombinant monoclonal antibodies using IdeS proteoloytic digestion and electrospray mass spectrometry. Anal Biochem 415:212–214
29. Boyd PN, Lines AC, Patel AK (1995) The effect of the removal of sialic acid, galactose and total carbohydrate on the functional activity of Campath-1H. Mol Immunol 32:1311–1318
30. Scallon BJ et al (2007) Higher levels of sialylated Fc glycans in immunoglobulin G molecules can adversely impact functionality. Mol Immunol 44:1524–1534

# Chapter 14

# Cloning, Expression, and Purification of Monoclonal Antibodies in scFv-Fc Format

**Jiahui Yang and Christoph Rader**

## Abstract

This protocol describes the generation of monoclonal antibodies in single-chain variable fragment (scFv)-Fc format. It includes the cloning of the scFv-Fc expression cassette into a mammalian expression vector followed by transient transfection of mammalian cells and purification by protein A affinity chromatography. The protocol is intended for applications in basic and preclinical research that require rapid access to milligram amounts of protein.

**Key words:** Monoclonal antibodies, scFv-Fc format, Hemagglutinin tag, FreeStyle 293F cells, Protein A affinity chromatography

## 1. Introduction

The success of monoclonal antibodies (mAbs) as research reagents and as diagnostic, preventative, and therapeutic drugs in medicine is based on the ability to bind to virtually any molecule of interest with high affinity and specificity. The most common format of mAbs is the natural ~150-kDa IgG molecule which consists of two identical light chains and two identical heavy chains that assemble into a Y-shaped configuration with two Fab arms and one Fc stem. The Fab portion consists of the light chain with variable ($V_L$) and constant ($C_L$) domain and the N-terminal half of the heavy chain with variable ($V_H$) and first constant ($C_H1$) domain. The Fc portion consists of the C-terminal half of the heavy chain with second ($C_H2$) and third ($C_H3$) constant domain. Fab and Fc portions are connected by a hinge region that also stabilizes the four-chain assembly with disulfide bridges. Antibody engineering has been instrumental in the generation of mAbs that deviate from the IgG format, in particular antibody molecules that maintain high affinity

Gabriele Proetzel and Hilmar Ebersbach (eds.), *Antibody Methods and Protocols*, Methods in Molecular Biology, vol. 901, DOI 10.1007/978-1-61779-931-0_14, © Springer Science+Business Media, LLC 2012

and specificity at smaller size and lower complexity (1, 2). For example, the ~25-kDa single-chain variable fragment (scFv) molecule fuses a single $V_L$ and $V_H$ domain through a polypeptide linker and does not contain any constant domains. The smaller size and lower complexity of the scFv format facilitate expression in bacteria and on phage without, in general, compromising high affinity and specificity. Nonetheless, many applications require the presence of the Fc portion through which the antibody molecule acquires extended circulatory half-life and mediates effector functions such as antibody-dependent cellular cytotoxicity (ADCC) and complement-dependent cytotoxicity (CDC). In addition, the presence of an Fc portion permits purification of the antibody molecule by protein A affinity chromatography. The ~110 kDa scFv-Fc format (3) is an antibody molecule that combines the simplicity of the scFv format with the necessity of the Fc portion. In contrast to the IgG molecule, which requires separate light- and heavy-chain expression cassettes on the same or on separate plasmids, the scFv-Fc molecule can be produced from a single expression cassette (Fig. 1) which is easier to clone and typically gives higher protein yields. In addition, the smaller size of the scFv-Fc molecule compared to the conventional IgG molecule may be advantageous for penetrating tissues in vivo and for binding to recessed epitopes on cell surface antigens. Several mAbs in scFv-Fc format, also referred

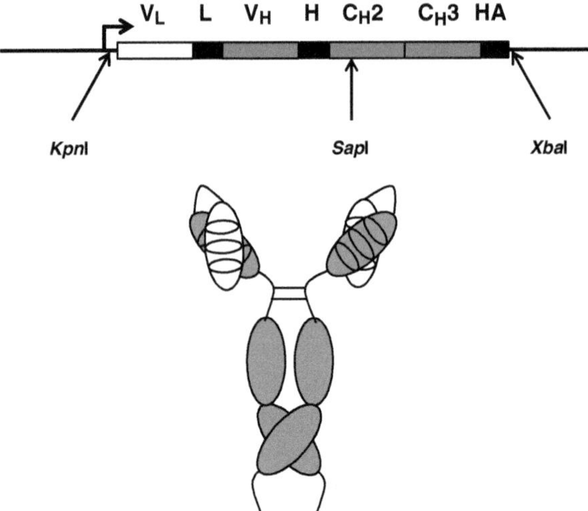


Fig. 1. Expression cassette of pCEP4/scFv-Fc-HA. The variable domain of the light chain ($V_L$) is show in *white*. The variable domain ($V_H$), second constant domain ($C_H2$), and third constant domain ($C_H3$) of the heavy chain are shown in *gray*. Linker (L), hinge (H), and hemagglutinin (HA) tag are shown in *black*. The positions of *Kpn*I, *Sap*I, and *Xho*I restriction sites used for cloning are indicated. Pointed out in the homodimeric scFv-Fc-HA protein depicted at the bottom are the three complementarity-determining regions (CDRs) of $V_L$ and $V_H$, the linker connecting $V_L$ and $V_H$, the hinge connecting $V_H$ and $C_H2$ with two disulfide bridges stabilizing the homodimer, and the HA tag at the C-terminus.

to as SMIPs for Small Modular ImmunoPharmaceuticals, are currently under preclinical and clinical investigation for the treatment of autoimmune diseases and cancer (4–7). We here provide a protocol for the cloning, expression, and purification of mAbs in scFv-Fc format. We have successfully applied this protocol to the production of scFv-Fc proteins with mouse, rabbit, or human scFv portion fused to a human Fc portion with IgG1 isotype. In addition to these chimeric mouse/human, chimeric rabbit/human, and fully human scFv-Fc proteins, our protocol can be easily adapted to incorporate Fc portions from other species and isotypes or engineered Fc portions that modulate effector functions and circulatory half-life. Whereas our protocol is based on expression in mammalian cells, scFv-Fc proteins have also been expressed in insect (8), yeast (9), and plant (10) cells, as well as in bacteria (11).

The protocol encompasses the cloning of the scFv-Fc expression cassette that encodes a C-terminal hemagglutinin (HA) tag for detection of scFv-Fc-HA protein (Fig. 1). The expression cassette is generated by custom synthesis of scFv-Fc-HA or scFv encoding DNA with flanking *Kpn*I/*Xho*I or *Kpn*I/*Sap*I restriction sites, respectively, and cloning into mammalian expression vector pCEP4. Following transient transfection of a commercially available human embryonic kidney cell line (FreeStyle 293F) adapted to grow in suspension and protein-free medium, scFv-Fc-HA protein is purified from the supernatant by Protein A affinity chromatography. Using this protocol, we reformatted the chimeric mouse/human anti-human CD20 mAb rituximab from IgG1 to scFv-Fc-HA format (Fig. 2). Purified rituximab scFv-Fc-HA (Fig. 3) was recovered with a yield of up to 10 mg/L and was found to be equivalent to rituximab IgG1 with respect to antigen binding (Fig. 4), ADCC, and CDC. Taken together, our protocol provides rapid access to a simplified mAb molecule tailored for applications in basic and preclinical research.

## 2. Materials

All steps in this protocols can be successfully executed in a laboratory with standard molecular and cell biology equipment, including autoclave, digital balance with 0.01-g readability, freezers (−20 and −80°C), incubator (37°C; e.g., VWR Signature General Purpose Incubator, www.vwr.com), shaker (e.g., Innova 4000 Benchtop Incubator Shaker, New Brunswick Scientific, www.nbsc.com), heat blocks, laminar flow hood, light microscope, UV photometer (e.g., Eppendorf BioPhotometer, www.eppendorf.com), liquid nitrogen tank with cryoboxes, microfuge (e.g., Eppendorf 5415D), microwave oven, refrigerated benchtop centrifuge with

```
GGTACCGGCGCGCCACC   17

ATGGACTGGACCTGGCGAATCCTTTTCCTGGTCGCCGCAGCAACAGGGGCCCACTCGCAAATTGTGCTCTCGCAGAGCCCGGCTATTCTCTCCGCCTCGCCTGGT  122
 M  D  W  T  W  R  I  L  F  L  V  A  A  A  T  G  A  H  S  Q  I  V  L  S  Q  S  P  A  I  L  S  A  S  P  G
GAAAAAGTGACAATGACCTGTCGCGCCTCCAGCTCAGTATCGTACATTCACTGGTTCCAACAGAAACCCGGATCATCGCCGAAACCCTGGATCTACGCAACGAGC  227
 E  K  V  T  M  T  C  R  A  S  S  S  V  S  Y  I  H  W  F  Q  Q  K  P  G  S  S  P  K  P  W  I  Y  A  T  S
AATCTGGCGTCGGGAGTCCCGGTGAGATTTTCGGGATCGGGCTCAGGGACCTCATATTCGCTTACTATCTCACGGGTAGAAGCGGAGGATGCCGCGACCTACTAC  332
 N  L  A  S  G  V  P  V  R  F  S  G  S  G  S  G  T  S  Y  S  L  T  I  S  R  V  E  A  E  D  A  A  T  Y  Y
TGCCAACAGTGGACAAGCAATCCCCCAACCTTTGGGGGAGGGACTAAGTTGGAGATCAAAGGGGGAGGCGGGTCAGGAGGGGGTGGATCAGGTGGCGGTGGATCG  437
 C  Q  Q  W  T  S  N  P  P  T  F  G  G  G  T  K  L  E  I  K  G  G  G  G  S  G  G  G  G  S  G  G  G  G  S
CAAGTCCAGTTGCAGCAGCCAGGAGCAGAATTGGTCAAGCCTGGCGCGTCCGTCAAAATGTCATGCAAGGCCTCCGGATATACGTTCACGTCCTACAACATGCAT  542
 Q  V  Q  L  Q  Q  P  G  A  E  L  V  K  P  G  A  S  V  K  M  S  C  K  A  S  G  Y  T  F  T  S  Y  N  M  H
TGGGTGAAACAGACACCGGGACGGGGGTTGGAATGGATCGGGGCGATCTACCCTGGTAACGGAGACACGTCGTATAACCAGAAGTTTAAGGGAAAGGCGACGCTT  647
 W  V  K  Q  T  P  G  R  G  L  E  W  I  G  A  I  Y  P  G  N  G  D  T  S  Y  N  Q  K  F  K  G  K  A  T  L
ACGGCAGATAAGAGCTCGTCGACAGCGTACATGCAGCTGTCCTCGCTCACTTCAGAGGATAGCGCTGTCTACTATTGTGCTAGGTCGACGTACTATGGCGGTGAC  752
 T  A  D  K  S  S  S  T  A  Y  M  Q  L  S  S  L  T  S  E  D  S  A  V  Y  Y  C  A  R  S  T  Y  Y  G  G  D
TGGTACTTCAATGTATGGGGAGCGGGGACTACGGTGACAGTGTCCGCGGAGCCCAAGTCATCGGACAAGACACACACTTGCCCTCCCTGTCCCGCACCGGAATTG  857
 W  Y  F  N  V  W  G  A  G  T  T  V  T  V  S  A  E  P  K  S  S  D  K  T  H  T  C  P  P  C  P  A  P  E  L
CTGGGAGGACCCTCCGTGTTTCTCTTTCCCCCGAAACCCAAGGATACCTTGATGATCTCGCGAACCCCGGAGGTGACGTGTGTGGTAGTAGATGTGTCCCACGAG  962
 L  G  G  P  S  V  F  L  F  P  P  K  P  K  D  T  L  M  I  S  R  T  P  E  V  T  C  V  V  V  D  V  S  H  E
GACCCTGAAGTAAAGTTCAACTGGTATGTGGACGGTGTGGAGGTCCATAACGCGAAAACCAAGCCACGGGAAGAGCAGTACAATTCGACATACAGAGTCGTGTCG 1067
 D  P  E  V  K  F  N  W  Y  V  D  G  V  E  V  H  N  A  K  T  K  P  R  E  E  Q  Y  N  S  T  Y  R  V  V  S
GTCCTTACAGTCCTCCATCAGGACTGGCTTAACGGGAAGGAATACAAGTGCAAAGTATCAAACAAAGCCCTCCCAGCCCCGATTGAAAAGACGATCTCGAAAGCC 1172
 V  L  T  V  L  H  Q  D  W  L  N  G  K  E  Y  K  C  K  V  S  N  K  A  L  P  A  P  I  E  K  T  I  S  K  A
AAAGGACAACCACGCGAGCCGCAAGTCTATACTCTGCCGCCGTCCCGCGACGAACTCACAAAGAATCAGGTGTCCCTCACATGCCTGGTAAAAGGATTCTATCCT 1277
 K  G  Q  P  R  E  P  Q  V  Y  T  L  P  P  S  R  D  E  L  T  K  N  Q  V  S  L  T  C  L  V  K  G  F  Y  P
TCCGATATCGCGGTCGAATGGGAAAGCAATGGTCAGCCGGAGAACAACTACAAAACAACACCGCCGGTGTTGGACTCCGATGGGTCATTCTTTCTCTATTCGAAG 1382
 S  D  I  A  V  E  W  E  S  N  G  Q  P  E  N  N  Y  K  T  T  P  P  V  L  D  S  D  G  S  F  F  L  Y  S  K
CTGACTGTAGACAAGTCCCGCTGGCAGCAAGGCAATGTGTTTTCGTGCTCAGTGATGCATGAGGCCCTGCATAATCACTACACGCAGAAATCACTAAGCTTGTCT 1487
 L  T  V  D  K  S  R  W  Q  Q  G  N  V  F  S  C  S  V  M  H  E  A  L  H  N  H  Y  T  Q  K  S  L  S  L  S
CCGGGTGCTGCTAGCTACCCGTACGACGTTCCGGACTACGCTTCTTGA 1535
 P  G  A  A  S  Y  P  Y  D  V  P  D  Y  A  S  *

CTCGAG 1541
```

Fig. 2. DNA and amino acid sequence of rituximab scFv-Fc-HA. Using custom DNA synthesis, the variable domains of chimeric mouse/human anti-human CD20 mAb rituximab linked with a $(G_4S)_3$ linker were fused to the hinge-$C_H2$-$C_H3$ portion of human IgG1 followed by a C-terminal HA tag. The DNA sequence was custom optimized for expression in human cells. Flanking sequences with *Kpn*I and *Asc*I restriction sites (*bold*) at the 5′ end and *Xho*I restriction site at the 3′ end are shown in *italics*. Internal *Sap*I, *Hin*dIII, and *Nhe*I restriction sites are shown in *bold*. *Underlined* amino acid sequences indicate signal peptide, $(G_4S)_3$ linker, hinge, and HA decapeptide. Note that the amino acid sequence of the hinge (EPKS<u>S</u>DKTHTCPPCP) contains a C-to-S mutation compared to the wild-type hinge (EPKS<u>C</u>DKTHTCPPCP) to remove the cysteine that forms a disulfide bridge with $C_L$ in the IgG1 molecule.

swinging bucket rotor and microplate carriers (e.g., Sorvall Legend RT, Thermo Scientific, www.thermoscientific.com), refrigerated microfuge (e.g., Eppendorf 5417R), refrigerator (4°C), Bunsen burner, water bath, and vortexer. General disposables such as 0.5-, 1.5-mL microfuge tubes, 50-mL centrifuge tubes, filtered 10-μL, 20-μL, 100-μL, 200-μL, 1-mL pipette tips (e.g., ART, Molecular BioProducts, www.mbpinc.com), disposable pipettes, and cell culture flasks are not specially listed.

### 2.1. Cloning of pCEP4/scFv-Fc-HA Plasmid via KpnI and XhoI

1. Glass spreading rod.
2. Razor blades.
3. 14-mL round-bottom tubes with snap caps.
4. 50–2,000-μL UVette disposable single sealed cuvettes (Eppendorf, cat. no. 952010051).
5. Model B1A EasyCast Mini Gel Electrophoresis System with B1A-10 and B1A-6 combs (Owl Separation Systems, www.owlsci.com).
6. EC 105 Compact Power Supply (Owl Separation Systems).

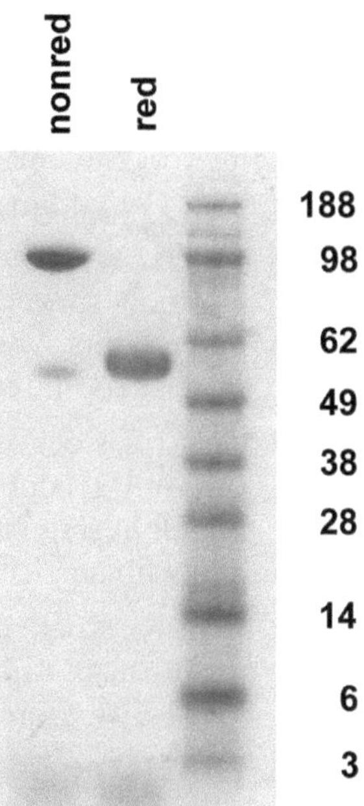


Fig. 3. SDS-PAGE analysis of rituximab scFv-Fc-HA purified by Protein A affinity chromatography. For each lane, 4 μg of protein in NuPAGE LDS Sample Buffer with (*red for reducing*) or without (*nonred for nonreducing*) NuPAGE Sample Reducing Reagent was separated by electrophoresis on a 1.5-mm, 10-well NuPAGE Novex 4–12% Bis-Tris gel using NuPAGE MES SDS Running Buffer followed by staining with SimplyBlue SafeStain based on Coomassie Brilliant Blue G-250 (see Note 22). A molecular weight standard (SeeBlue Plus2 Pre-Stained Standard) is given on the right in kDa. The figure shows that reducing conditions split the ~110-kDa homodimeric scFv-Fc-HA protein into ~55-kDa monomeric scFv-hinge-$C_H2$-$C_H3$-HA polypeptides.

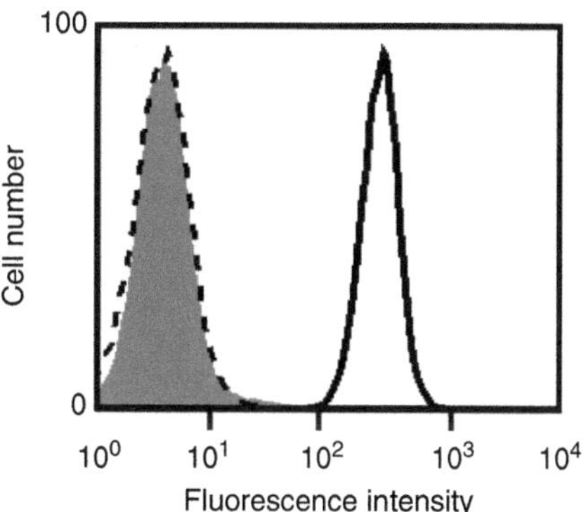


Fig. 4. Flow cytometry analysis of the binding of rituximab scFv-Fc-HA to human cells expressing CD20. Human mantle cell lymphoma cell line HBL-2 was incubated with 1 μg/mL rituximab scFv-Fc-HA (*bold line*), control scFv-Fc-HA (*dashed line*), or no antibody (*gray shade*) for 1 h. After washing twice, the cells were incubated with 5 μg/mL biotinylated rat anti-HA mAb 3F10 for 1 h, washed twice, and incubated with 2 μg/mL Streptavidin–Phycoerythrin for 30 min. For all dilutions and washings, ice-cold 1% (vol/vol) fetal bovine serum in PBS was used, and all incubations were done on ice. Stained cells were analyzed with an FACSCalibur instrument and FlowJo analytical software. The *y*-axis gives the cell number in linear scale and the *x*-axis the fluorescence intensity in logarithmic scale. The figure shows that rituximab scFv-Fc-HA maintains its recognition of cells expressing CD20. Further experiments demonstrated that rituximab scFv-Fc-HA is equivalent to rituximab IgG1 with respect to antigen binding, ADCC, and CDC.

7. Safe Imager blue-light transilluminator (Invitrogen, www.invitrogen.com).
8. Water purified by, e.g., a Picopure 2 UV Plus system (Hydro Service and Supplies, www.hydroservice.com); sterilize by filtration through a 0.22-µm filter (e.g., Millipore Steriflip Filter Units, www.millipore.com, cat. no. SCGP00525) and store at room temperature.
9. Glycerol stock of *E. coli* strain TOP10 (Invitrogen, cat. no. C4040-03) containing a custom synthesized scFv-Fc-HA encoding DNA fragment (e.g., DNA2.0, Menlo Park, CA) in a plasmid with ampicillin resistance gene (Fig. 1). Store at −80°C.
10. Glycerol stock of *E. coli* strain TOP10 (Invitrogen) containing mammalian expression vector pCEP4 (Invitrogen, cat. no. V044-50). Store at −80°C.
11. LB + 100 µg/mL carbenicillin plates (Teknova, www.teknova.com, cat. no. L1010); store at 4°C.
12. LB medium: Dissolve 20 g NaCl (Mallinckrodt Baker, www.fishersci.com, cat. no. 758112; store at room temperature), 20 g Bacto tryptone (BD Biosciences, www.bd.com, cat. no. 211705; store at room temperature), and 10 g Bacto yeast extract (BD Biosciences, cat. no. 212750; store at room temperature) in 1.9 L total volume with water. Bring to pH 7.0 with 1 N NaOH (Fisher Scientific, cat. no. AC12426-0010; store at room temperature). Bring to 2 L total volume with water. Sterilize by autoclaving in two 1-L or four 500-mL glass bottles. Store at room temperature.
13. 100 µg/µL Carbenicillin: Dissolve 1 g carbenicillin disodium (Duchefa, www.duchefa.com, cat. no. C0109.0005; store at 4°C) in 10 mL water. Sterilize by filtration through a 0.22-µm filter. Store 1-mL aliquots in 1.5-mL microfuge tubes at −20°C.
14. QIAprep Spin Miniprep Kit (Qiagen, www.qiagen.com, cat. no. 27106); store at room temperature.
15. 10 U/µL KpnI, 10× NEBuffer 1, and 100× BSA (New England Biolabs, www.neb.com, cat. no. R0142S); store at −20°C. Prepare 10× BSA freshly by mixing 10 µL 100× BSA with 90 µL water in a 1.5-mL microfuge tube.
16. 20 U/µL XhoI (New England Biolabs, cat. no. R0146S); store at −20°C.
17. 6× Gel loading dye solution (Fermentas, www.fermentas.com, cat. no. R0611); store at room temperature.
18. Agarose (Invitrogen, cat. no. 16500500); store at room temperature.
19. TAE buffer [40 mM Tris-acetate (pH 8.0), 1 mM EDTA; diluted in water from 50× TAE] (Quality Biological, www.qualitybiological.com, cat. no. 351-008-131); store at room temperature.

20. SYBR Safe DNA gel stain (Invitrogen, cat. no. S33102); store at room temperature.
21. 1-kb DNA ladder (Fermentas, cat. no. SM0314); store at room temperature.
22. Qiagen MinElute Gel Extraction Kit (Qiagen, cat. no. 28606); store at room temperature.
23. Isopropanol (Sigma-Aldrich, www.sigmaaldrich.com, cat. no. I9516); store at room temperature.
24. 2,000 U/μL T4 DNA ligase and 10× T4 DNA ligase buffer (New England Biolabs, cat. no. M0202M); store at −20°C.
25. One Shot TOP10 Chemically Competent *E. coli* (Invitrogen, cat. no. C4040-10); store at −80°C.
26. SOC medium (Invitrogen, cat. no. 15544-034); store at room temperature.
27. 95% (vol/vol) Ethanol (The Warner Graham Company, www.warnergraham.com, cat. no. 190 proof); store at room temperature in a fire safety cabinet.
28. DNA sequencing primers:

    pCEP forward (5′-AGCAGAGCTCGTTTAGTGAACCG-3′).

    CH2 reverse (5′-GCAATTCCGGTGCGGGACAG-3′).

    EBV reverse (5′-GTGGTTTGTCCAAACTCATC-3′).

### 2.2. Cloning into pCEP4/scFv-Fc-HA Plasmid via KpnI and SapI

In addition to all materials listed in Subheading 2.1:

1. Model D2 Spider Wide Gel Electrophoresis System with D1-20C combs (Owl Separation Systems).
2. 10 U/μL *Sap*I (New England Biolabs, cat. no. R0569M); store at −20°C. For *Sap*I troubleshooting, see www.neb.com/nebecomm/products/faqproductR0569.asp.

### 2.3. Transient Transfection of Mammalian Cells with pCEP4/scFv-Fc-HA

1. Glass spreading rod.
2. Refrigerated floor centrifuge (e.g., Sorvall Evolution RC, Thermo Scientific) with fixed-angle rotor for 500-mL centrifuge bottles (e.g., Sorvall SLA-3000 Super-Lite, Thermo Scientific).
3. Savant SpeedVac concentrator (Thermo Scientific, cat. no. DNA120-115).
4. Cell culture incubator with humidified atmosphere containing 8% $CO_2$ at 37°C (e.g., Heracell 150i, Thermo Scientific).
5. Hemocytometer (e.g., Hausser Scientific, www.hausserscientific.com).
6. CELLSPIN system with stirring platform and separate control unit (INTEGRA Biosciences, www.integra-biosciences.com, cat. no. 183001).

7. 14-mL round-bottom tubes with snap caps.
8. 500-mL Erlenmeyer flask.
9. 500-mL centrifuge bottles (e.g., Sorvall Dry-Spin Polypropylene Bottles, Fisher Scientific, cat. no. 50-866-922).
10. 0.22-μm/33-mm Millex-GV PVDF Filter Unit (Millipore, cat. no. SLGV033RS).
11. 3-mL Luer Lok syringe.
12. CELLSPIN 500-mL spinner flask with two pendula (INTEGRA Biosciences, cat. no. 182051).
13. 250-mL polycarbonate Erlenmeyer flasks (Corning, www.corning.com, cat. no. 430183).
14. Water (see Subheading 2.1).
15. One Shot TOP10 Chemically Competent *E. coli* (see Subheading 2.1).
16. SOC medium (see Subheading 2.1).
17. 95% (vol/vol) Ethanol (see Subheading 2.1).
18. LB + 100 μg/mL carbenicillin plates (see Subheading 2.1).
19. LB medium (see Subheading 2.1).
20. 100 μg/μL Carbenicillin (see Subheading 2.1).
21. GenElute HP Endotoxin-Free Plasmid Maxiprep Kit (Sigma-Aldrich, cat. no. NA0400); store at room temperature.
22. 3 M Sodium acetate (pH 5.2) (Quality Biological, cat. no. 351-035-721); store at room temperature.
23. Isopropanol (Sigma-Aldrich); store at room temperature.
24. 70% (vol/vol) Ethanol: Mix 35 mL ethanol (Sigma-Aldrich, cat. no. E7023; store at room temperature) with 15 mL Endotoxin-Free Water from the GenElute HP Endotoxin-Free Plasmid Maxiprep Kit in a 50-mL centrifuge tube. Store at room temperature.
25. FreeStyle 293F cells (Invitrogen, cat. no. R790-07); store in 10% (vol/vol) DMSO in FreeStyle 293 Expression Medium at −196°C (liquid nitrogen).
26. ~70% (vol/vol) Ethanol: Dilute ~3 vol 95% (vol/vol) ethanol (see Subheading 2.1) with ~1 vol water.
27. Phosphate-buffered saline (PBS): 9,000 mg/L (155.17 mM) NaCl, 795 mg/L (2.97 mM) $Na_2HPO_4 \times 7H_2O$, 144 mg/Lf (1.06 mM) $KH_2PO_4$, pH 7.4; (Invitrogen, cat. no. 10010-023); store at room temperature.
28. FreeStyle 293 Expression Medium (protein-free; Invitrogen, cat. no. 12338-026); store protected from light at 4°C.
29. Trypan Blue (Lonza, www.lonza.com, cat. no. 17-942E); store at room temperature.

30. Opti-MEM I Reduced Serum Medium (Invitrogen, cat. no. 31985-062); store protected from light at 4°C.
31. 293fectin Transfection Reagent (Invitrogen, cat. no. 12347-019); store protected from light at 4°C.

### 2.4. Purification of scFv-Fc-HA by Protein A Affinity Chromatography

1. Water (see Subheading 2.1).
2. 50-mL 0.45-μm Steriflip Sterile Disposable Vacuum Filtration System (Millipore, cat. no. SE1M003M00).
3. 500-mL 0.45-μm Stericup-HV Filter Unit (Millipore, cat. no. SCHVU05RE).
4. 1,000-mL 0.45-μm Stericup-HV Filter Unit (Millipore, cat. no. SCHVU11RE).
5. 76-mm Amicon Ultrafiltration Membranes with 10-kDa MWCO (Millipore, cat. no. PBGC07610).
6. 400-mL Amicon Stirred Cell 8400 (Millipore, cat. no. 5124).
7. Compressed nitrogen gas bottle with pressure regulator.
8. PBS (see Subheading 2.3).
9. Peristaltic Pump P-1 (GE Healthcare, www.gelifesciences.com, cat. no. 18-1110-91) with 1.0-mm (i.d.) silicone tubing (GE Healthcare, cat. no. 19-4692-01), Peristaltic Pump P-1 tubing connectors (GE Healthcare, cat. no. 19-2150-01), and 0.75-mm (i.d.) 1/16″ PEEK tubing (GE Healthcare, cat. no. 18-1112-53).
10. Polyacrylamide gel electrophoresis equipment: Owl P8DS Vertical Electrophoresis System (Owl Separation Systems).
11. EC 105 Compact Power Supply (Owl Separation Systems).
12. 15-mL Amicon Ultra Centrifugal Filter Device with 30-kDa MWCO (Millipore, cat. no. UFC903024).
13. 50–2,000-μL UVette disposable single sealed cuvettes (see Subheading 2.1).
14. 14-mL round-bottom tube with snap cap.
15. Slide-A-Lyzer Dialysis Cassettes with 10-kDa MWCO and 3-mL capacity (Thermo Scientific, www.piercenet.com, cat. no. 66380).
16. 4-L beaker (optional).
17. 10-mL syringe with 21-G needle (optional).
18. 1-mL HiTrap Protein A HP columns (GE Healthcare, cat. no. 17-0402-01).
19. 1-M Tris–HCl (pH 8.0) (Mediatech, www.cellgro.com, cat. no. 46-031-CM); store at room temperature.

20. 0.5 M Acetic acid: Dilute 286 μL glacial (17.47 M) acetic acid (Mallinckrodt Baker through Fisher Scientific, cat. no. 250414; store at room temperature in a cabinet for acids) in water to a total volume of 10-mL. Store at room temperature.
21. 20% (vol/vol) Ethanol: Mix 10 mL ethanol (see Subheading 2.3) with 40 mL water in a 50-mL centrifuge tube. Store at room temperature.
22. NuPAGE Novex 4–12% Bis-Tris Gel 1.5 mm, 10 well (Invitrogen, cat. no. NP0335BOX); store at room temperature.
23. NuPAGE MES SDS Buffer Kit with MES SDS Running Buffer, Sample Reducing Agent, Antioxidant, and LDS Sample Buffer (Invitrogen, cat. no. NP0060); store at room temperature.
24. SeeBlue Plus2 Pre-Stained Standard (Invitrogen, cat. no. LC5925); store at room temperature.
25. SimplyBlue SafeStain based on Coomassie Brilliant Blue G-250 (Invitrogen, cat. no. LC6060); store at room temperature.
26. Biotinylated rat anti-HA mAb 3F10 (Roche Applied Science, www.roche-applied-science.com, cat. no. 12158167001) (optional).
27. Streptavidin–Phycoerythrin (BD Biosciences, cat. no. 349023) (optional).
28. Fetal bovine serum (Invitrogen, cat. no. 26140-111) (optional).
29. FACSCalibur instrument (BD Biosciences) (optional).
30. FlowJo analytical software (TreeStar, www.flowjo.com) (optional).

## 3. Methods

### 3.1. Cloning of pCEP4/scFv-Fc-HA Plasmid via Restriction Sites

This protocol takes about 6 days.

1. From frozen glycerol stocks, streak out (1) *E. coli* strain TOP10 containing a custom synthesized scFv-Fc-HA encoding DNA fragment with flanking *Kpn*I and *Xho*I restriction sites (Fig. 1) in a plasmid with ampicillin resistance gene encoding β-lactamase and (2) *E. coli* strain TOP10 containing mammalian expression vector pCEP4 (carrying ampicillin resistance gene) on LB + 100 μg/mL carbenicillin plates and incubate overnight at 37°C (see Note 1).
2. Pick six single colonies from each plate to inoculate 3 mL LB medium with 100 μg/mL carbenicillin in twelve 14-mL round-bottom tubes with snap caps, and shake at 37°C and 250 rpm overnight.

3. Centrifuge at 3,000×$g$ for 10 min at 4°C. Decant the supernatant and absorb residual liquid by storing the inverted tubes on a paper towel for a few minutes.
4. Resuspend the bacterial pellets in 250 μL Qiagen buffer P1 from the QIAprep Spin Miniprep Kit, transfer the suspension into 1.5-mL microfuge tubes, and then proceed with reagents and protocols supplied by the QIAprep Spin Miniprep Kit using 50 μL water for elution. Pool the six preparations of each plasmid (scFv-Fc-HA and pCEP4) in a 1.5-mL microfuge tube and measure the absorbance at 260 nm with a disposable cuvette in a UV photometer. Use the absorbance at 260 nm to calculate the plasmid concentration based on the assumption that 50 μg/mL DNA gives an absorbance of 1. Dilute with water to a final concentration of 100 ng/μL.
5. For *Kpn*I/*Xho*I digestion of both plasmids, combine 30 μL 100 ng/μL (3 μg) plasmid with 5 μL 10× NEBuffer 1, 5 μL 10× BSA, 6 μL water, 2 μL 10 U/μL *Kpn*I, and 2 μL 20 U/μL *Xho*I (Σ 50 μL). Incubate at 37°C for 2 h.
6. Directly add 10 μL 6× gel loading dye solution and separate by electrophoresis on a 1% (wt/vol) agarose gel in 1× TAE buffer using a B1A-6 comb and as reference a 1-kb DNA ladder (see Note 2). The excised scFv-Fc-HA encoding DNA fragment and the double cut pCEP4 vector are visible as bright bands of ~1.5 and ~10 kb, respectively.
7. Separately cut out the 1.5- and 10-kb bands with a razor blade, dissect them further into smaller pieces, and transfer ~0.3-g portions into 1.5-mL microfuge tubes. Purify the scFv-Fc-HA encoding DNA fragment and the double cut pCEP4 vector using reagents and protocols supplied by the Qiagen MinElute Gel Extraction Kit. Pool each DNA sample in 15 μL water and measure the absorbance at 260 nm with a disposable cuvette in a UV photometer. Use the absorbance at 260 nm to calculate the DNA concentration based on the assumption that 50 μg/mL DNA gives an absorbance of 1. Dilute with water to a final concentration of 100 ng/μL (double cut pCEP4 vector) or 50 ng/μL (excised scFv-Fc-HA encoding DNA fragment). Store at −20°C.
8. For ligation, combine 2 μL of 100 ng/μL double cut pCEP4 vector (200 ng) with 2 μL of 50 ng/μL excised scFv-Fc-HA encoding DNA fragment (100 ng), 2 μL 10× T4 DNA ligase buffer, 13 μL water, and 1 μL 2,000 U/μL T4 DNA ligase in a 1.5-mL microfuge tube (Σ 20 μL). Prepare a ligation mixture in parallel with double cut pCEP4 vector alone as background control. Incubate at room temperature for 30 min.
9. For transformation, briefly spin the microfuge tubes containing ligation and background control reactions and place on ice.

Thaw two 50-μL vials of One Shot TOP10 Chemically Competent *E. coli* on ice for 10 min. Pipette 10 μL of the ligation reaction and background control reaction directly into the vial of competent cells and mix by tapping gently (see Note 3). Incubate the vials on ice for 30 min, followed by 30 s at 42°C, and then place on ice. Add 250 μL of SOC medium to each vial. Place the vials in two 50-mL centrifuge tubes and shake at 37°C and 225 rpm for 1 h.

10. Sterilize a glass spreading rod dipped in 95% (vol/vol) ethanol in the flame of a Bunsen burner, cool, and use to evenly distribute 200 μL from each vial on separate LB + 100 μg/mL carbenicillin plates. Incubate overnight at 37°C (see Note 4).
11. Randomly pick six colonies from the plate containing the scFv-Fc-HA encoding DNA fragment to inoculate 3 mL LB medium with 100 μg/mL carbenicillin in six 14-mL round-bottom tubes with snap caps, and shake at 37°C and 250 rpm overnight.
12. Centrifuge at 3,000 × *g* for 10 min at 4°C. Decant the supernatant and absorb residual liquid by storing the inverted tubes on a paper towel for a few minutes.
13. Resuspend the bacterial pellets in 250 μL Qiagen buffer P1 from the QIAprep Spin Miniprep Kit, transfer the suspension into 1.5-mL microfuge tubes, and then proceed with reagents and protocols supplied by the QIAprep Spin Miniprep Kit using 50 μL water for elution. Measure the absorbance at 260 nm with a disposable cuvette in a UV photometer. Use the absorbance at 260 nm to calculate the plasmid concentration based on the assumption that 50 μg/mL DNA gives an absorbance of 1. Dilute with water to a final concentration of 100 ng/μL.
14. In a 1.5-mL microfuge tube, prepare a *Kpn*I/*Xho*I digestion master mix sufficient for seven reactions: mix 7 μL 10× NEBuffer 1, 7 μL 10× BSA, 3.5 μL 10 U/μL *Kpn*I, 3.5 μL 20 U/μL *Xho*I, and 14 μL water (Σ 35 μL). In six 1.5-mL microfuge tubes, mix 5 μL of the master mix with 5 μL of the 100 ng/μL plasmid mini-preparations (Σ 10 μL) and incubate at 37°C for 2 h.
15. Directly add 2 μL 6× gel loading dye solution, and separate by electrophoresis on a 1% (wt/vol) agarose gel in 1× TAE buffer using a B1A-10 comb and as reference a 1-kb DNA ladder. Clones that have the scFv-Fc-HA encoding DNA fragment correctly inserted in the pCEP4 vector reveal two bright bands of ~10 and ~1.5 kb. The insert can be further confirmed by DNA sequencing using primers pCEP forward (upstream from *Kpn*I), CH2 reverse (internal; Fig. 1), and EBV reverse (downstream from *Xho*I).
16. Pool confirmed pCEP4/scFv-Fc-HA plasmid mini-preparations and store at –20°C.

#### *3.2. Cloning into pCEP4/scFv-Fc-HA Plasmid via KpnI and SapI*

This protocol takes about 6 days.

1. From a frozen glycerol stock, streak out *E. coli* strain TOP10 containing a custom synthesized scFv encoding DNA fragment with flanking *Kpn*I and *Sap*I restriction sites (Fig. 1) in a plasmid with ampicillin resistance gene on LB + 100 μg/mL carbenicillin plates and incubate overnight at 37°C.
2. Pick six single colonies from the plate to inoculate 3 mL LB medium with 100 μg/mL carbenicillin in six 14-mL round-bottom tubes with snap caps, and shake at 37°C and 250 rpm overnight.
3. Centrifuge at 3,000 × *g* for 10 min at 4°C. Decant the supernatant and absorb residual liquid by storing the inverted tubes on a paper towel for a few minutes.
4. Resuspend the bacterial pellets in 250 μL Qiagen buffer P1 from the QIAprep Spin Miniprep Kit, transfer the suspension into 1.5-mL microfuge tubes, and then proceed with reagents and protocols supplied by the QIAprep Spin Miniprep Kit using 50 μL water for elution. Pool the six preparations in a 1.5-mL microfuge tube and measure the absorbance at 260 nm with a disposable cuvette in a UV photometer. Use the absorbance at 260 nm to calculate the plasmid concentration based on the assumption that 50 μg/mL DNA gives an absorbance of 1. Dilute with water to a final concentration of 100 ng/μL.
5. For *Kpn*I/*Sap*I digestion, combine 30 μL 100 ng/μL (3 μg) plasmid with 5 μL 10× NEBuffer 1, 5 μL 10× BSA, 6 μL water, 2 μL 10 U/μL *Kpn*I, and 2 μL 10 U/μL *Sap*I (Σ 50 μL). Incubate at 37°C for 2 h.
6. In parallel, *Kpn*I/*Sap*I digest pCEP4/scFv-Fc-HA prepared in Subheading 3.1 by combining 30 μL 100 ng/μL (3 μg) plasmid with 5 μL 10× NEBuffer 1, 5 μL 10× BSA, 6 μL water, 2 μL 10 U/μL *Kpn*I, and 2 μL 10 U/μL *Sap*I (Σ 50 μL) and incubating at 37°C for 2 h.
7. Directly add 10 μL 6× gel loading dye solution to both reactions and separate by electrophoresis on a 1% (wt/vol) agarose gel in 1× TAE buffer using a B1A-6 comb and as reference a 1-kb DNA ladder (see Note 2). The excised scFv encoding DNA fragment and the double cut pCEP4 vector with the Fc-HA insert are visible as bright bands of ~1 and ~10.5 kb, respectively.
8. Separately cut out the 1- and 10.5-kb bands with a razor blade, dissect them further into smaller pieces, and transfer ~0.3-g portions into 1.5-mL microfuge tubes. Purify the excised scFv encoding DNA fragment and the double cut pCEP4/Fc-HA vector using reagents and protocols supplied by the Qiagen

MinElute Gel Extraction Kit. Pool each DNA sample in 25 μL water and measure the absorbance at 260 nm with a disposable cuvette in a UV photometer. Use the absorbance at 260 nm to calculate the DNA concentration based on the assumption that 50 μg/mL DNA gives an absorbance of 1. Dilute with water to a final concentration of 100 ng/μL (double cut pCEP4/Fc-HA vector) or 50 ng/μL (excised scFv encoding DNA fragment). Store at −20°C.

9. For ligation, combine 2 μL 100 ng/μL double cut pCEP4/Fc-HA vector (200 ng) with 2 μL 50 ng/μL excised scFv encoding DNA fragment (100 ng), 2 μL 10× T4 DNA ligase buffer, 13 μL water, and 1 μL 2,000 U/μL T4 DNA ligase in a 1.5-mL microfuge tube (Σ 20 μL). Prepare a ligation mixture in parallel with double cut pCEP4/Fc-HA vector alone as background control. Incubate at room temperature for 30 min.
10. For transformation, briefly spin the microfuge tubes containing ligation and background control reactions and place on ice. Thaw two 50-μL vials of One Shot TOP10 Chemically Competent *E. coli* on ice for 10 min. Pipette 10 μL of ligation reaction and background control reaction directly into the vial of competent cells and mix by tapping gently (see Note 3). Incubate the vials on ice for 30 min, followed by 30 s at 42°C, and then place on ice. Add 250 μL of SOC medium to each vial. Place the vials in two 50-mL centrifuge tubes and shake at 37°C and 225 rpm for 1 h.
11. Sterilize a glass spreading rod dipped in 95% (vol/vol) ethanol in the flame of a Bunsen burner, cool, and use to evenly distribute 200 μL from each vial on separate LB + 100 μg/mL carbenicillin plates and incubate overnight at 37°C (see Note 5).
12. Randomly pick eight colonies from the plate containing the scFv encoding DNA fragment to inoculate 3 mL LB medium with 100 μg/mL carbenicillin in eight 14-mL round-bottom tubes with snap caps, and shake at 37°C and 250 rpm overnight.
13. Centrifuge at 3,000 × *g* for 10 min at 4°C. Decant the supernatant and absorb residual liquid by storing the inverted tubes on a paper towel for a few minutes.
14. Resuspend the bacterial pellets in 250 μL Qiagen buffer P1 from the QIAprep Spin Miniprep Kit, transfer the suspension into 1.5-mL microfuge tubes, and then proceed with reagents and protocols supplied by the QIAprep Spin Miniprep Kit using 50 μL water for elution. Measure the absorbance at 260 nm with a disposable cuvette in a UV photometer. Use the absorbance at 260 nm to calculate the plasmid concentration based on the assumption that 50 μg/mL DNA gives an absorbance of 1. Dilute with water to a final concentration of 100 ng/μL.

15. In a 1.5-mL microfuge tube, prepare a *Kpn*I/*Sap*I digestion master mix sufficient for ten reactions: mix 10 μL 10× NEBuffer 1, 10 μL 10× BSA, 5 μL 10 U/μL *Kpn*I, 5 μL 10 U/μL *Sap*I, and 20 μL water (Σ 50 μL). In twenty-four 1.5-mL microfuge tubes, mix 5 μL of the master mix with 5 μL of the100 ng/μL plasmid mini-preparations (Σ 10 μL) and incubate at 37°C for 2 h.
16. Directly add 2 μL 6× gel loading dye solution, and separate by electrophoresis on a 1% (wt/vol) agarose gel in 1× TAE buffer using a B1A-10 comb and as reference a 1-kb DNA ladder. Clones that have the scFv encoding DNA fragment correctly inserted in the pCEP4 vector reveal two bright bands of ~10.5 and ~1 kb. However, to distinguish clones with the new *Kpn*I/*Sap*I insert from background clones with the original *Kpn*I/*Sap*I insert, further confirmation by DNA sequencing using primers pCEP forward (upstream from *Kpn*I), CH2 reverse (internal; Fig. 1), and EBV reverse (downstream from *Sap*I) is required.
17. Store confirmed pCEP4/scFv-Fc-HA plasmid mini-preparations at −20°C.

### 3.3. Transient Transfection of Mammalian Cells

1. *Plasmid maxi-preparation (required time: ~3 days)*. Thaw a confirmed pCEP4/scFv-Fc-HA plasmid mini-preparation at room temperature. Thaw one 50-μL vial of One Shot TOP10 Chemically Competent *E. coli* on ice for 10 min. Pipette 0.5 μL (50 ng) of the mini-preparation directly into the vial of competent cells and mix by tapping gently. Incubate the vial on ice for 30 min, followed by 30 s at 42°C, and then place on ice. Add 250 μL of SOC medium to the vial. Place the vial in a 50-mL centrifuge tube and shake at 37°C and 225 rpm for 1 h. Remove 10 μL and combine with 90 μL SOC in a 1.5-mL microfuge tube. Sterilize a glass spreading rod dipped in 95% (vol/vol) ethanol in the flame of a Bunsen burner, cool, and use to evenly distribute the 100-μL dilution on an LB + 100 μg/mL carbenicillin plate and incubate overnight at 37°C. Pick one colony from the plate to inoculate 3 mL LB medium with 100 μg/mL carbenicillin in a 14-mL round-bottom tube with snap cap, and shake at 37°C and 250 rpm for 8 h. Transfer 150 μL of the 3-mL bacterial culture into 150 mL LB medium with 100 μg/mL carbenicillin in a 500-mL Erlenmeyer flask and shake at 37°C and 250 rpm overnight (see Note 6). Transfer the bacterial supernatant to a 500-mL centrifuge tube and centrifuge at 3,000 × *g* for 10 min at 4°C in a refrigerated floor centrifuge with fixed-angle rotor. Decant the supernatant and absorb residual liquid by storing the inverted tube on a paper towel for a few minutes. Resuspend the bacterial pellet in 12 mL of Resuspension/RNase A Solution from the GenElute

HP Endotoxin-Free Plasmid Maxiprep Kit, transfer the suspension into a 50-mL centrifuge tube, and then proceed with reagents and protocols supplied by the GenElute HP Endotoxin-Free Plasmid Maxiprep Kit using 3 mL Endotoxin-Free Water for elution by centrifugation at 3,000 × *g* for 5 min at 4°C in a refrigerated benchtop centrifuge with swinging bucket rotor.

2. Measure the absorbance at 260 nm with a disposable cuvette in a UV photometer. Use the absorbance at 260 nm to calculate the plasmid concentration based on the assumption that 50 μg/mL DNA gives an absorbance of 1. The plasmid concentration is typically ~250 μg/mL but can be higher or lower.
3. To achieve an optimal plasmid concentration of 500 ± 100 μg/mL, transfer three ~700-μL aliquots into 1.5-mL microfuge tubes and concentrate with open lids in a Savant SpeedVac concentrator at the medium heat setting to ~350-μL (see Note 7). Pool the concentrated plasmid maxi-preparation in a 1.5-mL centrifuge tube and repeat measuring the absorbance at 260 nm with a disposable cuvette in a UV photometer (see Note 8).
4. In a laminar flow hood, sterilize the plasmid maxi-preparation by filtration through a 0.22-μm/33-mm Millex-GV PVDF Filter Unit using a 3-mL Luer Lok syringe, and store ~500-μL (~250-μg) aliquots in 1.5-mL microfuge tubes at −20°C (see Note 9).
5. *Preparation of FreeStyle 293F cells (required time: ~2 weeks).* Remove a 1-mL cryovial with at least $5 \times 10^6$ cells from liquid nitrogen and thaw quickly in a 37°C water bath. Just before the cells are completely thawed, decontaminate the outside of the vial with ~70% (vol/vol) ethanol, move to the laminar flow hood, and transfer the entire content of the vial into a 14-mL centrifuge tube containing 10 mL of PBS pre-warmed to 37°C. Centrifuge the tube at 300 × *g* for 10 min at room temperature in a refrigerated benchtop centrifuge with swinging bucket rotor. In the laminar flow hood, aspirate and discard the supernatant, gently resuspend the pellet with a 5-mL pipette in 5 mL fresh FreeStyle 293 Expression Medium pre-warmed to 37°C, and transfer the cell suspension into a 175-$cm^2$ cell culture flask containing 25 mL fresh FreeStyle 293 Expression Medium pre-warmed to 37°C. Shake the flask gently to mix the cell suspension and incubate for 3–5 days in a cell culture incubator with humidified atmosphere containing 8% $CO_2$ at 37°C (see Note 10). Once the cells are ~90% confluent (~$3 \times 10^7$ viable cells/30 mL/flask), shake and tap the flask to resuspend attached cells. (The number of viable cells can be determined by Trypan Blue staining using a hemocytometer or an electronic counting device.) In the laminar

flow hood, use a 25-mL pipette to transfer the cell suspension into a 50-mL centrifuge tube and centrifuge at 300 × *g* for 10 min at room temperature in a refrigerated benchtop centrifuge with swinging bucket rotor. In the laminar flow hood, aspirate and discard the supernatant and resuspend the cell pellet in 25 mL fresh FreeStyle 293 Expression Medium pre-warmed to 37°C. Vortex vigorously for 10–30 s to get a single cell suspension. Distribute the single cell suspension among five 175-$cm^2$ cell culture flasks containing 25 mL fresh FreeStyle 293 Expression Medium pre-warmed to 37°C (5 mL/flask, 1:5 dilution) and incubate for 2–3 days in the cell culture incubator with humidified atmosphere containing 8% $CO_2$ at 37°C. Repeat these passaging steps as necessary to maintain or expand the cells prior to transfection (see Note 11).

6. The day before transfection, prepare eight 175-$cm^2$ cell culture flasks with FreeStyle 293F cells at ~60% confluence (~$2 \times 10^7$ viable cells/30 mL/flask) as described before and continue incubation for 24 h in the cell culture incubator with humidified atmosphere containing 8% $CO_2$ at 37°C. The cells should be ~90% confluent (~$3 \times 10^7$ viable cells/30 mL/flask) when harvested for transfection (see Note 12).
7. To harvest the cells, shake and tap the flasks to resuspend attached cells. Determine the number of viable cells by Trypan Blue staining using a hemocytometer or an electronic counting device. The viability must be >90% at the time of transfection (see Note 13).
8. *Transfection (required time: ~1 h).* In the laminar flow hood, first dilute and mix 8 × 30 μg (Σ 240 μg) from the prepared plasmid maxi-preparation in Opti-MEM I Reduced Serum Medium to a total volume of 8 mL in a 50-mL centrifuge tube. Subsequently, dilute 8 × 60 μL (Σ 480 μL) 293fectin Transfection Reagent (a cationic lipid) in Opti-MEM I Reduced Serum Medium to a total volume of 8 mL in a separate 50-mL centrifuge tube, mix gently by swirling, and incubate for 5 min at room temperature. Add the diluted plasmid to the diluted 293fectin Transfection Reagent (Σ 16 mL), mix gently by swirling, and incubate for 30 min at room temperature. Proceed with the preparation of the cells during this incubation.
9. In the laminar flow hood, shake and tap the flasks again to keep the cells resuspended. Use a 25-mL pipette to transfer the cell suspensions from the eight prepared flasks into separate 50-mL centrifuge tubes and centrifuge at 300 × *g* for 10 min at room temperature in a refrigerated benchtop centrifuge with swinging bucket rotor. In the laminar flow hood, aspirate and discard the supernatants and resuspend each cell pellet in 25 mL fresh FreeStyle 293 Expression Medium pre-warmed to 37°C. Vortex vigorously for 10–30 s to get a single cell suspension.

Pool the 200-mL single cell suspension in a sterilized CELLSPIN 500-mL spinner flask and add fresh FreeStyle 293 Expression Medium pre-warmed to 37°C to a total volume of 224 mL.

10. In the laminar flow hood, use a 25-mL pipette to add the prepared 16-mL plasmid/cationic lipid complex in Opti-MEM I Reduced Serum Medium to the prepared 224-mL single cell suspension in the spinner flask. The spinner flask should contain a total volume of 240 mL with a final cell density of ~$1 \times 10^6$ viable cells/mL (Σ ~$2.4 \times 10^8$ viable cells).
11. Place the spinner flask on a CELLSPIN stirring platform in a cell culture incubator with humidified atmosphere containing 8% $CO_2$ at 37°C and rotate at 125 rpm for 72 h.
12. *Harvest of supernatant (required time: ~6–9 days)*. Move the spinner flask into the laminar flow hood. Use a 25-mL pipette to transfer the cell suspension into six 50-mL centrifuge tubes and centrifuge at 300 × *g* for 10 min at room temperature in a refrigerated benchtop centrifuge with swinging bucket rotor. In the laminar flow hood, use a 25-mL pipette to pool the supernatant in a 250-mL polycarbonate Erlenmeyer flask and store at −20°C.
13. Resuspend each cell pellet in 25 mL fresh FreeStyle 293 Expression Medium pre-warmed to 37°C. Vortex vigorously for 10–30 s to get a single cell suspension. Using a 25-mL pipette, transfer the 150-mL single cell suspension back into the same spinner flask, determine the number of viable cells in a small aliquot of the spinner flask culture by Trypan Blue staining using a hemocytometer or an electronic counting device, add fresh FreeStyle 293 Expression Medium pre-warmed to 37°C to achieve a cell density of ~$1 \times 10^6$ viable cells/mL, and continue incubation in humidified atmosphere containing 8% $CO_2$ at 37°C and 125 rpm for 72 h.
14. After determining the number of viable cells in a small aliquot of the spinner flask culture by Trypan Blue staining using a hemocytometer or an electronic counting device, harvest and store the second supernatant as described before. If the viability is >50%, bring the cells back into the spinner flask, add fresh FreeStyle 293 Expression Medium pre-warmed to 37°C to achieve a cell density of ~$1 \times 10^6$ viable cells/mL, and incubate for another 72 h as described before. Harvest and store the third and final supernatant as described before. The total volume of three harvested supernatants is ~1 L.

### 3.4. Purification of scFv-Fc-HA by Protein A Affinity Chromatography

This step takes about 2 days.

1. *Concentration of supernatant.* Thaw the harvested supernatant in a 37°C water bath, pool in a 500- or 1,000-mL 0.45-μm Stericup-HV Filter Unit, and filtrate under vacuum (see Note 14). Place a new 76-mm Amicon Ultrafiltration Membrane with

10-kDa MWCO in a 400 mL Amicon Stirred Cell 8400 ultrafiltration device. First rinse and then fill the ultrafiltration device with sterile water. Connect the device to a compressed nitrogen gas bottle through a pressure regulator and adjust the pressure to 50 psi until all water is drained from the device. Disconnect the device from the pressure source and add 350 mL of the filtrated culture supernatant. Reconnect the device to the pressure source, adjust the pressure to 50 psi, and leave the device at 4°C under constant stirring (~100 rpm) on a magnetic stirring plate. After the volume of the culture supernatant inside the device has dropped down to ~150 mL, stop the magnetic stirring plate, disconnect the pressure source, open the device, refill it with the remaining filtrated culture supernatant, and continue concentrating to a volume of ~25 mL in the device (see Note 15).

2. Collect the concentrate in two 50-mL centrifuge tubes. Rinse the ultrafiltration device with 40–50 mL sterile PBS and combine with the concentrate. Pass the prepared concentrate through two 50-mL 0.45-μm Steriflip Sterile Disposable Vacuum Filtration System under vacuum. Leave the concentrate under vacuum for an additional 15 min to remove nitrogen dissolved in the concentrate (see Note 16). Store the concentrate on ice or at 4°C to proceed with Protein A affinity chromatography on the same or next day, respectively, or freeze at −20°C.
3. Assemble the peristaltic pump and rinse the tubing with sterile water. Adjust the speed of the peristaltic pump to a flow rate of 1 mL/min.
4. Remove the upper screw cap on a 1-mL HiTrap Protein A HP column (see Note 17) and fill the column with sterile water before connecting to the peristaltic pump to avoid air bubbles in the column. For the same reason, the tubing of the peristaltic pump should be filled with water before connecting to the column. Remove the snap-off outlet of the column.
5. Rinse the column with 5 mL sterile water to remove all ethanol of the column storage buffer.
6. Equilibrate the column with 10 mL ice-cold PBS at a flow rate of 1 mL/min (see Note 18).
7. Reduce the flow rate to 0.5 mL/min. Load the prepared ice-cold concentrate (see Note 19).
8. Increase the flow rate to 1 mL/min and wash the column with 50 mL ice-cold PBS.
9. Prepare ten 1.5-mL microfuge tubes containing 0.65 mL 1 M Tris–HCl (pH 8.0) and place them under the column to collect the elution at 0.5 mL/tube. Elute the column with 5 mL 0.5 M ice-cold acetic acid at a flow rate of 1 mL/min.

10. Regenerate the column with 5 mL water followed by 5 mL 20% ethanol, seal the outlet, fasten the upper screw cap, and store at 4°C.
11. Identify the fractions that contain the eluted scFv-Fc-HA protein by measuring the absorbance at 280 nm with a disposable cuvette in a UV photometer [as blank sample use a mixture of 0.65 mL 1 M Tris–HCl (pH 8.0) and 0.5 mL 0.5 M acetic acid] (see Note 20).
12. Pool the fractions that contain the eluted scFv-Fc-HA protein in a 15-mL Amicon Ultra Centrifugal Filter Device with 30-kDa MWCO and concentrate by centrifugation at 3,000 × *g* for 30 min at 4°C in a refrigerated benchtop centrifuge with swinging bucket rotor. If necessary, continue the centrifugation until the volume of the concentrate is down to ~500 μL.
13. Discard the filtrate and add 15 mL PBS to the concentrate. Repeat the centrifugation as before until the volume of the concentrate is again down to ~500 μL.
14. Repeat step 13 (see Note 21).
15. Measure the concentration of the scFc-Fv protein preparation by measuring the absorbance at 280 nm with a disposable cuvette in a UV photometer. Use the absorbance at 280 nm to calculate the scFc-Fv protein concentration based on the estimation that 1 mg/mL of an immunoglobulin protein gives an absorbance of 1.4. Dilute the scFc-Fv protein sample with PBS to a suitable storage concentration (typically 0.5–1 mg/mL), and aliquot into several 1.5- or 0.5-mL microfuge tubes. Transfer tubes to 4°C and −80°C depending on short-term or long-term storage, respectively (see Note 22).
16. Analyze the purity and integrity of the scFv-Fc-HA protein on an SDS-PAGE gel run under reducing and nonreducing conditions and stained with Coomassie Brilliant Blue G-250 (Fig. 2) (see Note 23).

## 4. Notes

1. If the custom synthesized scFv-Fc-HA encoding DNA fragment is delivered in a plasmid with kanamycin resistance gene, use 50 μg/mL kanamycin for selection on LB plates and growth in LB medium. Carbenicillin is a semisynthetic analog of ampicillin susceptible to hydrolysis by β-lactamase. Carbenicillin is more stable than ampicillin and reduces the growth of satellite colonies.
2. For both DNA analysis and preparation by agarose gel electrophoresis, the use of SYBR Safe stain (see Subheading 2.1)

and blue light illumination rather than the hazardous combination of ethidium bromide and UV illumination is strongly recommended.

3. The remaining ligation mixture can be stored as a backup at −20°C or analyzed for ligation events by agarose gel electrophoresis.
4. Expect at least ten times more colonies on the plate containing the scFv-Fc-HA encoding DNA fragment compared to the control plate. Expect ~50% of colonies to contain the correct pCEP4/scFv-Fc-HA plasmid.
5. Expect more colonies on the plate containing the scFv-Fc-HA encoding DNA fragment compared to the control plate. Expect ~10% of colonies to contain the correct pCEP4/scFv-Fc-HA plasmid. As the efficiency of *Kpn*I/*Sap*I cloning is lower than the efficiency of *Kpn*I/*Xho*I cloning described in Subheading 2.1, more colonies may have to be picked to find the correct pCEP4/scFv-Fc-HA plasmid.
6. A healthy bacterial culture grown overnight in LB will generally reach an absorbance of >2 at 600 nm.
7. This concentration step may take several hours. The plasmid DNA will deposit on one side of the microfuge tubes; pipette up and down several times to completely collect the plasmid DNA. As an alternative to this concentration step, precipitate the plasmid DNA by adding 0.1 vol 3 M sodium acetate (pH 5.2) and 0.7 vol isopropanol, vortex, and centrifuge at 15,000 × *g* for 30 min at 4°C in a refrigerated microfuge. Carefully decant the supernatant, rinse the plasmid DNA pellet with 1 mL 70% (vol/vol) ethanol, and centrifuge as before for 10 min. Carefully decant the supernatant, air-dry the plasmid DNA pellet for up to 30 min, and resuspend in the desired volume of endotoxin-free water from the GenElute HP Endotoxin-Free Plasmid Maxiprep Kit.
8. Confirm the purified and concentrated pCEP4/scFv-Fc-HA plasmid by *Kpn*I/*Xho*I and *Kpn*I/*Sap*I digestion as described in Subheadings 3.1 and 3.2, respectively.
9. The holdup volume of the 0.22-μm/33-mm Millex-GV PVDF Filter Unit is ~100 μL. In order to avoid losing too much plasmid DNA in this filtration step, keep the total volume at or above 1 mL. Plasmid DNA for transfection into FreeStyle 293F cells must be pure, sterile, and free from phenol (toxic to cells) and salt (interferes with plasmid/cationic lipid complex formation) and potential ethanol (alternative concentration step in Note 7).
10. Put the flask horizontally in the incubator to allow the cells to distribute and attach to the bottom evenly. After 24–48 h, most of the cells will be attached.

11. FreeStyle 293F cells tend to grow in clusters with 2–10 cells each. Vigorous vortexing as described may be necessary in each of several passaging steps until the cultures grow predominantly as single cells and are suitable for transfection.
12. If the confluence is <90%, postpone the transfection to the next day.
13. For optimal transfection efficiency, a single cell suspension is required. If a significant portion of the cells is found in clusters, vortex for 20–30 s.
14. Cell debris that clogs the membrane of the filter unit will slow down the filtration rate and may make it necessary to use more than one filter unit. Alternatively, after thawing, centrifuge the harvested supernatant at 2,500×g for 10 min at room temperature in a refrigerated benchtop centrifuge with swinging bucket rotor before proceeding with the filtration.
15. After an initial burst in the first 1–2 min, the filtrate should come out of the device drop by drop while sterile water comes out as continuous stream. If the filtrate appears to come out of the device too fast, this could be due to a leakage in the sealing ring and requires reassembly of the device. The concentrate is typically darker and more viscous than the filtrate. It takes several hours to concentrate 500–750 mL and it is important not to let the ultrafiltration membrane dry out. If the concentrating cannot be finished in 1 day, the concentrate can be left at 4°C overnight inside the device and concentrating can be resumed the next day. For this, it is important to bleed the valve on the device after closing the pressure source because the residual pressure inside the device is sufficient to push out all the remaining concentrate and dry out the membrane.
16. Nitrogen dissolves into the concentrate under pressure. If the sample is not degassed before loading onto the affinity chromatography column, the dissolved nitrogen will be released from the sample and will form air bubbles in the column.
17. The Fc domain of human IgG1 strongly binds to both Protein A and Protein G. For the purification of scFv-Fc-HA proteins that contain Fc domains from other species or isotypes, the choice of either Protein A or Protein G is more critical. For example, mouse IgG1 and human IgG3 bind strongly to Protein G but only weakly to Protein A.
18. Placed in a bucket with ice during loading, equilibration buffer, concentrate, washing buffer, and elution buffer cool the column. A cold room is not necessary.
19. It is important to stop the peristaltic pump immediately after all the sample is taken up by the tubing. Transfer the tubing outlet to ice-cold PBS before restarting the peristaltic pump. Any delay in transferring the tubing while the peristaltic pump is running will result in air bubbles in the column.

20. Fractions 2, 3, and 4 typically contain the eluted scFv-Fc-HA protein, whereas the other fractions typically do not contain any detectable protein.
21. Alternative procedure to Subheading 3.4, steps 12–14: Pool the fractions that contain the eluted scFv-Fc-HA protein into a 14-mL round-bottom tube with snap cap. Load the collected eluate into a 10-mL syringe fitted with a 21-G needle and carefully inject into a Slide-A-Lyzer Dialysis Cassette with 10-kDa MWCO and 3-mL capacity. Remove needle and syringe after injection and fit the Slide-A-Lyzer dialysis cassette into a floatation support with the injection site facing upward. Place the dialysis cassette in a 4-L beaker with 2 L PBS prechilled to 4°C and leave at 4°C overnight under gentle stirring on a magnetic stirring plate. After dialysis, insert a new 10-mL syringe fitted with a new 21-G needle into the dialysis cassette, transfer the dialyzed sample into a 15-mL Amicon Ultra Centrifugal Filter Device with 30-kDa MWCO, and concentrate by centrifugation at 3,000 × *g* for 30 min at 4°C in a refrigerated benchtop centrifuge with swinging bucket rotor. If necessary, continue the centrifugation until the volume of the concentrate is down to ~500 μL.
22. For concentrations >1 mg/mL, buffers with lower salt concentration and/or slightly acidic or basic pH may provide higher solubility than PBS. Purified scFv-Fc-HA protein is stable at 4°C for several months.
23. Many SDS-PAGE systems and staining procedures are available. Suggested equipment and reagents are listed in Subheading 2.4.

## Acknowledgments

This work was supported by the Intramural Research Program of the Center for Cancer Research, National Cancer Institute, National Institutes of Health. We thank Marko Modric for comments.

## References

1. Holliger P, Hudson PJ (2005) Engineered antibody fragments and the rise of single domains. Nat Biotechnol 23:1126–1136
2. Kontermann RE (2010) Alternative antibody formats. Curr Opin Mol Ther 12:176–183
3. Shu L, Qi CF, Schlom J et al (1993) Secretion of a single-gene-encoded immunoglobulin from myeloma cells. Proc Natl Acad Sci USA 90:7995–7999
4. Zhao X, Lapalombella R, Joshi T et al (2007) Targeting CD37-positive lymphoid malignancies with a novel engineered small modular immunopharmaceutical. Blood 11: 2569–2577
5. Robak T, Robak P, Smolewski P (2009) TRU-016, a humanized anti-CD37 IgG fusion protein for the potential treatment of B-cell malignancies. Curr Opin Investig Drugs 10:1383–1390

6. Hayden-Ledbetter MS, Cerveny CG, Espling E et al (2009) CD20-directed small modular immunopharmaceutical, TRU-015, depletes normal and malignant B cells. Clin Cancer Res 15:2739–2746
7. Rubbert-Roth A (2010) TRU-015, a fusion protein derived from an anti-CD20 antibody, for the treatment of rheumatoid arthritis. Curr Opin Mol Ther 12:115–123
8. Brocks B, Rode HJ, Klein M et al (1997) A TNF receptor antagonistic scFv, which is not secreted in mammalian cells, is expressed as a soluble mono- and bivalent scFv derivative in insect cells. Immunotechnology 3:173–184
9. Powers DB, Amersdorfer P, Poul M et al (2001) Expression of single-chain Fv-Fc fusions in *Pichia pastoris*. J Immunol Methods 251:123–135
10. Van Droogenbroeck B, Cao J, Stadlmann J et al (2007) Aberrant localization and underglycosylation of highly accumulating single-chain Fv-Fc antibodies in transgenic Arabidopsis seeds. Proc Natl Acad Sci USA 104: 1430–1435
11. Cao P, Zhang S, Gong Z et al (2006) Development of a compact anti-BAFF antibody in *Escherichia coli*. Appl Microbiol Biotechnol 73:151–157

# Chapter 15

# PEGylation of Antibody Fragments for Half-Life Extension

Simona Jevševar, Mateja Kusterle, and Maja Kenig

## Abstract

Antibody fragments (Fab's) represent important structure for creating new therapeutics. Compared to full antibodies Fab' fragments possess certain advantages, including higher mobility and tissue penetration, ability to bind antigen monovalently and lack of fragment crystallizable (Fc) region-mediated functions such as antibody-dependent cell mediated cytotoxicity (ADCC) or complement-dependent cytotoxicity (CDC). The main drawback for the use of Fab's in clinical applications is associated with their short half-life in vivo, which is a consequence of no longer having the Fc region. To exert meaningful clinical effects, the half-life of Fab's need to be extended, which has been achieved by postproduction chemical attachment of polyethylene glycol (PEG) chain to protein using PEGylation technology. The most suitable approach employs PEG-maleimide attachment to cysteines, either to the free hinge cysteine or to C-terminal cysteines involved in interchain disulfide linkage of the heavy and light chain. Hence, protocols for mono-PEGylation of Fab via free cysteine in the hinge region and di-PEGylation of Fab via interchain disulfide bridge are provided in this chapter.

**Key words:** Fab' fragment, PEGylation, Conjugate, Half-life extension

## 1. Introduction

Full antibodies are not always optimal for therapeutic applications. Their size of about 150 kDa makes them unsuitable for intracellular targeting and tissue penetration. Their activating Fc domain may also cause unwanted side effects such as antibody-dependent cell mediated cytotoxicity (ADCC) or complement dependent cytotoxicity (CDC). Also, cross-linking by cells expressing Fc-region receptors (FcR-expressing cells) can lead to agonist effects. Inappropriate activation of FcR-expressing cells can lead to cytokine storm, a potentially fatal immune reaction caused by highly elevated levels of different cytokines. Activating the Fc domain may also contribute to platelet aggregation. Bivalency can cause potential cross-linking that can lead to activation followed

Gabriele Proetzel and Hilmar Ebersbach (eds.), *Antibody Methods and Protocols*, Methods in Molecular Biology, vol. 901, DOI 10.1007/978-1-61779-931-0_15, © Springer Science+Business Media, LLC 2012

by apoptosis, proliferation, or internalization—blocking antibodies can therefore act as agonist when used in bivalent format. A long half-life of ABs is also not desirable for certain applications, for example tumor imaging (1, 2).

Antibody fragments (Fab's) represent a potential solution to overcome unwanted properties of complete antibodies. Fab's are small (about 50 kDa) and therefore more suitable for applications where better tissue penetration is needed and a short half-life is not an issue. Use of Fab's for tumor imaging is one of such applications. Higher mobility and tissue penetration gives Fab's many advantages to whole antibodies, e.g., for intraocular injections or when used as antidotes, due to their wider and faster distribution. In this case, their decreased immunogenicity is also highly beneficial. When binding to the target molecule is sufficient for therapeutic efficacy, a nonactivating format such as Fab' can be advantageous as it avoids unwanted cytotoxicity (ADCC and CDC). The use of monovalent formats is preferred when bivalent binding can cause cross-linking of receptors and their activation (2). Short elimination half-life of Fab's is often considered a disadvantage for clinical applications, however for diagnostic purposes (e.g., tumor imaging) this fast clearance is beneficial, enabling short exposure of the body to active substance.

Fab's are usually produced in bacterial, high-yielding production process, resulting in lower production cost compared to whole antibody production. Currently six unmodified Fab's have been FDA approved and are on the market for different applications. ReoPro® (abciximab, a Fab fragment of a chimeric human–murine monoclonal antibody 7E3) binds to the glycoprotein II3/IIIa receptor on human platelets and inhibits platelet aggregation. It was approved in 1994 for the prevention of restenosis in patient undergoing coronary angioplasty. Lucentis® (ranibizumab, a Fab derived from bevacizumab) inhibits vascular endothelial growth factor A (VEGF-A) and was approved in 2006 for the treatment of wet age-related macular degeneration (AMD) and macular edema following retinal vein occlusion (3). CroFab® (crotalide polyvalent immune Fab) was approved in 2000 for the treatment of envenomation by four species of North American pit vipers. It is a standardized mixture of four different monospecific Fab fragments, obtained by papain digestion. One year later DigiFab® (anti-digoxin Fab fragment) was approved for the treatment of digoxin intoxication. Another digoxin immune Fab, marketed as Digibind®, is also approved as digoxin antidote, beside that it is currently undergoing clinical study to delay delivery in patients with severe preeclampsia. Fab's are also to be used for diagnostic purposes, e.g., CEA-Scan (arcitumomab—monoclonal mouse Fab labeled with $^{99m}$Tc) was approved for tumor imaging in diagnostics of colon cancer (3). Additionally to FDA approved unmodified Fab's, several different Fab's are in different preclinical and clinical development phases. CytoFab™, an anti-TNF-alpha polyclonal Fab product for the treatment of sepsis and other TNF-mediated diseases, is currently in clinical trials and has successfully completed Phase IIa (3).

The main drawback of smaller, nonglycosylated antibody fragments in comparison to whole antibodies is their drastically shorter elimination half-life, which is only a few hours in humans compared to 7–21 days reported for complete antibodies. In rat, elimination half-life is only 0.3–1 h for unmodified Fab, compared to 13 days for whole antibody where the FcRn recycle mechanism is responsible for the long half-life (4) (and own unpublished results).

Many technologies have been developed to improve the pharmacokinetic properties of Fab's. Such technologies can be grouped into genetic fusion to other proteins or protein domains (e.g., Fc domain, albumin) and post production modifications, by chemical conjugation with natural or synthetic polymers such as polysialylation, HESylation® (conjugation with hydroxyethyl starch) and PEGylation (5–7). The covalent attachment of polymer polyethylene glycol (PEG) to a protein, known as PEGylation is a well-established, widely used technology and fulfills many of the requirements for safe and efficacious drugs and most reports refer to use of PEGylation as half-life extension technology for Fab's (5, 8).

PEGylation can be done randomly (nonselective) or site-directed. In the case of nonselective PEGylation, PEG is predominately attached to primary amino groups of surface exposed lysines using activated esters or carbonates of a PEG chain. PEG attachment sites can be influenced to some extent by pH and PEG size; however, sufficient selectivity of reaction cannot be achieved when many surface-exposed lysines are present. N-terminal PEGylation has been reported by Kinstler et al. as an example of potentially more selective PEGylation (9).

However, for many of Fab' fragments random or N-terminal PEGylation is not the best choice due to the fact that the N terminus of Fab's being the epitope binding region. A different chemistry can be used targeting the thiol group of cysteine (Cys) in the hinge region, which can be selectively PEGylated using maleimide-activated PEG. By attachment of PEG to free hinge Cys far away from the epitope binding region the in vitro bioactivity of PEGylated Fab's are not significantly reduced compared to unmodified Fab's. SPR data show comparable values of dissociation constant, while the association constant is slightly reduced after PEG attachment, correlating to the in vitro bioactivity data (own unpublished data). The flexible nature of PEG chains shields the Fab and protects it from environmental effects, but also influences the interactions of the Fab fragment with the target molecules that are responsible for its biological function. This characteristic of PEG chains means that in vitro activities determined by cell-based bioassays and SPR equilibrium dissociation constant ($K_D$) for PEGylated proteins are not predictive for the in vivo therapeutic effect, because of the flexible PEG chains phenomenon cause steric hindrance and not conformational changes. Although steric hindrance can reduce the binding affinity to the receptor, this is in part compensated by the prolonged circulating half-life allowing sufficient receptor–ligand interactions to be therapeutically effective (10).

To date there are ten FDA approved PEGylated products, one of them being a PEGylated Fab fragment. Certolizumab pegol, registered as Cimzia® (UCB Pharma, Belgium) has been approved for the treatment of Crohn's disease in 2008 and rheumatoid arthritis in 2009. The PEGylated Fab fragment Cimzia® has been engineered to contain a free cysteine residue in the hinge region. This position is structurally located far from the antigen-binding region, and it is available for a specific conjugation with 40 kDa branched maleimide-activated PEG resulting in a well-defined PEG-protein conjugate (Fig. 1). According to published data, conjugation of a 40 kDa PEG chain to Fab fragment can prolong its elimination half-life to the extent approaching elimination half-life of full mAb's, allowing biweekly administration of Cimzia® (elimination half-life is 14 days) (1, 11).

Several PEGylated Fab' fragments can be found in different stages of preclinical and clinical development. A common feature of many Fab's is the requirement for monovalent binding to the antigen. CDP7657 is a monovalent PEGylated Fab' fragment

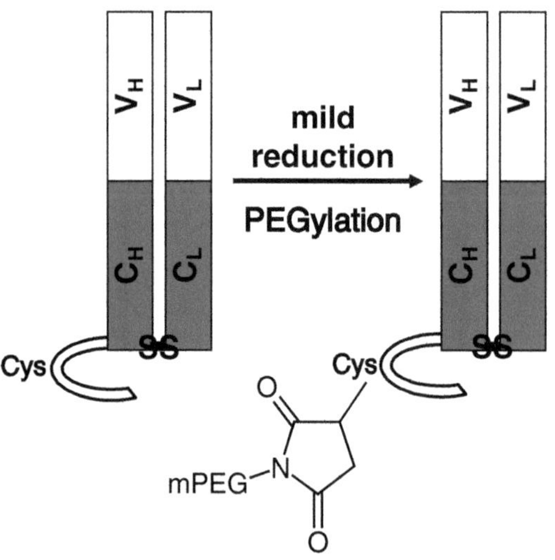


Fig. 1. PEGylation of Fab' fragment via free Cys in the hinge region.

directed against human CD40L protein, developed for the treatment of Systemic Lupus Erythematosus (SLE) and is in a phase I clinical study. In preclinical studies, it has been shown that treatment with monovalent PEGylated Fab' fragments efficiently inhibits CD40L function without causing thrombotic complications often associated with the treatment with whole IgG anti CD40L mAb (12, 13). Another example of PEGylated Fab in preclinical development is FR104; a PEGylated Fab' fragment of a humanized anti-CD28 monoclonal antibody with high affinity to CD28, thereby neutralizing its interaction with CD80/86 ligands. Due to its monovalent nature, the anti-CD28 blocks CD28–CD80/86 interactions without delivering any activation signal to T cells (14). FR104 is PEGylated on its C-terminal cysteine apparently applying the same PEGylation strategy as for preparation of Cimzia®. The PEGylated FR104 results in the serum half-life increasing by a factor 10.

An alternative approach for PEGylation is to target the interchain disulphide bridge between the light and heavy chain. After strong reduction of the Fab, PEG can be specifically attached to both heavy and light chain Cys residues (Fig. 2). This kind of modification requires highly stable Fab's; otherwise, heavy and light chain can be separated due to steric effects of PEG-chains. Based on published data PEGylated Fab's using the aforementioned approach often shows high chemical and thermal stability and good performance in PK and PD models. Attachment of a 20 kDa linear PEG chain to each Fab's chains has also been reported to result in a prolongation of half-lives to around 31 h in rats, while attachment of a 40 kDa branched PEG to free hinge cysteine can result in up to 51 h (11).

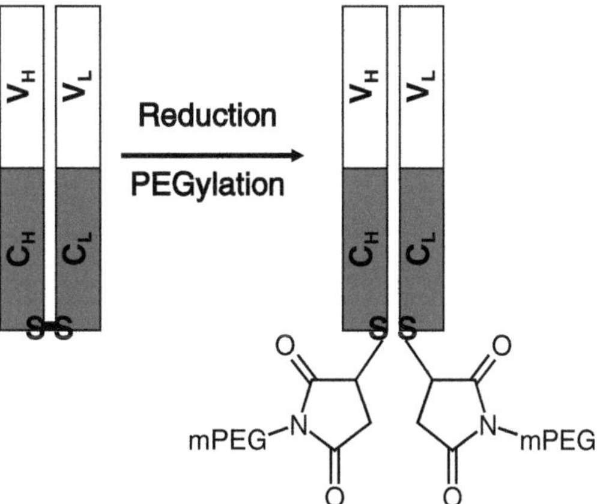


Fig. 2. Di-PEGylation of Fab' fragment via interchain disulfide bridge between light chain and heavy chain.

A novel PEGylation Technology was developed by PolyTherics (TheraPEG™). Using special PEG monosulfone reagents, site-specific bisalkylation of both sulfur atoms in the sufficiently exposed disulfide bond results in the insertion of the PEG linker into disulfide bonds and the formation of a PEGylated three-carbon bridge (15, 16).

The strategy is appropriate for site-specific PEGylation of Fab' fragments and it is similar to the aforementioned strategy employing interchain disulphide bridge between light and heavy chain which should be reduced prior to attachment of special PEG monosulfone reagent. The most obvious advantage of this strategy in comparison to traditional conjugation of two separate PEG chains to both cysteine residues at the C-termini of both Fab's chains, is thought to be the chemical linkage that is formed between both chains. The natural interchain disulfide bond is replaced by PEG-linkage. This is achieved via a special PEG reagent contributing to stabilization of the modified Fab molecule.

Based on published data for PEGylation of Fab and our own experience, the most suitable approaches employ PEG-maleimide attachment to cysteines, either to free hinge cysteines or to C-terminal cysteines involved in interchain disulfide linkage of the heavy and light chain. Hence, we describe below the mono-PEGylation of Fab via free cysteine in the hinge region and di-PEGylation of Fab via interchain disulfide bridge between light and heavy chains. Detailed protocols for lab scale production are also provided. Both protocols are fully scalable and can be transferred to pilot and then to industrial scale. However, in the case of mono-PEGylation of Fab via free cysteine in the hinge region, it is highly recommended to check reduction efficiency in lab scale tests first, since the efficiency of mild reduction directly influences overall process yield and should be considered as the most critical process step. On the other hand, reduction efficiency of interchain disulfide bridge is less problematic and PEGylation selectivity is high, resulting in a well defined product with high overall process yields.

## 2. Materials

All chemicals used for buffer preparation can be purchased from Sigma-Aldrich (St. Louis, MO, USA) unless otherwise noted. All buffers should be prepared using ultrapure water (purified deionized water, e.g., obtained with the Millipore Advantage A10 System), filtered through 0.22-μm polyethersulfone filters (e.g., Corning® 1,000-mL Bottle Top Vacuum Filter, 0.22-μm Pore 54.5 $cm^2$ PES Membrane, 431174) and stored at 4°C.

### 2.1. Fab Fragments

Fab fragments subjected to PEGylation in described protocols are produced in microbial expression system *E. coli* (see Note 1) (17).

It is highly recommended that Fab fragments are prepared in protein concentration above 5 mg/mL (around 8 mg/mL is optimal) enabling PEGylation at protein concentration of 5 mg/mL.

### 2.2. PEGylation

1. PEGylation Buffer 1: 20 mM sodium phosphate buffer, 50 mM NaCl, 10 mM EDTA, pH 7.5. Weigh into a glass container 2.76 g $NaH_2PO_4$ monohydrate, 2.92 g NaCl, and 3.72 g EDTA disodium salt dihydrate, add approximately 800 mL of water and adjust pH to 7.5 with 1 M NaOH. Transfer the solution to 1 L volumetric flask and fill with water to the mark. Filter the buffer through a 0.22-μm Corning filter.
2. PEGylation Buffer 2: 100 mM sodium phosphate buffer, 50 mM NaCl, 10 mM EDTA, pH 7.5 (see Note 2). Weigh into a glass container 13.8 g $NaH_2PO_4$ monohydrate, 2.92 g NaCl, and 0.74 g EDTA disodium salt dihydrate, add 800 mL of water and adjust pH to 7.5 with 1 M NaOH. Transfer the solution to 1 L volumetric flask and fill with water to the mark. Filter the buffer through a 0.22-μm Corning filter.
3. Tris(2-carboxyethyl)phosphine hydrochloride (TCEP) (cat. no. 20490, Pierce, Rockford, IL, USA).
4. 15 mM TCEP stock solution: Dissolve 4.3 mg of TCEP-HCl in 1 mL of PEGylation Buffer 1 (see Note 3).
5. 0.5 M TCEP stock solution: Dissolve 14.33 mg of TCEP-HCl in 100 μL of PEGylation Buffer 1 (see Note 3).
6. PEG reagent stock solution: Dissolve 30 mg of 20 kDa maleimide PEG-reagent (cat. no. SUNBRIGHT ME-200MA, NOF CORPORATION, Tokyo, Japan) in 600 μL of PEGylation Buffer 1 (see Note 4) to obtain PEG reagent stock solution with concentration 50 mg/mL (see Note 5).
7. Amicon® Ultra-4 Centrifugal Filter Unit with Ultracel-10 membrane (cat. no. UFC801024, Millipore, Billerica, MA, USA).
8. PD-10 Desalting Column (cat. no. 17-0851-01, GE Healthcare, UK).

### 2.3. Chromatographic Purification Components

1. Millex® GV (0.22 μm) filter unit with Durapore® PVDF membrane.
2. Chromatographic column: Tricorn 10/100 (GE Healthcare).
3. Chromatographic matrix: TSKgel SP-5PW (Tosoh, Tokyo, Japan). Pack the column according to producers' manual (see Note 6).
4. Equilibration buffer: 25 mM acetic acid, pH 4.0. Dilute 1.43 mL of glacial acetic acid in 0.9 L of water and adjust pH to 4.0 with 5 M NaOH. Transfer the solution to 1-L volumetric flask and fill with water to the mark. Filter the buffer through a 0.22-μm Corning filter.

5. Elution buffer: 25 mM acetic acid, 250 mM sodium chloride, pH 4.0. Weigh 14.61 g of sodium chloride, dissolve in 0.9 L of water, add 1.43 mL of glacial acetic acid, and adjust pH to 4.0 with 5 M NaOH. Transfer the solution to 1-L volumetric flask and fill with water to the mark. Filter the buffer through a 0.22-μm Corning filter.
6. ÄKTA purifier or similar chromatographic system equipped with fraction collector (GE Healthcare).

## 3. Methods

### *3.1. Mono-PEGylation of Fab Using the Single Hinge Cysteine*

1. Use 4 mL of Fab fragment solution in PEGylation Buffer 1 at the concentration 2.5 mg/mL (10 mg of Fab fragment).
2. Add 27 μL of 15 mM TCEP stock solution to achieve a final TCEP concentration of 0.1 mM.
3. Incubate at room temperature (RT) (see Note 7) for 90 min with gentle shaking.
4. Perform buffer exchange with PEGylation Buffer 1 using ultracentrifuge Amicon® Ultra-4 Centrifugal Filter Unit with Ultracel-10 membrane (10 kDa cutoff) to remove TCEP (see Note 8). Concentrate Fab solution at 3,220 *g* to approximately 0.5 mL (see Note 9) and add buffer to 4 mL. Repeat five times to achieve efficient removal of reducing agent. Final volume of Fab solution after buffer exchange should be around 4 mL.
5. Incubate reduced Fab at RT (see Note 7) for 24 h in order to achieve reconstitution of interchain disulfide bridge (see Note 10).
6. Prepare PEGylation mixture by adding 400 μL of PEG reagent stock solution (5 molar excess of PEG-maleimide) to the solution of reoxidized Fab.
7. Incubate overnight (16–18 h) at RT (see Note 7) with gentle shaking (see Note 11).
8. After incubation dilute PEGylation mixture by mixing one part of PEGylation mixture with three parts of equilibration buffer.
9. Filter diluted PEGylation mixture through Millex syringe driven filter unit.
10. Equilibrate column packed with TSK-GEL SP-5PW resin with three column volumes of equilibration buffer and load diluted and filtered sample onto the column (see Note 12).
11. Wash the column with two CV of equilibration buffer and elute PEGylated Fab fragment by applying linear gradient of

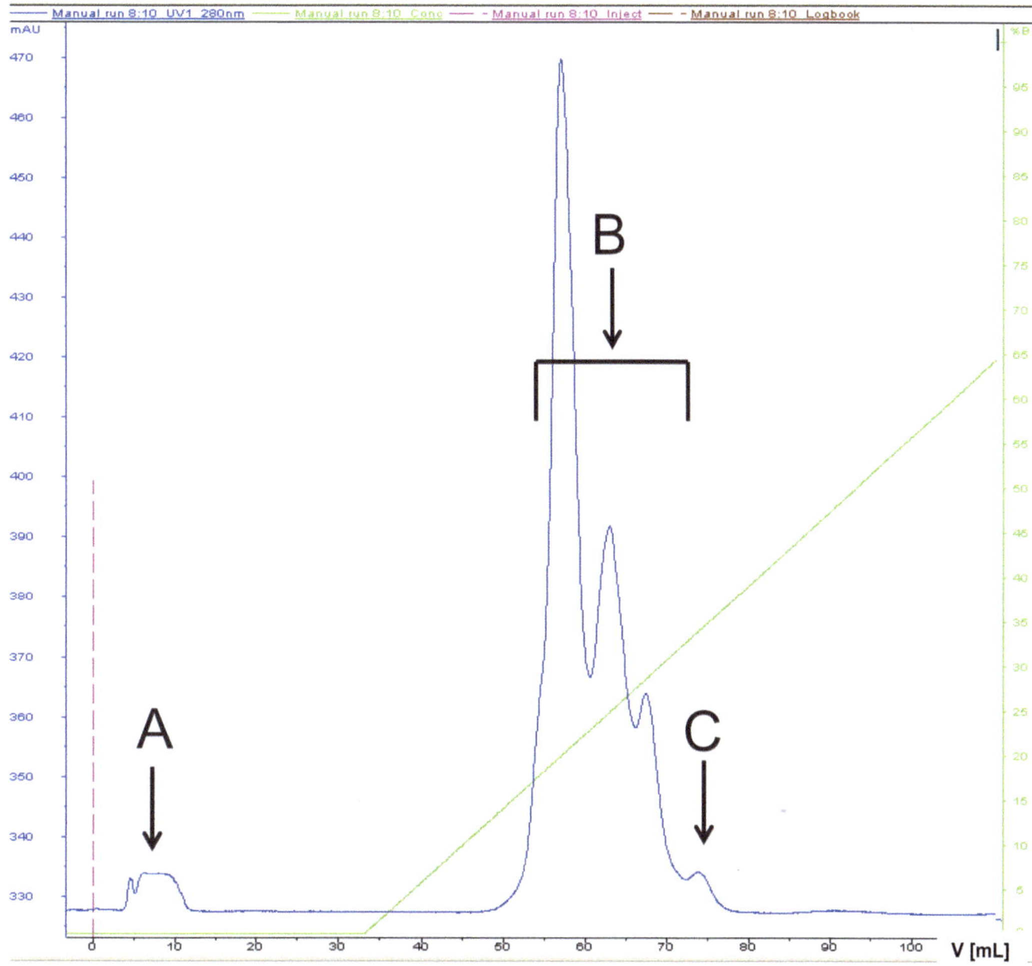


Fig. 3. Chromatographic purification of Fab' fragment di-PEGylated via interchain disulfide bridge between LC and HC with cation exchange chromatography; (**A**) PEG reagent and higher PEGylated Fab fragment, (**B**) Fab fragment di-PEGylated via interchain disulfide bridge, (**C**) non-PEGylated Fab fragment.

elution buffer (0–100% elution buffer in ten CV, see Note 12). Typical preparative cation exchange chromatogram of PEG-Fab's is shown in Fig. 3.

12. Use RP-HPLC-analysis and SDS-PAGE analysis for evaluation of PEGylation efficiency (see Note 13). Typical yields of PEGylation reaction performed by this procedure in lab scale are around 45% and overall process yield around 40%.

### 3.2. Di-PEGylation of Fab's

1. Use 2.3 mL of Fab solution in PEGylation Buffer 2 at the concentration of 5 mg/mL (11.5 mg of Fab fragment, see Note 14).
2. Add 0.2 mL of 0.5 M TCEP stock solution to achieve final TCEP concentration of 40 mM.
3. Incubate at RT (see Note 7) for 30 min with gentle shaking.

4. Remove reducing agent on PD-10 Desalting Column. Equilibrate the column with 25 mL of PEGylation Buffer 1. Apply 2.5 mL of Fab fragment solution and elute with 3.2 mL of the same buffer (see Note 15).
5. Immediately add 460 μL of PEG-maleimide stock solution (5 molar excess of PEG-maleimide) to prepare PEGylation mixture (see Note 16).
6. Incubate overnight (16–18 h) at RT (see Note 7) with gentle shaking.
7. Dilute PEGylation mixture by mixing one part of the PEGylation mixture with three parts of equilibration buffer.
8. Filter diluted PEGylation mixture through Millex syringe driven filter unit.
9. Equilibrate column packed with TSK-GEL SP-5PW resin with three column volumes of equilibration buffer and load diluted and filtered sample onto the column (see Note 12).
10. Wash the column with two column volumes of equilibration buffer and elute PEGylated Fab fragment by applying linear gradient of elution buffer (0–100% elution buffer in ten CV, see Note 12).
11. Use RP-HPLC analysis and SDS-PAGE analysis for evaluation of PEGylation efficiency (see Note 13). Using this procedure, PEGylation yield is typically around 90% and overall process yield is around 80%. Figure 4 shows a typical analytical RP-HPLC chromatogram of Fab and PEG-Fab, while Fig. 5 shows a SDS-PAGE of Fab and PEG-Fab (see Note 17).

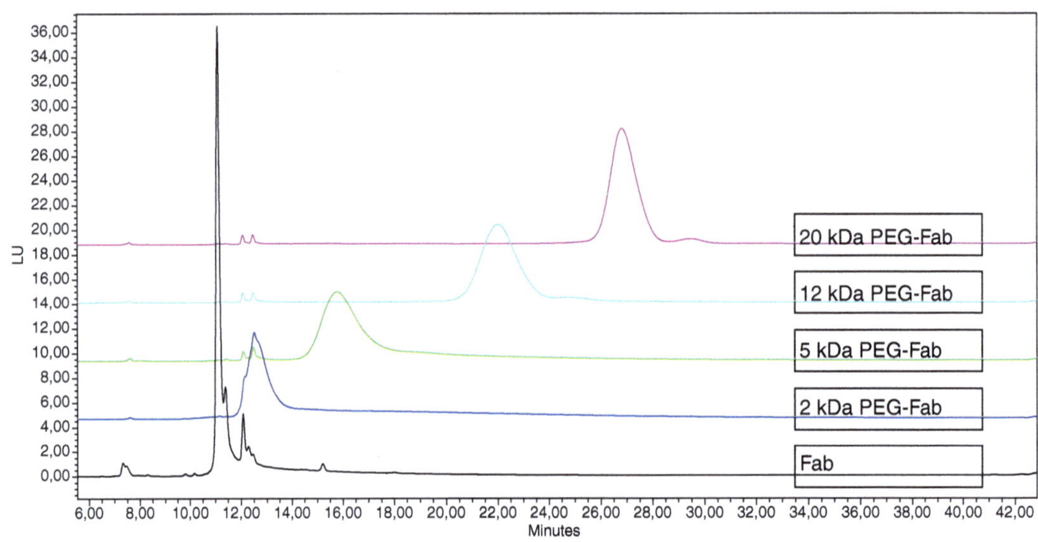


Fig. 4. Analytical RP-HPLC chromatogram of Fab and PEG-Fab's: 2 kDa PEG-Fab, 5 kDa PEG-Fab, 12 kDa PEG-Fab, and 20 kDa PEG-Fab.

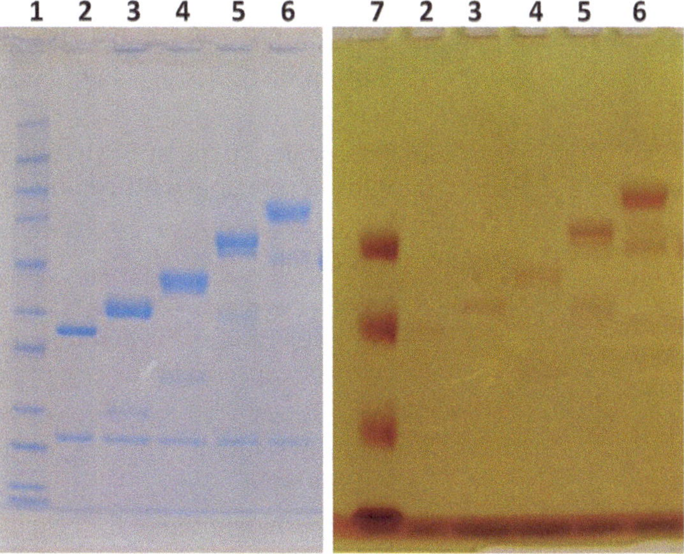


Fig. 5. SDS-PAGE analysis of non-PEGylated Fab (*lane 2*) and PEG-Fab's conjugates: 2 kDa PEG (*lane 3*), 5 kDa PEG-Fab (*lane 4*), 12 kDa PEG-Fab (*lane 5*), 20 kDa PEG-Fab (*lane 6*), Novex protein standards (*lane 1*), mix of PEG standards: 5 kDa, 12 kDa, 20 kDa, 30 kDa (*lane 7*). *Left* simply blue staining, *right* iodine staining.

## 4. Notes

1. Fab's from other alternative sources can also be used for PEGylation: e.g., Fab fragments produced in mammalian expression systems (18), in yeast *Pichia pastoris* (19), or even prepared with enzymatic digestion of whole mAbs with papain (20).
2. Higher buffer capacity is needed for the reduction of Fab in procedure 3.2 to maintain pH at 7.5, due to high concentration of TCEP.
3. Fresh TCEP stock solution must be prepared immediately before adding to Fab solution.
4. Use PEGylation Buffer 1 for the preparation of PEG reagent stock solution for both procedures (3.1 and 3.2).
5. PEG-reagent is usually stored frozen at –20°C. It is important to temperate PEG-reagent at RT before opening and weighing to reduce binding of water from air, which can cause PEG degradation. It is advised to use glass containers for more accurate weighing of PEG-reagent. When preparing PEG stock solutions at high concentrations (50–100 mg/mL), intensive mixing or shaking is needed. Afterwards, PEG solution should

be left for a few minutes to clarify before adding it to protein solution (highly concentrated PEG-reagent solution is viscous and can be opalescent due to many small air bubbles trapped in it).

6. To separate 10 mg of PEGylated Fab fragment, approximately 8-mL chromatographic column should be used.
7. RT is 22 ± 3°C. An incubator can be used to achieve this temperature.
8. Protein aggregation might occur at ultrafiltration as a result of supersaturation and high solvent flow rates. Higher aggregation could be expected in the case of proteins with low stability.
9. Approximately 10 min are needed to concentrate 4 mL of Fab fragment solution to 0.5 mL, when centrifugation is performed at 1,700 rcf.
10. The free thiol group of the cysteine residue in the hinge region of Fab's is usually cysteinylated during the cell disruption and needs to be selectively reactivated before conjugation with PEG-maleimide (18). Several reducing agents for selective reduction of the free hinge cysteine can be used: MEA, $Na_2SO_3$, TCEP, or THP. Since all aforementioned reducing agents are also able to disrupt disulfide bridge between the light and heavy chain of the Fab fragment, a certain time for reoxidation of the disulfide bridge is necessary after the removal of reducing agent and prior to addition of PEG-maleimide (18). Still, many reports can be found where PEGylation is performed immediately after the removal of the reducing agent, but this usually results in significantly lower PEGylation yields and low overall process yields (21, 22).
11. It is necessary to perform efficient mixing of the reaction mixture. Inefficient mixing may result in lower PEGylation yield.
12. It is advised to load the sample at lower flow-rate (0.5 mL/min), while for the other chromatographic steps higher flow-rates can be applied (e.g., 1 mL/min).
13. PEGylation efficiency is usually monitored by RP-HPLC. SDS-PAGE with Coomassie blue staining provides only nonquantitative monitoring. Iodine staining can be used to differentiate between PEGylated and non-PEGylated Fab fragments (23).
14. Mono-PEGylation of Fab fragment via free cysteine in the hinge region results in higher yields when the reaction is performed at higher protein concentration, ideally above 5 mg/mL, if the protein is stable at this level.
15. A PD-10 column is used instead of buffer exchange on Amicon® cells to shorten the time needed for the removal of the reducing agent. It is essential that the reducing agent removal is efficient and complete. We recommend to elute with a lower buffer volume: 3.2 mL instead of 3.5 mL.

16. In the process of di-PEGylation of Fab fragments via interchain disulfide bridge (Fab' without hinge cysteine), it is necessary to proceed with the PEGylation immediately after the removal of reducing agent to achieve higher yields.
17. One should be aware that the mobility of PEG-conjugates in SDS-PAGE is different than that of unmodified protein. The apparent MW of the PEG-protein conjugates is closer to the apparent MW of PEG standards than to the MW of protein standards.

## References


1. Liddell JM (2009) Production strategies for antibody fragment therapeutics. BioPharm Int 2:36–42
2. Labrijn AF, Aalberse RC, Schuurman J (2008) When binding is enough: nonactivating antibody formats. Curr Opin Immunol 20:479–485
3. Rader C (2009) Overview on concepts and applications of Fab antibody fragments. Curr Protoc Protein Sci. Chapter 6, 6.9.1–6.9.14
4. Chapman AP, Antoniw P, Spitali M et al (1999) Therapeutic antibody fragments with prolonged in vivo half-lives. Nat Biotechnol 17:780–783
5. Chen C, Constantinou A, Deonarain M (2011) Modulating antibody pharmacokinetics using hydrophilic polymers. Expert Opin Drug Deliv 8:1221–1236
6. Kontermann RE (2009) Strategies to extend plasma half-lives of recombinant antibodies. BioDrugs 23:93–109
7. Constantinou A, Epenetos AA, Hreczuk-Hirst D et al (2008) Modulation of antibody pharmacokinetics by chemical polysialylation. Bioconjug Chem 19:643–650
8. Jevsevar S, Kunstelj M, Porekar VG (2010) PEGylation of therapeutic proteins. Biotechnol J 5:113–128
9. Kinstler O, Molineux G, Treuheit M et al (2002) Mono-N-terminal poly(ethylene glycol)-protein conjugates. Adv Drug Deliv Rev 54:477–485
10. Bailon P, Won CY (2009) PEG-modified biopharmaceuticals. Expert Opin Drug Deliv 6:1–16
11. Humphreys DP, Heywood SP, Henry A et al (2007) Alternative antibody Fab' fragment PEGylation strategies: combination of strong reducing agents, disruption of the interchain disulphide bond and disulphide engineering. Protein Eng Des Sel 20:227–234
12. Wakefield I, Peters C, Burkly L et al (2010) CDP7657, a monovalent Fab PEG anti-CD40L antibody, inhibits immune responses in both HuSCID mice and non-human primates. Arthritis Rheum 62:1245
13. Vugler A, Sutton D, Marshall D et al (2010) Blockade of CD40L with a monovalent Fab' PEG monoclonal antibody inhibits disease in the murine collagen-induced arthritis model. Arthritis Rheum 62:1244
14. Poirier N, Azimzadeh AM, Zhang T et al (2010) Inducing CTLA-4-dependent immune regulation by selective CD28 blockade promotes regulatory T cells in organ transplantation. Sci Transl Med 2:17ra10
15. Balan S, Choi JW, Godwin A et al (2007) Site-specific PEGylation of protein disulfide bonds using a three-carbon bridge. Bioconjug Chem 18:61–76
16. Shaunak S, Godwin A, Choi JW et al (2006) Site-specific PEGylation of native disulfide bonds in therapeutic proteins. Nat Chem Biol 2:312–313
17. Kwong KY, Rader C (2009) *E. coli* expression and purification of Fab antibody fragments. Curr Protoc Protein Sci. Chapter 6, 6.10
18. Pepinsky RB, Walus L, Shao Z et al (2011) Production of a PEGylated Fab' of the anti-LINGO-1 Li33 antibody and assessment of its biochemical and functional properties in vitro and in a rat model of remyelination. Bioconjug Chem 22:200–210
19. Gach JS, Maurer M, Hahn R et al (2007) High level expression of a promising anti-idiotypic antibody fragment vaccine against HIV-1 in *Pichia pastoris*. J Biotechnol 128:735–746
20. Zhao Y, Gutshall L, Jiang H et al (2009) Two routes for production and purification of Fab fragments in biopharmaceutical discovery research: papain digestion of mAb and transient expression in mammalian cells. Protein Exp Purif 67:182–189
21. Lu Y, Harding SE, Turner A et al (2008) Effect of PEGylation on the solution conformation of antibody fragments. J Pharm Sci 97:2062–2079

22. Leong SR, DeForge L, Presta L et al (2001) Adapting pharmacokinetic properties of a humanized anti-interleukin-8 antibody for therapeutic applications using site-specific pegylation. Cytokine 16:106–119

23. Kurfurst MM (1992) Detection and molecular-weight determination of polyethylene glycol-modified hirudin by staining after sodium dodecyl-sulfate polyacrylamide-gel electrophoresis. Anal Biochem 200:244–248

# Chapter 16

# Bispecific Antibody Derivatives Based on Full-Length IgG Formats


## Michael Grote, Alexander K. Haas, Christian Klein, Wolfgang Schaefer, and Ulrich Brinkmann



## Abstract

Monoclonal antibodies have emerged as an effective therapeutic modality, and numerous antibodies have been approved for the treatment of several severe diseases or are currently in clinical development. To improve their therapeutic potential, monoclonal antibodies are constantly evolved by protein engineering. Particularly, the generation of bispecific antibodies raised special interest because of their ability to bind two different antigens at the same time, and the efficiency of these formats has been demonstrated in several clinical and preclinical studies. Up to now, the major drawbacks in using bispecific antibodies as a therapeutic agent have been difficult design and low-yield expression of homogeneous antibody populations. However, major technological improvements were made in protein engineering during the last years. This allows the design of several new IgG-based bispecific antibody formats that can be prepared in high yields and high homogeneity using conventional expression and purification techniques. Especially, recent development of IgG-fusions with disulfide-stabilized Fv fragments and of CrossMab-technologies facilitates the generation of bispecific antibodies with IgG-like architectures. Here we describe design principles and methods to express and purify different bispecific antibody formats derived from full-length IgGs.



**Key words:** Bispecific antibody, Single-chain variable fragment (scFv), Disulfide-stabilized Fv antibody fragment (dsFv), CrossMab, Knobs-into-holes


## 1. Introduction

Since the invention of hybridoma technology in 1975 (1), monoclonal antibodies have been constantly developed to improve them for clinical application. Antibody chimerization, humanization, and the later development of monoclonal antibodies from human origin paved the way for an effective new therapeutic modality in the treatment of cancer, as well as inflammatory, metabolic, viral, and autoimmune diseases (2–4). In recent years, significant progress


Gabriele Proetzel and Hilmar Ebersbach (eds.), *Antibody Methods and Protocols*, Methods in Molecular Biology, vol. 901,
DOI 10.1007/978-1-61779-931-0_16, © Springer Science+Business Media, LLC 2012

has been made in protein engineering techniques, enabling the design of completely new formats of antibodies and antibody-based molecules with improved therapeutic properties (5). In particular, bispecific antibodies have raised special interest because of their ability to simultaneously bind two separate antigens or different epitopes of the same antigen. In contrast to combination therapy using two individual monoclonal antibodies, bispecific antibodies offer the opportunity of dual targeting with a single molecule and benefit from synergistic or additive effects. The dual targeting strategy has been explored in numerous preclinical studies using several different antigen pairs (e.g., VEGFR1 and VEGFR2 (6), Her2 and VEGF (7), EGFR and IGF-1R (8, 9), or IL-1α and IL-1β (7, 10, 11)). These studies consistently demonstrate that simultaneous targeting with bispecific antibodies was more efficient than monotherapies against the same target.

The effectiveness of monoclonal antibodies often requires engagement of the cellular immune system via induction of antibody-dependent cell-mediated cytotoxicity (ADCC). However, triggering ADCC with monoclonal antibodies depends on a strong interaction between the Fc domain and Fcγ receptors (FcγRs) on effector cells and still faces several limitations (2, 4). Thus, retargeting effector cells of the immune system (e.g., cytotoxic T-cells, natural killer cells, neutrophils or macrophages) to target cells (e.g., cancer cells) is perhaps the most exciting application of bispecific antibodies. Most successfully, retargeting of cytotoxic T-cells to tumor cells via the CD3 co-receptor and a tumor cell-specific antigen (e.g., CD19 or EpCAM) was evaluated in several clinical studies demonstrating considerable potential of these molecules (12). In addition, stimulation of ADCC was achieved by retargeting of natural killer cells via specific targeting of FcγRIIIA, thereby avoiding activation of inhibitory receptors (e.g., FcγRIIB) via natural Fc/FcγR interactions (13, 14).

Monoclonal antibodies have also been evaluated for payload delivery to target cells. For example, the Her2-binding antibody trastuzumab coupled to the chemotherapy agent DM1 showed promising results in clinical trials (15, 16). So far, most targeting concepts are based on chemical conjugation of payloads or generation of protein fusions (17–20). However, bispecific antibodies can also be applied for this task. In a recent study it was shown that bispecific antibodies that bind cell-surface targets (e.g., Her2, IGF1R, CD22, or LeY), as well as digoxigenin (DIG), efficiently delivered digoxigeninylated payloads (e.g., DIG-Cy5, DIG-Doxorubicin, or DIG-GFP) to cancer cells (21). Additionally, bispecific antibodies can be applied for two-step pre-targeting therapies (22). In the first step, the bispecific antibody is injected and binds to the target cells in the body. After clearance of unbound antibodies from the organism, the payload is administered and immediately captured by the pre-targeted bispecific antibodies.

This approach significantly reduces toxic side effects of the payload compared to antibody conjugates, because the plasma half-life of the payload alone is usually significantly lower compared to antibody–payload conjugates. Thus, unbound payloads are rapidly cleared from the body after injection and do not harm normal tissues.

Until now, the major hindrance in the development of bispecific antibodies as a therapeutic agent has been the production of sufficient yields of homogenous bispecific antibody populations by traditional technologies like quadroma or chemical conjugation. In quadroma technology, two different murine hybridoma cell lines are fused to generate a hybrid hybridoma (23). Within these cells the heavy and light chains of both antibodies randomly assemble into a variety of different immunoglobulins leading to the undesired formation of heavy-chain homodimers and mispairing of light and heavy chains. As a consequence, the desired bispecific antibody statistically accounts for only 12.5% of all assembly products, and purification from the other products is hardly possible (24). However, hybrid bispecific antibodies have been designed via fusion of murine and rat hybridomas (25). The resulting IgGs are preferentially composed of one mouse γ2a and one rat γ2b heavy chain, targeting with one arm an antigen on the tumor cell and with the other arm the CD3 co-receptor on cytotoxic T cells. Additionally, the hybrid Fc portion of these antibodies efficiently binds to activating human FcγRs expressed on macrophages, dendritic cells, and natural killer cells (26, 27). Thus, these antibodies are referred to as trifunctional triomabs and show promising results in clinical studies (28). Alternatively, bispecific antibodies have been produced by chemical conjugation of two different monoclonal antibodies or antibody fragments after purification and some of these molecules have been evaluated in the clinic (29, 30). However, chemically cross-linked antibodies often suffer from low product homogeneity, poor stability, and antibody inactivation.

### 1.1. Bispecific Antibody Derivatives Generated by Recombinant Gene Fusions

Because of their modular architecture, antibodies are especially accessible to protein engineering. Genes of IgG molecules can be subcloned into mammalian expression vectors and are thus target for numerous modifications. In this way, a variety of different bispecific antibody formats have been developed during the last years, including IgG-like molecules, as well as recombinant antibody fragments (3, 31, 32). The latter are characterized by their small size, and a plethora of different assemblies were designed, for example tandem single-chain Fv (scFv) fragments, diabodies, tandem single-domain antibodies and variations thereof (33). The small size of recombinant bispecific formats gives rise to improved tissue and solid tumor penetration rates, and several of these molecules have already entered clinical studies aiming cancer therapy (34). Moreover, bispecific antibody fragments do not require glycosylation and thus can be efficiently produced in bacteria like

*Escherichia coli* (35). However, the small size and the lack of constant regions also results in a short in vivo half-life of these formats due to rapid clearing from circulation, as well as complete loss of Fc-related effector functions (e.g., ADCC or binding to neonatal Fc receptors), respectively. In some cases, prolonged in vivo half-life and effector functions were reconstituted by addition of polyethylene glycol or direct coupling to human serum albumin and by inclusion of Fc regions, respectively (36, 37).

### 1.2. IgG-Derived Bispecific Antibody Derivatives Containing Fv Fragments as Additional Binding Modules

In contrast to bispecific antibody fragments, bispecific antibody derivatives based on full-length IgG formats are large molecules with intact Fc portions. This offers the possibility of binding to neonatal Fc receptors and leads to long serum half-lives (38). An increasing repertoire of bispecific antibodies with IgG-like features has been created by recombinant permutation of antigen-binding building blocks (e.g., scFv or single-domain antibodies) with IgG-type antibodies (Fig. 1a). Several of these antibody formats are both bispecific and bivalent for each antigen (2+2 format). For example, C- or N-terminal fusions of scFv fragments with either heavy or light chains directly add the antigen-binding specificity of two scFv fragments to a fully functional IgG antibody (31). The same method was also adopted for recombinant IgG-fusions with single-domain antibodies (3, 39). The dual variable domain (DVD) IgG format was designed by attaching VL and VH domains to the N termini of the same domains of a second antigen-binding specificity (10, 11). Furthermore, a bispecific format was described that is bivalent for one antigen but monovalent for the second antigen (2+1 format) (40). In these molecules, a VL domain is coupled to the CH3 domain of an IgG heavy chain, whereas the corresponding VH domain is attached to the CH3 domain of the second heavy chain. Co-expression of both heavy chains results in formation of an IgG-like antibody with an additional Fv domain attached to its Fc part.

However, bispecific antibody formats containing additional Fv modules often suffer from low stability and are prone to aggregation as a result of weak VH–VL binding interfaces in single Fv fragments (41). Stable Fv modules can be produced by connecting the VH and VL domains by a peptide linker regenerating the antigen-binding site in a single molecule (42–44). Alternatively, VH–VL heterodimers can be stabilized by an interchain disulfide bond which requires introduction of two cysteine residues at positions VH44 and VL100 (Kabat numbering scheme) (45–47).

### 1.3. IgG-Derived Bispecific Antibodies Generated by Domain Exchanges and Knobs-into-Holes Technologies

To avoid the problems of heavy chain homodimerization and mispairing of light and heavy chains, the abovementioned IgG-like bispecific antibody formats deviate from the native IgG molecular architecture. However, two elegant approaches were made to effectively induce heterodimerization of the two heavy chains and to discriminate between the two light chain/heavy

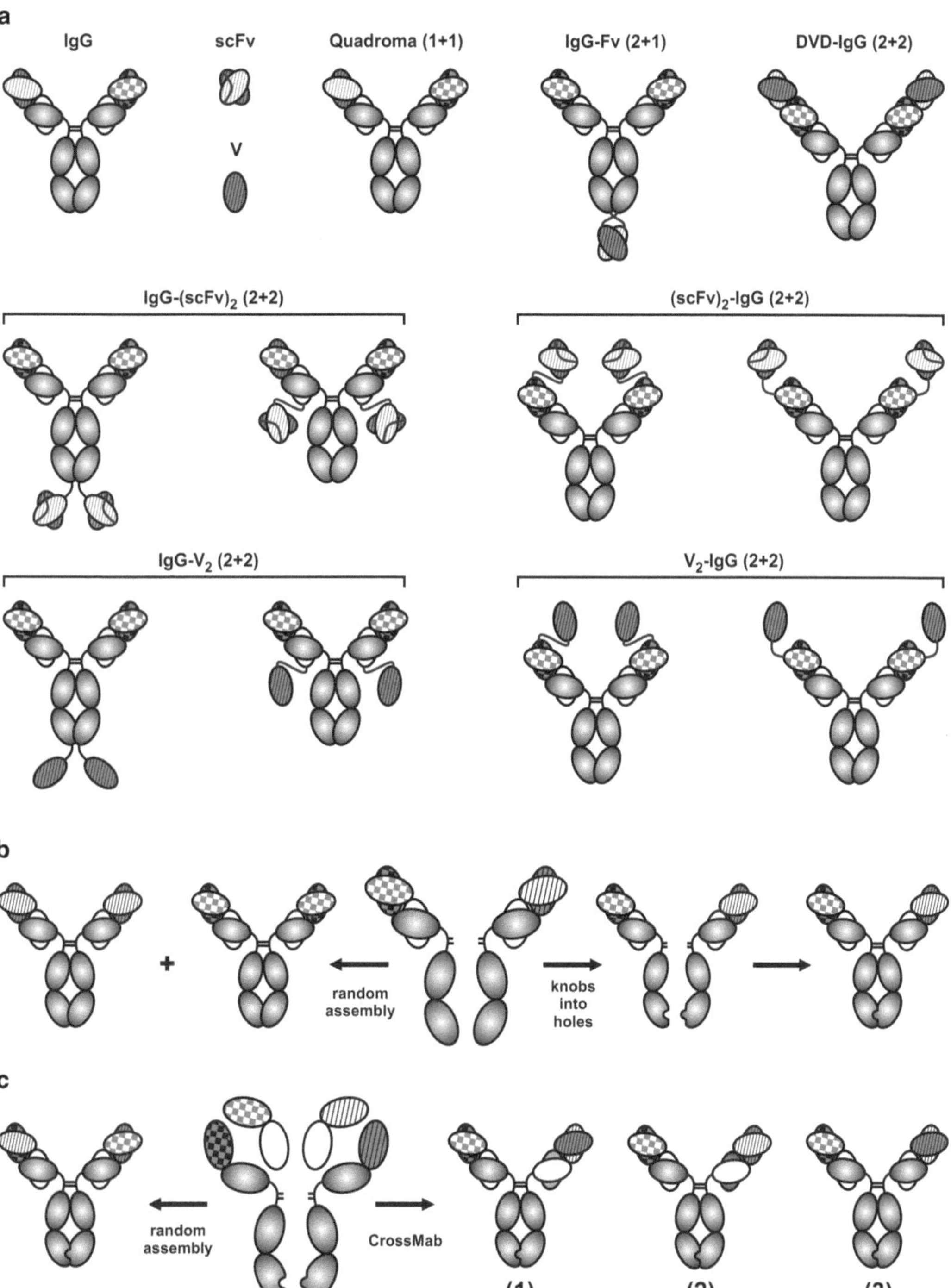


Fig. 1. Bispecific antibody formats derived from full-length IgGs. Heavy chain constant domains are represented in *dark gray color*. Light chain constant domains are shown in *white color*. Variable domains of the two different antigen-binding specificities are indicated with *dashed lines* or *boxes*, respectively. Heavy and light chains variable domains are distinguished by *dark* and *pale* contrasting, respectively. (**a**) C-terminal scFv-fusions are shown on the left [IgG-(scFv)$_2$ and IgG-V$_2$] and N-terminal fusions on the right [(scFv)$_2$-IgG and V$_2$-IgG]. A detailed description of each format is presented in the text. (**b**) The "Knobs-into-holes" method prevents bispecific antibodies from heavy chain homodimerization due to reengineering of the CH3 domain. (**c**) The "CrossMab" technology combines the "knob-into-holes" method with a Fab domain exchange. The domain exchange can comprise the complete VH-CH1 and VL-Cκ domains (1) or only the CH1 and Cκ domains (2) or the VH and VL domains (3), respectively.

chain interactions, respectively. Firstly, Carter et al. developed the "knobs-into-holes" technique that relies on reengineering the CH3 domain of the antibody's Fc portion (48). Based on the crystal structure of the antibody's Fc domain, the authors introduced a "knob" mutation (e.g., T366Y) into one heavy chain and a "hole" mutation (e.g., Y407T) into the other heavy chain. As shown schematically in Fig. 1b, co-expression of both heavy chains in a single host cell thermodynamically favors the formation of the heterodimeric over the homodimeric product. While the "knobs-into-holes" technique provided a tool for preferential heavy chain heterodimerization, the potential light chain/heavy chain mispairing remained challenging for a long time. Just recently, Schaefer et al. described a generic approach to solve the problem also of mispairing between heavy and light chains (49). The "CrossMab" technology utilizes a simple domain crossover in one arm of the antibody to diversify the interfaces of both antibody arms. As shown in Fig. 1c, the domain exchange can encompass the complete VH-CH1 and VL-Cκ domains or only the VH and VL domains or the CH1 and Cκ domains, respectively. In combining both, the "knobs-into-holes" and the "CrossMab" technology, it is possible to generate IgG-like bispecific antibodies of defined composition. The resulting bispecific antibodies possess monovalent binding sites for each antigen (1 + 1 format) and Fc parts identical to natural IgGs with knobs/holes and thus benefit from IgG-like pharmacokinetic properties and effector functions (49).

Taken together, major technological improvements have been made to design and produce new bispecific antibody formats over the last two decades. Because methods like "CrossMab" and "knobs-into-holes" do not change the antigen-binding sites of the antibody, they allow the conversion of basically any IgG antibody into a bispecific format. In addition, these new technologies hold the potential to routinely express high levels of homogenous bispecific antibodies required to launch clinical studies. Importantly, an increasing understanding of the biology involved in human diseases is detrimental for the selection of the right targets for efficient bispecific antibody-based therapies and to reduce side-effects during therapy. In this regard, cell-type specific retargeting of certain effector cells or molecules via bispecific antibodies is capable to overcome current limitations in monoclonal antibody-based therapies and may deliver effective new drug formats.

## 2. Materials

### 2.1. Transient Production of Bispecific Antibodies in Mammalian Cells

1. Human embryonic kidney 293 cells (ATCC, Manassas, VA, USA).
2. Synthetic or complex medium that is suitable for propagation of mammalian cells: e.g., MEM supplemented with 10% fetal bovine serum.
3. Plasmid DNAs that encode components of bispecific antibody derivatives, such as modified heavy chains and corresponding light chains.
4. 293-Transfection Reagent (EMD Chemicals or Merck KGaA, Darmstadt, Germany).
5. 0.22-μm filter.

### 2.2. Purification of Bispecific Antibodies

1. Protein-A-Sepharose™ (GE Healthcare, UK).
2. Superdex200™ (GE Healthcare).
3. HiTrap Protein-A HP (5 mL) column (GE Healthcare).
4. PBS buffer: 10 mM $Na_2HPO_4$, 1 mM $KH_2PO_4$, 137 mM NaCl, and 2.7 mM KCl, pH 7.4.
5. 0.1 M citrate buffer, pH 2.8.
6. 1 M Tris–HCl, pH 8.5.
7. Concentrating filter unit (Amicon Ultra centrifugal filter device 30 K, Millipore, Billerica, MA, USA).
8. Superdex200 HiLoad 120 mL 16/60 gel filtration column (GE Healthcare).

### 2.3. Characterization of Bispecific Antibodies

1. 4–20% Tris–glycine gels (NuPAGE®, Invitrogen, Carlsbad, CA, USA).
2. Peptide-N-Glycosidase F (Roche Molecular Biochemicals, Indianapolis, USA).
3. Biacore™ (GE Healthcare).

## 3. Methods

So far, the production of bispecific antibodies as therapeutic agents was hampered by low expression yields and difficulties in purification of bispecific antibodies. Improvements made to design and express new bispecific antibody formats during the last years now facilitates purification to homogeneity and high-rate recovery. Depending on the application (e.g., the biology of the target antigens), it may be necessary to specifically select for the valency of bispecific antibody formats (e.g., 1+1, 2+1, or 2+2 formats) (see Note 1). Here we describe the design and generation of three bispecific antibody formats that are based on full-length IgG molecules. These molecules can be produced in high yield within robust transient mammalian expression systems. Furthermore, IgG-like bispecific antibodies allow the application of generic production processes and analytical procedures that are already established for natural IgGs, including standard protein-A-based downstream processing.

### 3.1. Design Principles of Different Bispecific Antibody Formats

#### 3.1.1. C-terminal IgG-$(scFv)_2$ fusion (2+2 format)

To generate bispecific antibodies of the 2+2 format, a scFv fragment is attached to the C-terminus of a natural IgG (21). This results in a bispecific antibody format with two identical heavy chains that is bivalent for each antigen-binding site (Fig. 1). Consequently, this format does not require the "knobs-into-holes" technique, and heavy chain heterodimerization is not necessary. In addition, only one light chain construct is needed for both antibody arms, thereby avoiding the problem of light chain/heavy chain mispairing. To generate such molecules, gene segments that encode scFv fragments flanked by endonuclease cleavage sites (for cloning purposes) can be generated by various technologies, including automated gene synthesis or PCR-derived methods as described elsewhere (40, 50). The composition of expression cassettes that encode components of such bispecific antibody derivatives is shown in Fig. 2. In these bispecific heavy chain constructs, the CH3 of IgG and VH domain of the scFv fragment (VH*) as well as the VH* and the VL domain of the scFv fragment (VL*) are separated by $(G_4S)_2$ and $(G_4S)_3$ peptide linkers, respectively. The linker length is optimized to allow correct pairing of both domains. Furthermore, VH* and VL*, which carry the second binding specificity contain cysteine residues at positions 44 and 100 (Kabat numbering scheme), respectively. These positions can be mutated to cysteines without interfering with the structural integrity of the individual domains and induces the formation of an interchain disulfide bond between both domains, which stabilizes the scFv fragment (see Note 2). For expression of the bispecific antibodies in mammalian cells, both DNA fragments are placed into appropriate mammalian expression vectors which contain all features required for propagation in *E. coli* (e.g., ori for replication in bacteria and beta-lactamase gene), as well as for expression in mammalian cells. For the latter purpose, the vector contains immediate early enhancer and promoter sequences from human cytomegalovirus ($P_{CMV}$), as well as polyadenylation signals. The resulting bispecific heavy chain construct contains the scFv fragment attached to the C-terminus of the CH3 domain of a natural IgG (Fig. 2). To complete the bispecific antibody, the corresponding light chain is encoded in a similar manner on a second expression plasmid. Both,

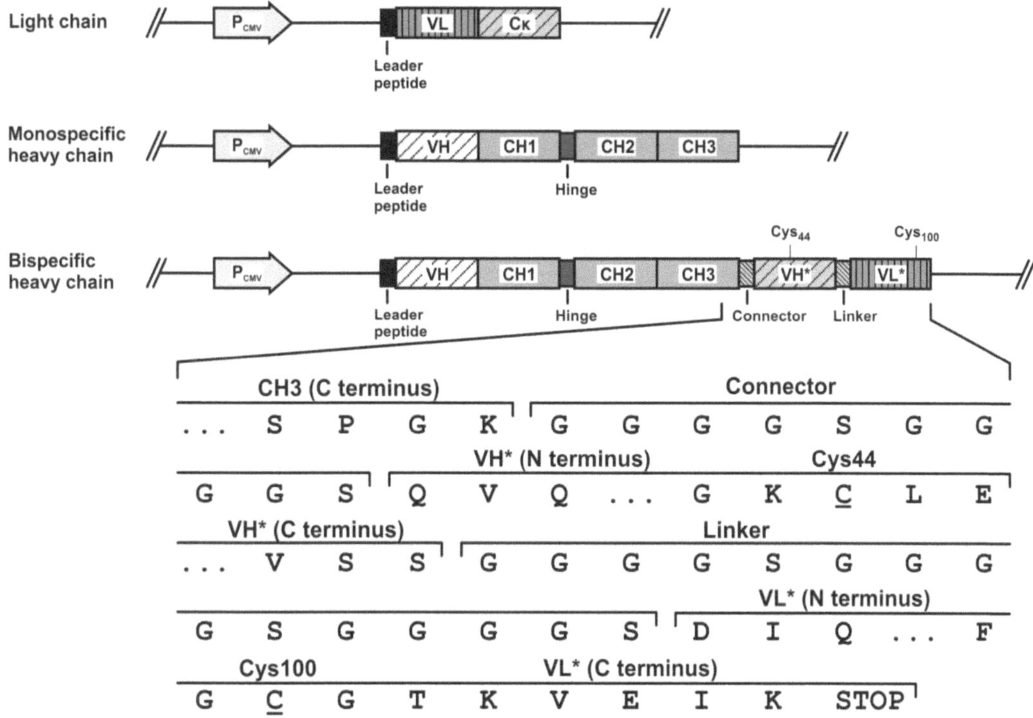


Fig. 2. Design principle of bispecific antibodies via C-terminal IgG-(scFv)2 fusion (2 + 2 format). Primary sequences for critical linker sites are presented on the *bottom*. Mutated residues in VH* and VL* to generate Cys44 and Cys100 for scFv disulfide stabilization are also indicated. Sequences of the variable domains that encode the second specificity were adopted from a Dig-binding antibody derivative (21).

heavy and light chain plasmids are used for transient expression of the bispecific antibody in mammalian cells as described below (see Subheading 3.2). To facilitate purification of the bispecific antibodies without cell lysis, both heavy and light chains are preceded by a leader peptide. The leader peptide enables co-translational transport of the nascent polypeptide into the endoplasmic reticulum and is thus important for antibody folding and secretion into the cell culture medium (see Note 3). Thereby, the antibody is readily available for protein-A affinity chromatography (see Subheading 3.3).

*3.1.2. C-terminal IgG-Fv fusion (2 + 1 format)*

In contrast to the IgG-$(scFv)_2$ format described above, bispecific antibodies of the 2 + 1 format containing C-terminal IgG-Fv fusions require two different heavy chains (Fig. 1a). In the first heavy chain, an additional VH* domain is fused to the CH3 domain of a natural IgG, whereas the second heavy chain contains an additional VL* domain at the same position (Fig. 3). Thus, heavy chain homodimerization is theoretically possible, although the additional VH*–VL* interaction thermodynamically favors

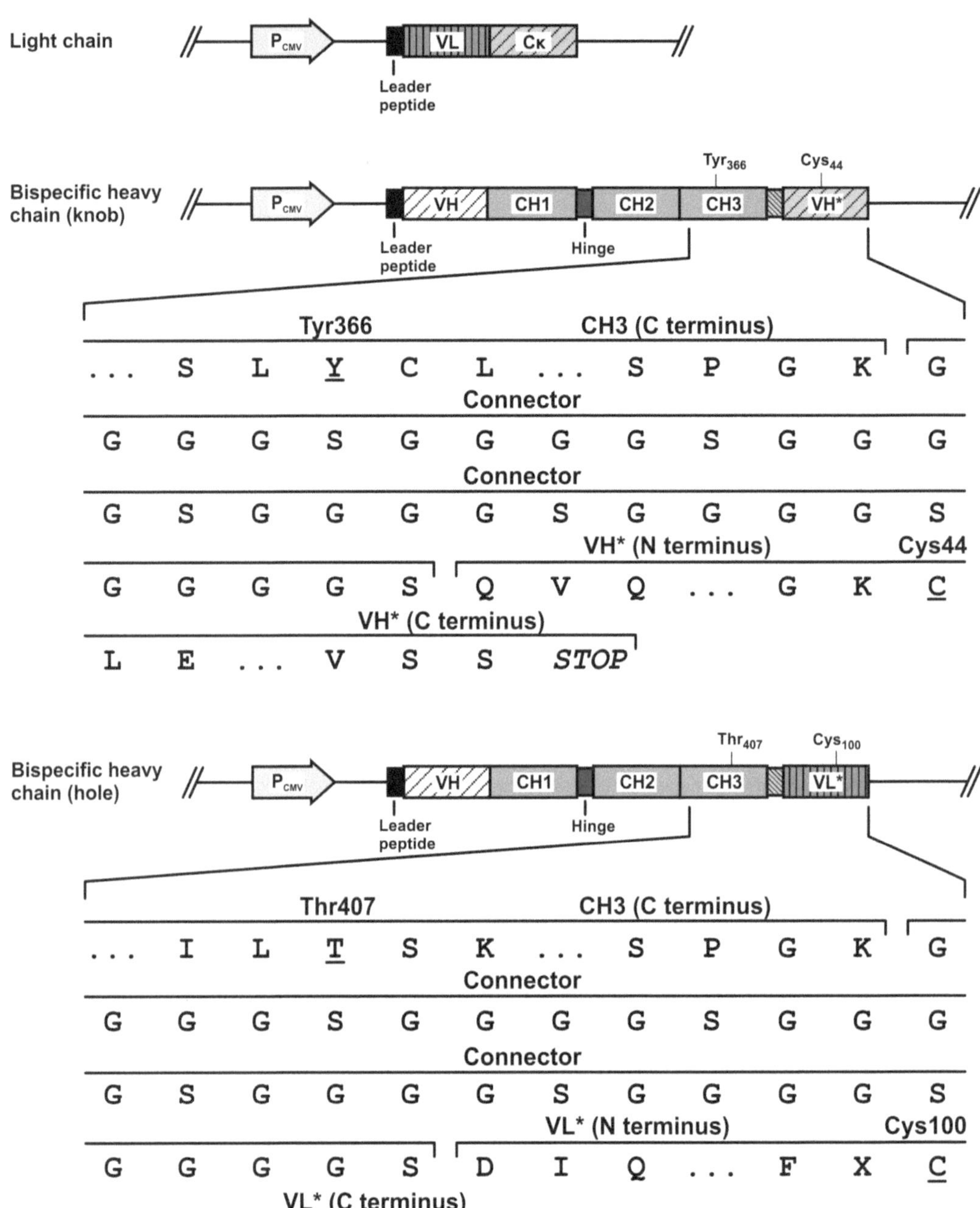


Fig. 3. Design principle of bispecific antibodies via C-terminal IgG-Fv fusion (2 + 1 format). Primary sequences for critical linker sites are presented on the *bottom* of each map. Mutated residues in VHII and VLII to generate Cys44 and Cys100 for Fv disulfide stabilization are indicated. In addition, "knobs-into-holes" mutations in both CH3 domains are shown (Tyr366 and Thr407, respectively). Alternatively, knob mutations can be comprised of T366W and S354C and hole mutations by Y349C, T366S, L368A, and Y407V amino acid replacement (51). Sequences of the variable domains that encode the second specificity were adopted from a Dig-binding antibody derivative (21).

heterodimerization of both heavy chains. However, introduction of "knobs-into-holes" mutations into the CH3 domains of the natural IgG heavy chains reduces remaining homodimerization (e.g., T366Y and Y407T, respectively; Fig. 3) (see Note 4). For mammalian expression of bispecific IgG-Fv fusions, both bispecific heavy chain constructs are cloned into expression vectors as described above. As shown in detail in Fig. 3, the VH* and VL* domains are preceded by long linker peptides. This is necessary, as antigen binding occurs at the N-termini of the variable domains and a shorter linker might lead to steric hindrance of antigen binding due to the CH3 domain, dependent on the nature of the antigen. Furthermore, the Fv fragment is stabilized by the intermolecular disulfide bond that bridges Cys44 of VH* with Cys100 of VL* (Fig. 3). As described already for the 2 + 2 format, bispecific antibodies of the 2 + 1 format are expressed and purified by routine cell culture and biochemical procedures (see Subheadings 3.2 and 3.3).

#### 3.1.3. CrossMab IgGs (1 + 1 format)

Various CrossMab derivatives can be applied to generate bispecific antibodies. This chapter covers three different CrossMabs that have previously been described by Schaefer et al. (49): (1) $\text{CrossMab}^{\text{Fab}}$ in which the complete light chain and the Fab domains of the heavy chain are exchanged; (2) $\text{CrossMab}^{\text{VH-VL}}$ with exchanged VH and VL domains, and (3) $\text{CrossMab}^{\text{CH1-C}\kappa}$ containing exchanged CH1 and Cκ domains. In addition to Cκ, this approach may equally be applied to lambda light chains. These CrossMabs consist of two different heavy chains and two different light chains. Heterodimerization of the heavy chains is accomplished by use of the "knobs-into-holes" methodology (see Note 4). In the case of the $\text{CrossMab}^{\text{Fab}}$, one arm of the bispecific antibody is taken directly from the unmodified Fab of the starting antibody. On the opposite side, the VH and CH1 domains are used as the new light chain; VL and Cκ are connected to the Fc part to form the new heavy chain. The sequences that define the crossover position of the Fab-exchanged CrossMab are listed in detail in Fig. 4a. The two other described molecules ($\text{CrossMab}^{\text{VH-VL}}$ and $\text{CrossMab}^{\text{CH1-C}\kappa}$) contain crossovers between light-chain and heavy-chain domains as well as between variable and constant domains (Fig. 4b, c). These crossovers provide a good structural overlap, do not lead to predicted immunogenic epitopes (50) and provide distances between the variable and constant domains that do not lead to repulsive contacts. The architectures of the CrossMabs that are described in Fig. 4 may be summarized as follows: in all cases, the disulfide bridges connecting the heavy and light chains at the C-terminal ends of the Fab domains remain intact; the choice of the non-crossed side for the "knob" is arbitrary.

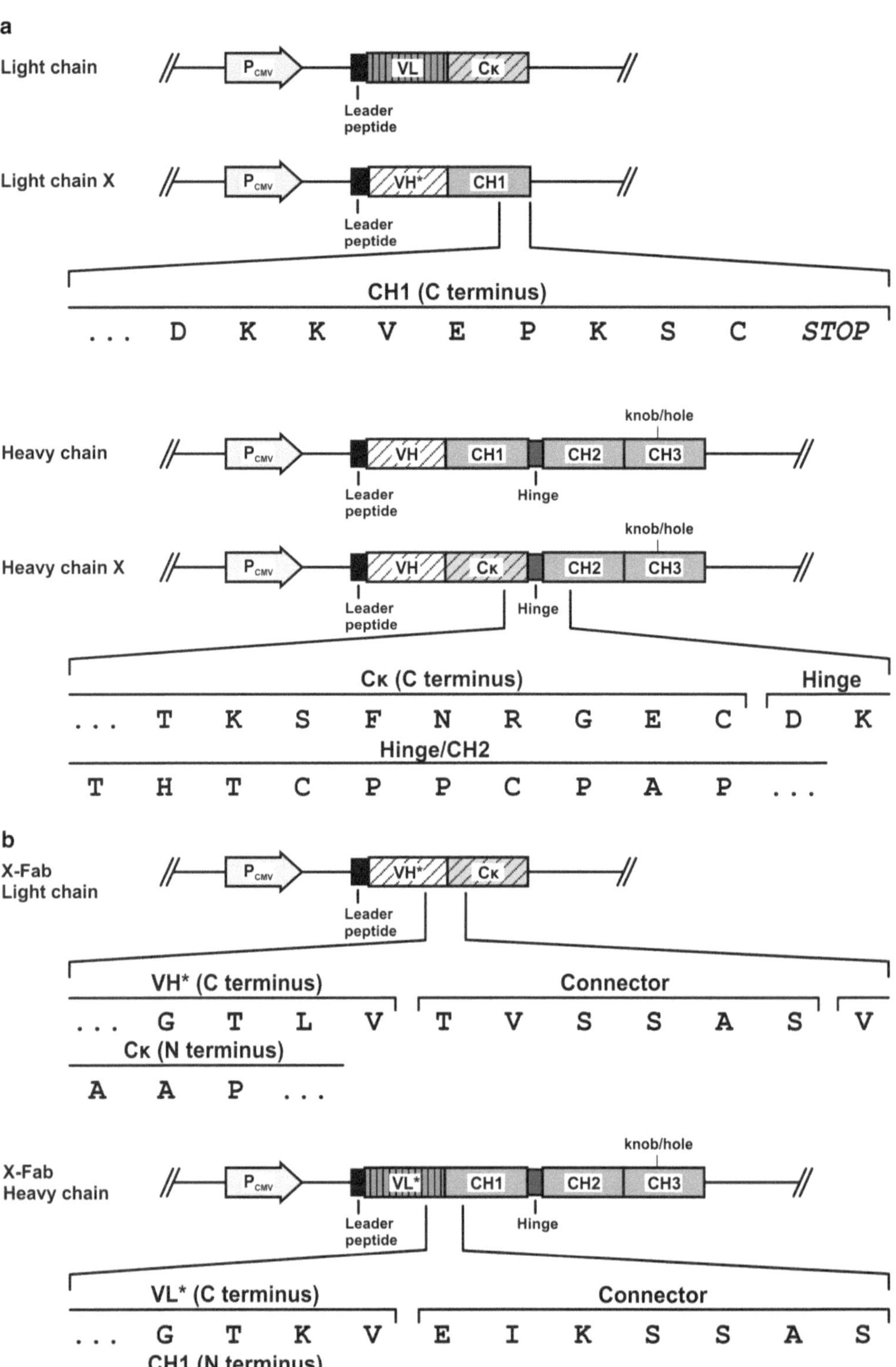


Fig. 4. Design principle of bispecific antibodies via CrossMab technology. Primary sequences for critical crossover sites are presented on the *bottom* of each map. The "knobs-into-holes" mutations in both CH3 domains are indicated and described in Fig. 3.

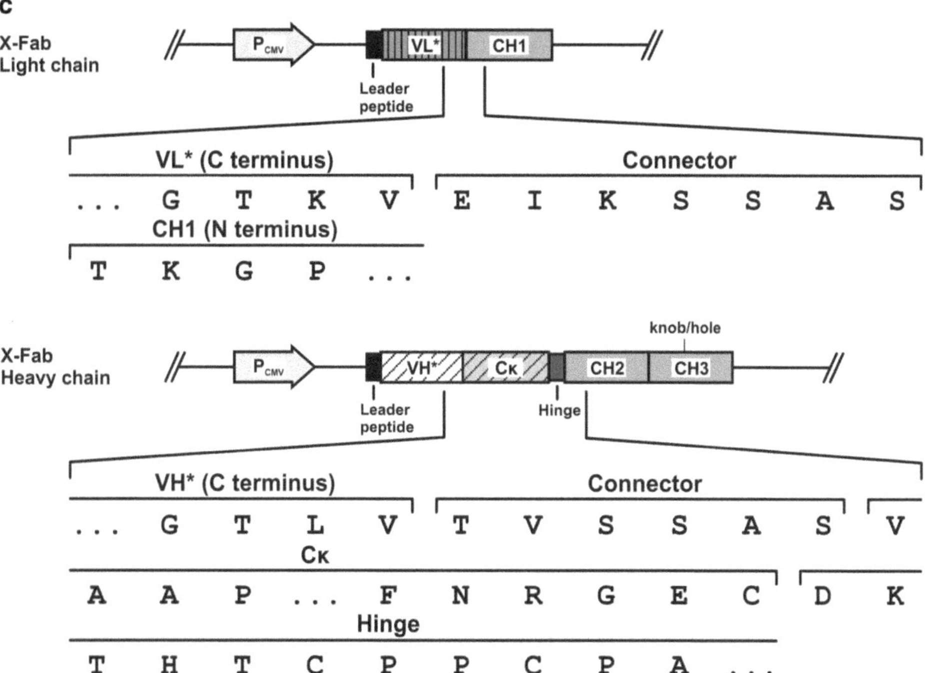


Fig. 4. (continued)

| | |
|---|---|
| *CrossMab*$^{Fab}$ | |
| Non-crossed arm | |
| LC | VL-Cκ* |
| HC | VH-CH1*-hinge-CH2-CH3(knob) |
| Crossed arm | |
| LC | VH-CH1* |
| HC | VL-Cκ*-hinge-CH2-CH3(hole) |
| *CrossMab*$^{VH-VL}$ | |
| Non-crossed arm | |
| LC | VL-Cκ* |
| HC | VH-CH1*-hinge-CH2-CH3(knob) |
| Crossed arm | |
| LC | VH-Cκ* |
| HC | VL-CH1*-hinge-CH2-CH3(hole) |
| *CrossMab*$^{CH1-C\kappa}$ | |
| Non-crossed arm | |
| LC | VL-Cκ* |
| HC | VH-CH1*-hinge-CH2-CH3(knob) |
| Crossed arm | |
| LC | VL-CH1* |
| HC | VH-Cκ*-hinge-CH2-CH3(hole) |

### 3.2. Transient Production of Bispecific Antibodies in Mammalian Cells

IgG-derived bispecific antibodies are expressed by transient transfection of non-adherent human embryonic kidney 293 suspension cells.

1. On the day of transfection, cells are seeded in fresh cell culture medium suitable for propagation of mammalian HEK293 cells at a density of $1–2 \times 10^6$ viable cells/mL.
2. Expression plasmids are co-transfected into the cells using 293-transfection reagents according to the manufacturer's instructions.
3. For transfection, equimolar ratios of both, heavy- and light-chain plasmid DNAs are used.
4. Cell culture supernatants containing the bispecific antibodies are harvested on day 7 after transfection.
5. The cell culture suspension is centrifuged at $14{,}000 \times g$ for 45 min at 4°C and subsequently filtrated through a 0.22-μm filter.
6. After filtration, supernatants can be stored at −20°C until protein-A-purification.

### 3.3. Purification of Bispecific Antibodies

Bispecific antibodies based on full-length IgG formats can be purified from cell culture supernatants with Protein-A-Sepharose™ and Superdex200™ size exclusion chromatography.

1. The sterile filtered cell culture supernatants are applied on a HiTrap Protein-A HP (5 mL) column equilibrated with PBS buffer.
2. Unbound proteins are removed by washing the column with equilibration buffer and the desired bispecific antibodies are recovered with 0.1 M citrate buffer, pH 2.8.
3. After elution, the fractions are immediately neutralized with 1 M Tris–HCl, pH 8.5, pooled and concentrated via centrifugation through a concentrating filter unit.
4. Subsequently, the concentrated material is loaded on a Superdex200 HiLoad 120 mL 16/60 gel filtration column.
5. Fractions containing purified bispecific antibodies in correct (monomeric) form can be separated from high molecular weight aggregates. Thereafter, they are pooled and stored at −80°C in aliquots. Once purified, correctly folded bispecific antibody derivatives have a low propensity to aggregate. Nevertheless, we recommend storage in aliquots to prevent repeated freeze–thawing.

### 3.4. Characterization of Bispecific Antibodies

1. Initial characterization of the antibody's purity and molecular weight can be determined by reducing and nonreducing SDS-PAGE analysis using 4–20% Tris–glycine gels.

2. The integrity of bispecific antibodies can be further determined by NanoElectrospray Q-TOF mass spectrometry. Prior to this, *N*-glycans should be removed by enzymatic treatment with Peptide-*N*-Glycosidase F.
3. Finally, evaluation of binding specificities, kinetics, and affinities of bispecific antibodies can be performed by label-free surface plasmon resonance analysis (see also Chapters 11 and 12).

## 4. Notes

1. Due to the modular composition of bispecific antibody derivatives, the choice of appropriate bispecific antibody formats should be based on the desired features of the molecule. For example, multivalency for one or both binding sites is applicable in cases where avidity or antigen crosslinking is desired. In contrast, monovalency of binding units (e.g., the CrossMab format), is advantageous when avidity effects or crosslinking needs to be avoided.
2. In some cases, stability of Fv domains can be increased by adding a linker peptide between the VH and VL domain. However, the weak binding affinity between VH and VL domains in its hydrophobic interface often requires additional stabilization of scFv domains. The described disulfide bond between VH44 and VL100 is a generic tool that works for most Fv domains and can be applied in prokaryotic, as well as eukaryotic expression systems. In addition, the stability of Fv domains can be improved by mutations in the VH–VL interface that increase the affinity between both domains or by selection of Fv domains with increased stability via display technologies. Both approaches can also be combined to further improve Fv domain stability.
3. Leader peptides for secretion of recombinant antibodies into the culture medium may include sequences that naturally precede murine or human heavy- or light-chain polypeptides.
4. Knob-and-hole mutations in the CH3 domains of natural IgG heavy chains strongly favor heterodimerization of heavy chains. The knob amino acids in the first heavy chain fill a cavity formed by the hole amino acids in the second heavy chain. Steric hindrance between knob amino acids in two identical heavy chains interferes with and thereby strongly reduces the formation of heavy chain homodimers. Association of two heavy chains with hole mutations leads to low-affinity interfaces between both the heavy chains and therefore represent only a minor side product. Thus, the knobs-into-holes approach usually generates defined heterodimers with high yields.

## References


1. Kohler G, Milstein C (1975) Continuous cultures of fused cells secreting antibody of predefined specificity. Nature 256:495–497
2. Chames P, Van Regenmortel M, Weiss E, Baty D (2009) Therapeutic antibodies: successes, limitations and hopes for the future. Br J Pharmacol 157:220–233
3. Chan AC, Carter PJ (2010) Therapeutic antibodies for autoimmunity and inflammation. Nat Rev Immunol 10:301–316
4. Weiner LM, Surana R, Wang S (2010) Monoclonal antibodies: versatile platforms for cancer immunotherapy. Nat Rev Immunol 10:317–327
5. Kontermann RE (2010) Alternative antibody formats. Curr Opin Mol Ther 12:176–183
6. Lu D, Jimenez X, Zhang H et al (2001) Complete inhibition of vascular endothelial growth factor (VEGF) activities with a bifunctional diabody directed against both VEGF kinase receptors, fms-like tyrosine kinase receptor and kinase insert domain-containing receptor. Cancer Res 61:7002–7008
7. Bostrom J, Yu SF, Kan D et al (2009) Variants of the antibody herceptin that interact with HER2 and VEGF at the antigen binding site. Science 323:1610–1614
8. Lu D, Zhang H, Ludwig D et al (2004) Simultaneous blockade of both the epidermal growth factor receptor and the insulin-like growth factor receptor signaling pathways in cancer cells with a fully human recombinant bispecific antibody. J Biol Chem 279: 2856–2865
9. Lu D, Zhang H, Koo H et al (2005) A fully human recombinant IgG-like bispecific antibody to both the epidermal growth factor receptor and the insulin-like growth factor receptor for enhanced antitumor activity. J Biol Chem 280:19665–19672
10. Wu C, Ying H, Grinnell C et al (2007) Simultaneous targeting of multiple disease mediators by a dual-variable-domain immunoglobulin. Nat Biotechnol 25:1290–1297
11. Wu C, Ying H, Bose S et al (2009) Molecular construction and optimization of anti-human IL-1alpha/beta dual variable domain immunoglobulin (DVD-Ig) molecules. MAbs 1:339–347
12. Lum LG, Davol PA (2005) Retargeting T cells and immune effector cells with bispecific antibodies. Cancer Chemother Biol Response Modif 22:273–291
13. Behar G, Siberil S, Groulet A et al (2008) Isolation and characterization of anti-FcgammaRIII (CD16) llama single-domain antibodies that activate natural killer cells. Protein Eng Des Sel 21:1–10
14. Muller D, Kontermann RE (2007) Recombinant bispecific antibodies for cellular cancer immunotherapy. Curr Opin Mol Ther 9:319–326
15. Krop IE, Beeram M, Modi S et al (2010) Phase I study of trastuzumab-DM1, an HER2 antibody-drug conjugate, given every 3 weeks to patients with HER2-positive metastatic breast cancer. J Clin Oncol 28:2698–2704
16. Burris HA, Rugo HS, Vukelja SJ et al (2011) Phase II study of the antibody drug conjugate trastuzumab-DM1 for the treatment of human epidermal growth factor receptor 2 (HER2)-positive breast cancer after prior HER2-directed therapy. J Clin Oncol 29:398–405
17. Wu AM, Senter PD (2005) Arming antibodies: prospects and challenges for immunoconjugates. Nat Biotechnol 23:1137–1146
18. Ronca R, Sozzani S, Presta M, Alessi P (2009) Delivering cytokines at tumor site: the immunocytokine-conjugated anti-EDB-fibronectin antibody case. Immunobiology 214:800–810
19. Kreitman RJ (2006) Immunotoxins for targeted cancer therapy. AAPS J 8:E532–E551
20. Goldsmith SJ (2010) Radioimmunotherapy of lymphoma: Bexxar and Zevalin. Semin Nucl Med 40:122–135
21. Metz S, Haas AK, Daub K et al (2011) Bispecific digoxigenin-binding antibodies for targeted payload delivery. Proc Natl Acad Sci U S A 108:8194–8199
22. Goldenberg DM, Chatal JF, Barbet J et al (2007) Cancer imaging and therapy with bispecific antibody pretargeting. Update Cancer Ther 2:19–31
23. Milstein C, Cuello AC (1983) Hybrid hybridomas and their use in immunohistochemistry. Nature 305:537–540
24. Suresh MR, Cuello AC, Milstein C (1986) Bispecific monoclonal antibodies from hybrid hybridomas. Methods Enzymol 121:210–228
25. Lindhofer H, Mocikat R, Steipe B, Thierfelder S (1995) Preferential species-restricted heavy/light chain pairing in rat/mouse quadromas. Implications for a single-step purification of bispecific antibodies. J Immunol 155:219–225
26. Zeidler R, Mysliwietz J, Csanady M et al (2000) The Fc-region of a new class of intact bispecific antibody mediates activation of accessory cells and NK cells and induces direct phagocytosis of tumour cells. Br J Cancer 83:261–266
27. Morecki S, Lindhofer H, Yacovlev E et al (2008) Induction of long-lasting antitumor immunity by concomitant cell therapy with

allogeneic lymphocytes and trifunctional bispecific antibody. Exp Hematol 36:997–1003

28. Burges A, Wimberger P, Kumper C et al (2007) Effective relief of malignant ascites in patients with advanced ovarian cancer by a trifunctional anti-EpCAM x anti-CD3 antibody: a phase I/ II study. Clin Cancer Res 13:3899–3905
29. Lum LG, Davol PA, Lee RJ (2006) The new face of bispecific antibodies: targeting cancer and much more. Exp Hematol 34:1–6
30. Repp R, van Ojik HH, Valerius T et al (2003) Phase I clinical trial of the bispecific antibody MDX-H210 (anti-FcgammaRI x anti-HER-2/ neu) in combination with Filgrastim (G-CSF) for treatment of advanced breast cancer. Br J Cancer 89:2234–2243
31. Marvin JS, Zhu Z (2005) Recombinant approaches to IgG-like bispecific antibodies. Acta Pharmacol Sin 26:649–658
32. Muller D, Kontermann RE (2010) Bispecific antibodies for cancer immunotherapy: current perspectives. BioDrugs 24:89–98
33. Kipriyanov SM, Le Gall F (2004) Recent advances in the generation of bispecific antibodies for tumor immunotherapy. Curr Opin Drug Discov Dev 7:233–242
34. Fischer N, Leger O (2007) Bispecific antibodies: molecules that enable novel therapeutic strategies. Pathobiology 74:3–14
35. Schirrmann T, Al-Halabi L, Dubel S, Hust M (2008) Production systems for recombinant antibodies. Front Biosci 13:4576–4594
36. Kubetzko S, Balic E, Waibel R et al (2006) PEGylation and multimerization of the anti-p185HER-2 single chain Fv fragment 4D5: effects on tumor targeting. J Biol Chem 281:35186–35201
37. Muller D, Karle A, Meissburger B et al (2007) Improved pharmacokinetics of recombinant bispecific antibody molecules by fusion to human serum albumin. J Biol Chem 282: 12650–12660
38. Roopenian DC, Akilesh S (2007) FcRn: the neonatal Fc receptor comes of age. Nat Rev Immunol 7:715–725
39. Demarest SJ, Glaser SM (2008) Antibody therapeutics, antibody engineering, and the merits of protein stability. Curr Opin Drug Discov Dev 11:675–687
40. Bossenmaier B, Brinkmann U, Dormeyer W et al (2010) Bispecific Anti ErbB3/Anti cMet antibodies. Patent no. 120100256339
41. Glockshuber R, Malia M, Pfitzinger I, Pluckthun A (1990) A comparison of strategies to stabilize immunoglobulin Fv-fragments. Biochemistry 29:1362–1367
42. Bird RE, Hardman KD, Jacobson JW et al (1988) Single-chain antigen-binding proteins. Science 242:423–426
43. Huston JS, Mudgett-Hunter M, Tai MS et al (1991) Protein engineering of single-chain Fv analogs and fusion proteins. Methods Enzymol 203:46–88
44. Huston JS, Levinson D, Mudgett-Hunter M et al (1988) Protein engineering of antibody binding sites: recovery of specific activity in an anti-digoxin single-chain Fv analogue produced in Escherichia coli. Proc Natl Acad Sci U S A 85:5879–5883
45. Reiter Y, Brinkmann U, Lee B, Pastan I (1996) Engineering antibody Fv fragments for cancer detection and therapy: disulfide-stabilized Fv fragments. Nat Biotechnol 14:1239–1245
46. Jung SH, Pastan I, Lee B (1994) Design of interchain disulfide bonds in the framework region of the Fv fragment of the monoclonal antibody B3. Proteins 19:35–47
47. Reiter Y, Brinkmann U, Jung SH, Pastan I, Lee B (1995) Disulfide stabilization of antibody Fv: computer predictions and experimental evaluation. Protein Eng 8:1323–1331
48. Ridgway JB, Presta LG, Carter P (1996) 'Knobs-into-holes' engineering of antibody CH3 domains for heavy chain heterodimerization. Protein Eng 9:617–621
49. Schaefer W, Regula JT, Bahner M et al (2011) Immunoglobulin domain crossover as a generic approach for the production of bispecific IgG antibodies. Proc Natl Acad Sci U S A 108: 11187–11192
50. Sturniolo T, Bono E, Ding J et al (1999) Generation of tissue-specific and promiscuous HLA ligand databases using DNA microarrays and virtual HLA class II matrices. Nat Biotechnol 17:555–561
51. Merchant AM, Zhu Z, Yuan JQ et al (1998) An efficient route to human bispecific IgG. Nat Biotechnol 16:677–681

# Chapter 17

# Generation of Fluorescent IgG Fusion Proteins in Mammalian Cells

**Alexander K. Haas, Klaus Mayer, and Ulrich Brinkmann**

## Abstract

The generation of recombinantly produced fluorescent antibody derivatives that are derived from full-length immunoglobulin G (IgG) has until now been problematic. One major reason for that lies in different and partially incompatible secretion- and folding-requirements of antibodies and green fluorescent protein (GFP) derived fluorescent entities in mammalian cells. The use of citrine as fluorescent fusion entity can overcome this limitation. Citrine is a modified yellow fluorescent protein (YFP) derivative which in contrast to GFP and yellow fluorescent protein (YFP) folds effectively and properly in the endoplasmic reticulum (ER) of mammalian cells. Provided that proper design parameters regarding fusion positions and linker/connector sequences are applied, citrine can be fused to different positions of IgGs and be expressed without interfering with secretion capability or functionality of IgG–citrine derivatives. Because IgG–citrine fusions are stable and retain biophysical properties of IgGs, they can be expressed and purified in the same manner as regular antibodies. IgG–citrine fusions not only retain the binding properties (affinity and specificity) of antibodies but also contain Fc-regions (useful for immunoassay applications), and are fully defined molecules (in contrast to antibody conjugates with fluorophores).

**Key words:** Immunoglobulin G, Multifunctional antibody, Citrine, Antibody-fusion protein, Green fluorescent protein, Enhanced green fluorescent protein, Yellow fluorescent protein, Fluorobodies, Fluorescent antibodies

## 1. Introduction

Fluorescent antibodies are widely used for research and analytical applications and can be generated by different technologies. These include chemical conjugation of fluorophores to antibodies, or the generation of recombinant fusion proteins that harbor antibody

Gabriele Proetzel and Hilmar Ebersbach (eds.), *Antibody Methods and Protocols*, Methods in Molecular Biology, vol. 901, DOI 10.1007/978-1-61779-931-0_17, © Springer Science+Business Media, LLC 2012

fragments as well as fluorescent proteins. The first method, chemical coupling to antibodies, is an established and robust technology. The resulting fluorescent entities contain in most cases full-length IgGs. This facilitates handling and applications because IgGs are stable and enable assay versatility due to the presence of Fc regions. On the other hand, such molecules possess the disadvantage that as chemical conjugates they are rather undefined molecules, in terms of number of fluorophores per antibody and position of coupling (which may affect binding).

Recombinant fusion proteins can overcome these limitations inherent in chemical conjugates of fluorescent molecules to antibodies. They have the fluorescent entities fused to antibody fragments at defined positions and in defined quantities (in most cases one per molecule). A variety of such fusion proteins have been produced by coupling small recombinant antibody fragments to fluorescent proteins (1–4). However, a disadvantage of such molecules is that they are difficult to produce in large quantities, and in the case of antibody fragment fusions they do not contain Fc-regions. This limits their stability, their serum half-life in vivo and makes purification and handling rather difficult.

The combination of the best of both approaches would be the generation of full-length IgG fusions with fluorescent proteins. Unfortunately, this turned out to be quite challenging, mainly because of different folding requirements of antibodies and GFP-derived proteins: antibodies are secreted proteins that contain many inter and intramolecular disulfide bonds. These molecules require the redox environment and chaperone assisted folding environment in the ER to correctly assemble. In contrast, GFP originates from the cytosol of eukaryotic jellyfish and hence needs a completely different environment for proper folding (5, 6). The procedure that we describe in this protocol overcomes these limitations, permitting the effective generation of full-length IgG fusion with fluorescent protein. The "trick" is to utilize a fluorescent entity as fusion partner that can be secreted in mammalian cells in the same manner as normal antibodies. This also enables the application of "standard" expression and purification procedures that are already well established for IgGs. Because of this, general expression and purification protocols are only briefly covered in this review. The most important aspect (which we have therefore covered in detail) is the choice of the correct fluorescent fusion partner, the choice of proper fusion positions, and the use of optimized connector/linker sequences between IgGs and fluorescent entities. These aspects are therefore covered in more detail in the following protocols.

## 2. Material

### *2.1. Transient Expression and Purification of IgG–Citrine Fusion Proteins*

1. Expression vectors, e.g., based on pUC18, with beta-lactamase for ampicillin resistance and cassettes for protein expression in mammalian cells.
2. Human embryonic kidney HEK 293 cells (ATCC, Manassas, VA, USA).
3. 0.22-μm filter.

### *2.2. Purification of IgG-Derived Fluorescent Antibodies*

1. Protein-A-Sepharose™ (GE Healthcare, UK).
2. Superdex200™ (GE Healthcare).
3. HiTrap Protein-A HP (5 mL) column (GE Healthcare).
4. Equilibration buffer.
5. PBS buffer: 10 mM $Na_2HPO_4$, 1 mM $KH_2PO_4$, 137 mM NaCl, and 2.7 mM KCl, pH 7.4.
6. 0.1 M citrate buffer, pH 2.8.
7. 1 M Tris–HCl, pH 8.5.
8. Concentrating filter unit (Amicon Ultra centrifugal filter device 30 K, Millipore, Billerica, MA, USA).
9. Superdex200 HiLoad 120 mL 16/60 gel filtration column (GE Healthcare).
10. 4–20% Tris–glycine gels (NuPAGE®, Invitrogen, Carlsbad, CA, USA).

### *2.3. Microscopic Characterization of IgG-Derived Fluorescent Antibodies*

1. Glass coverslips.
2. Citrine antibody fusion proteins.
3. MCF7 Cells (ATCC).
4. PBS.
5. Paraformaldehyde.
6. Blocking reagent Goat Serum Dilution Buffer (GSDB): 16% goat serum, 20 mM sodium phosphate pH 7.4, 0.3% Triton X-100, 450 mM NaCl.
7. Anti-human kappa-light chains antibodies (Dako Inc., Carpinteria, CA, USA).
8. Cy3-labeled secondary antibodies.

### *2.4. FACS Characterization of IgG-Derived Fluorescent Antibodies*

1. FACS buffer: PBS containing 5% fetal bovine serum (FCS).
2. Cells.
3. Accutase for attached cells.

4. 96-Well rounded bottom microtiter plates.
5. Antibody–citrine fusion protein.
6. Isotype control antibodies.
7. Secondary Cy5 labeled antibodies.

## 3. Methods

So far, the production of fluorescent antibodies was hampered by low expression yields and difficulties in purification. Improvements made to design and in particular the use of a GFP variant (7) that is compatible with mammalian secretion systems now facilitates expression, purification, and handling of IgG fusions. The following protocols describe the design and generation of bivalent IgG-like antibody formats that contain citrine as fluorescent entity. These molecules can be produced in good yields with robust transient mammalian expression systems. They can be used for FACS analyses, microscopy, and other techniques that are aimed at visualization and/or tracking of antigen binding.

### 3.1. Design of IgG-Derived Fluorescent Fusion Proteins that Contain Two Citrine Entities

Generally, fluorescent proteins can be coupled to N or C termini of the heavy (H) or light (L) chains of antibodies. The procedure that we describe here in detail covers their attachment to the C termini of antibody chains (Fig. 1). One important feature for the design of IgG–citrine fusions is the allowance of sufficient flexibility between antibody domains and the fluorescent proteins (Fig. 2). This minimizes interference between the different domains during protein folding and assures good expression yields and benign biophysical properties of the resulting fusion protein. Expression plasmids were generated by gene synthesis of the desired protein and linker modules, followed by subcloning with standard molecular biology techniques.

We found that the placement of a doubled Glycine–Glycine–Glycine–Glycine–Serine [$(G_4S)_2$] linker at the C termini of both light chains (or heavy chains) is sufficient to fulfill this requirement (Fig. 2). We found that this flexible sequence stretch is necessary because direct fusion (without linker) or introduction of different linker sequences (including the linker sequences from commercially available eGFP expression vectors) interfered with expression and purification of the fusion proteins (8). Figure 3a, b display the composition of the expression cassette(s) for generation of IgG–citrine fusions. These figures also show in detail the critical sequence composition (and linker) at the positions where antibody domains are connected to the citrine.

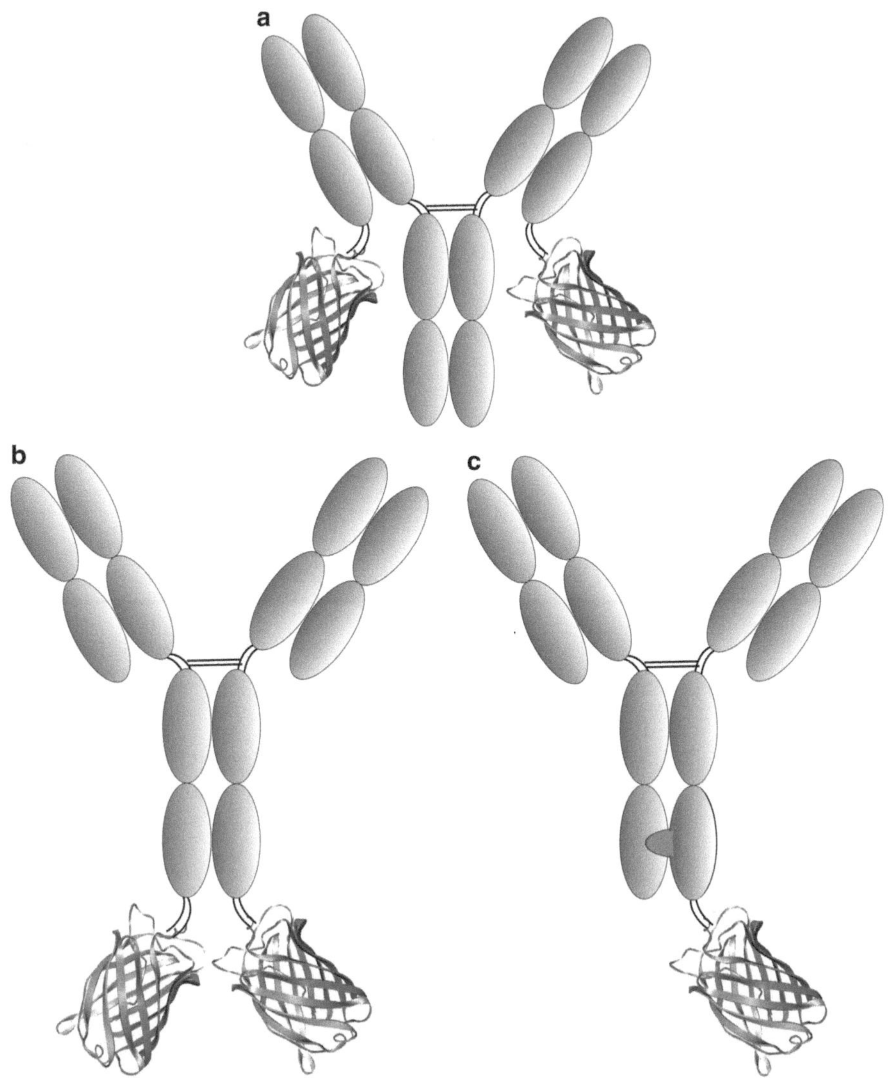


Fig. 1. Composition of antibody–citrine fusion proteins: citrine can be added to (**a**) the C termini of the light chains or to (**b**) the C termini of the heavy chains. (**c**) Using the knobs-into-holes (k-i-h) technology, it is also possible to have only one citrine fused to the IgG.

### *3.2. Design of Antibody Fusion Proteins that Contains One Citrine Entity*

IgG-fusions can also be produced which contain only one fluorescent protein. For that, one citrine entity can be fused to the C terminus of one heavy chain via the flexible linker peptide in the same manner as described above for the double-citrine molecules (Fig. 1c). To attach a second heavy chain (without citrine) to this modified H-chain, the "knobs into holes" technology (9, 10) can be applied. This technique allows the directed heterodimeric association of two different heavy chains in one antibody. We have generated a format that is composed of one heavy chain with "hole" mutations Y349C, T366S, L368A and Y407V, a corresponding heavy chain carrying the "knob" mutations S354C and T366W and, via a

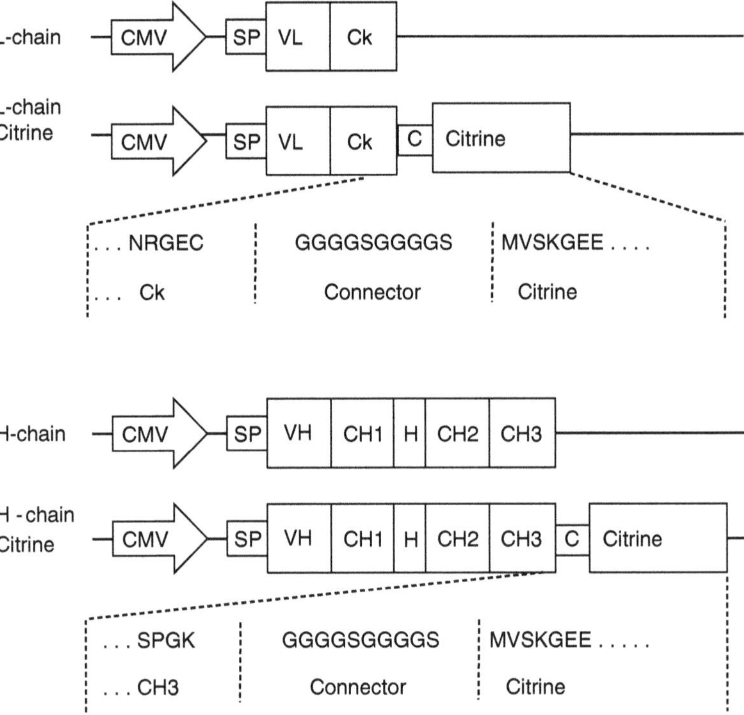


Fig. 2. Expression cassettes for production of antibody-fusions with two citrines. CMV: promoter derived from CMV; SP: signal peptide; H: hinge region; C: connecting peptide.

$(G_4S)_2$ linker, a single citrine molecule. The composition of the expression cassette(s) including its critical sequence composition at the positions for generation of these knobs-into-holes containing mono-IgG–citrine fusions (Fig. 3). Knob-into-hole IgGs with citrine are produced by coexpression of three components in HEK 293 cells. These are encoded by plasmids that have the expression cassettes that are listed in Fig. 3. Figure 3a shows the L-chain expression cassette, Fig. 3b encodes H-chain "hole" without citrine, and Fig. 3c shows the cassette for H-chain "knob" with C-terminally fused citrine.

### 3.3. Design of Antibody Fusions Composed of Two Complementary Half-Citrines

Another approach to generate an antibody that contains just one fluorescent entity combines the "knobs into holes" technique with a protein complementation approach. It has previously been shown that citrine can be split into two halves which (even though made as separate entities) can assemble to a fluorescent enzyme if they are in close proximity (11, 12). To apply this principle for the generation of IgG fusion proteins, separate halves of citrine are connected (via flexible linkers) to H-chains which contain either "knob" or "hole" mutations to force heterodimerization. The principle of this approach is shown in Fig. 4. When the antibody is produced and enters the secretory pathway, it becomes folded in

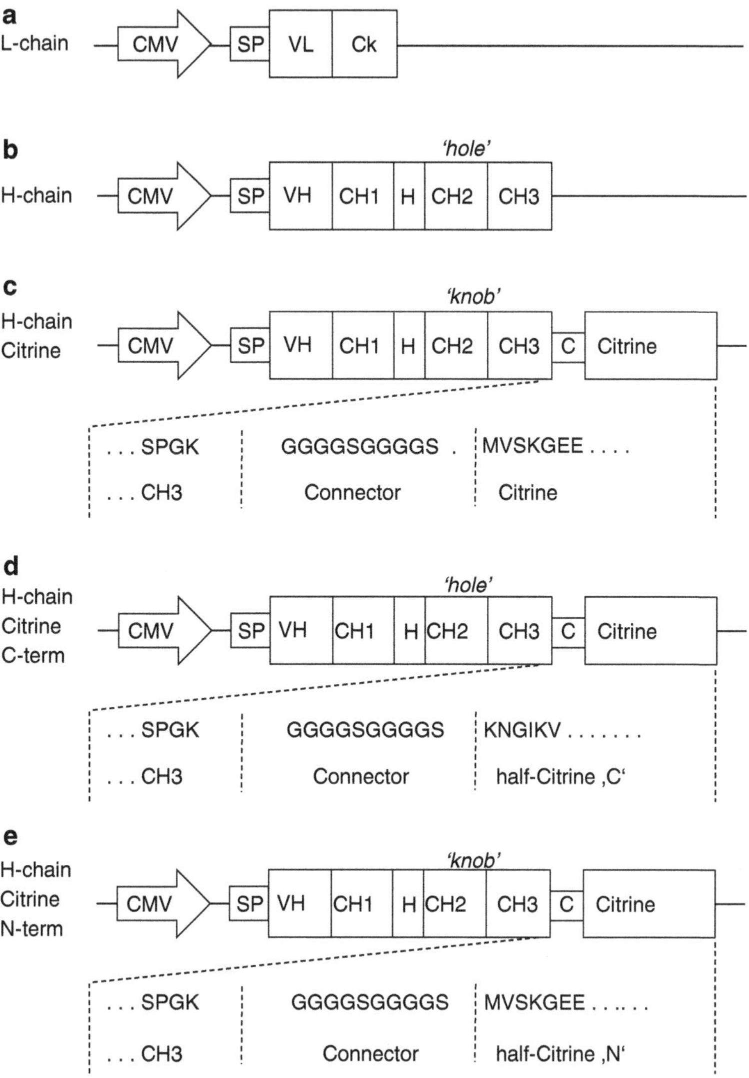


Fig. 3. Expression cassettes for production of antibody-fusions that are composed of knobs-into-holes H-chains and contain only one citrine. CMV: promoter derived from CMV; SP: signal peptide; H: hinge region; C: connecting peptide.

the ER where both heavy chains come in close contact. This enables both halves of citrine to come together and to assemble into one fluorescent molecule. The composition of the expression cassette(s) including critical sequence composition at the positions for generation of these knobs-into-holes containing mono-IgG–citrine fusions is shown in Fig. 3: knob-into-hole IgGs with citrine are produced by coexpression of three components. Figure 3a shows the L-chain expression cassette, Fig. 3d encodes H-chain "hole" that contains the N-terminal portion of citrine, and Fig. 3e shows the cassette for H-chain "knob" with the C-terminal half of citrine.

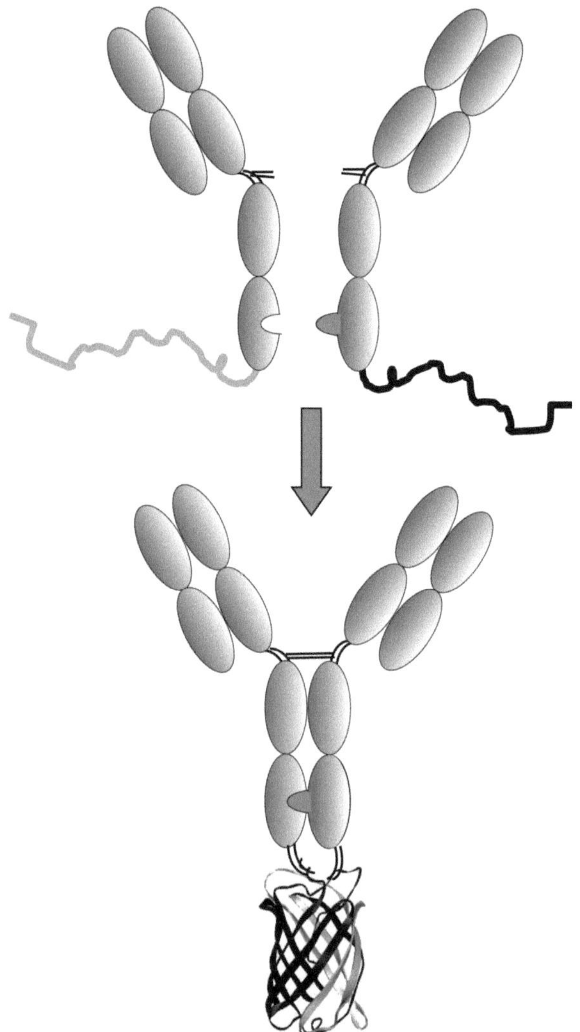

Fig. 4. Composition of antibody–citrine fusion proteins generated by complementation of half-citrines.

### 3.4. Transient Expression of IgG–Citrine Fusion Proteins

Protein encoding sequences as defined above are generated by gene syntheses or PCR technologies and placed into vectors that enable selection and propagation in *E. coli* (origin of replication from the vector pUC18, beta-lactamase gene to confer ampicillin resistance). These vectors additionally contain modules that enable effective expression in mammalian cells (origin of replication, oriP, of Epstein-Barr Virus (EBV), the immediate early enhancer and promoter from the human cytomegalovirus (HCMV) and a poly-adenylation sequence). All gene segments that code for antibody light and heavy chains (with and without additionally fused entities) include at the 5′-end a DNA sequence coding for a leader peptide (MGWSCIILFLVATATGVHS). This enables secretion in eukaryotic cells. Fluorescent IgG-derived antibody fusion proteins can be expressed by transient transfection of nonadherent human embryonic kidney HEK 293 cells in suspension. These cells are cultivated in a cell culture medium suitable for propagation of mammalian cells at 37°C and 8% $CO_2$. On the day of transfection, cells are seeded in fresh medium at a density of $1–2 \times 10^6$ viable cells/mL. Equimolar amounts of both heavy and light chain plasmid DNAs (with or without fused citrine coding regions) are cotransfected into the cells. Cell culture supernatants containing the fluorescent antibody derivatives are harvested 7 days after transfection, centrifuged to remove the producer cells (14,000 × *g* for 45 min at 4°C), and subsequently filtrated through a 0.22-μm filter. After filtration, supernatants can be stored at -20°C.

### 3.5. Purification of IgG-Derived Fluorescent Antibodies

The described fluorescent antibody derivatives contain functional Fc regions and therefore can be purified from cell culture supernatants using the same procedures as for IgGs.

1. Protein-A-Sepharose™ and Superdex200™ size exclusion chromatography can be applied for lab scale production and also for larger batches.
2. As an example, sterile filtered cell culture supernatants are applied on a HiTrap Protein-A HP (5 mL) column equilibrated with PBS buffer.
3. Unbound proteins are removed by washing the column with equilibration buffer and the desired fluorescent antibodies are recovered with 0.1 M citrate buffer, pH 2.8.
4. After elution, the fractions are immediately neutralized with 1 M Tris–HCl, pH 8.5, pooled, and concentrated via centrifugation through a concentrating filter unit.
5. Subsequently, the concentrated material is loaded on a Superdex200 HiLoad 120 mL 16/60 gel filtration column.
6. The protein concentration of purified antibodies and derivatives can be determined via optical density (OD) at 280 nm with the OD at 320 nm as the background correction, using the molar extinction coefficient calculated on the basis of the amino acid sequence.
7. Protein fractions were pooled, snap-frozen, and stored at -80°C.
8. The purity and molecular weight of the fluorescent antibody derivatives can be assessed by SDS-PAGE analysis using 4–20% Tris–glycine gels (see Note 1).

### 3.6. Characterization of IgG-Derived Fluorescent Antibodies

Evaluation of binding specificities, kinetics, and affinities are performed by surface plasmon resonance in the same manner as normal IgG's are assessed. Functionality (and pH dependence) of the fluorophore portion of the molecule can be assessed by spectrometric methods. For example, using a microtiter plate fluorescence reader, fluorescence at different pH levels of the fusion proteins can be assessed. Citrine fluorescence requires excitement at 516 nm and its emission can be measured at 529 nm. In our analyses, both emission and excitation bandwidth were 5 nm and each read was performed ten times with an integration time of 40 μs.

The combined functionality of antibody-mediated binding as well as fluorescence can be assessed on cells which carry antigens that are recognized the IgG portion of the fusion proteins. FACS analyses and fluorescence microscopy are well suited for that. Here we describe an example for microscopic analyses:

1. Cells that express the cell surface antigen, or control cells without said antigen, are grown on glass coverslips to a density of about 50–70%.
2. The cells are then exposed to the citrine antibody fusion proteins in a concentration of 5 nM for 2 h on ice, or for 2 h at 37°C.
3. The cells are washed in cold PBS, and fixed with paraformaldehyde (or subjected to temperature shifts for internalization studies). An example for the results of such studies is shown in Fig. 5 with cell surface localization in panel A and internalization in panel B.

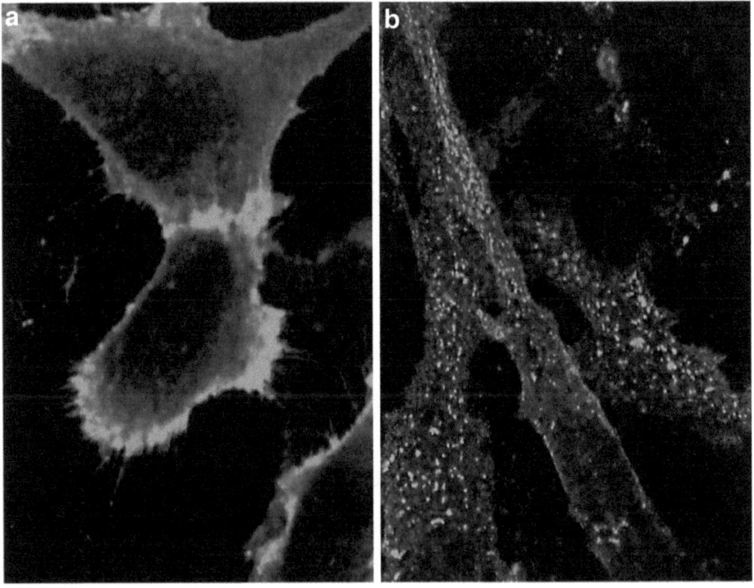


Fig. 5. Cell surface binding and internalization of IgG–citrine fusions insulin-like growth factor 1 (IGF-1) receptor binding antibodies binds to and internalize the receptor into the endocytic pathway (13, 14). Because the antibody remains bound to its target, it becomes cointernalized. This can be visualized with the IgG–citrine fusion protein. In *panel a* (*left*) application of the IgG–citrine fusion protein at 4°C followed by fixation shows cell surface localization due to antibody binding. On the *right* (*panel b*) shows the application of the IgG–citrine fusion protein at 37°C for 18 h and subsequent fixation reveals internalization of the majority of the bound antibody.

4. For costaining of the antibody portion, the fixed cells are washed in PBS, incubated with the blocking reagent GSDB and incubated with anti-human kappa-light chains antibodies at a concentration of 6.5 μg/mL for 1.5–2 h in a humidity chamber.
5. Thereafter, the antibodies can be detected with Cy3-labeled secondary antibodies.

### 3.7. Characterization of IgG-Derived Fluorescent Antibodies by FACS

For FACS analysis, either nonattached cells are used or adherent cells are detached by 15-min incubation in Accutase.

1. Cultured cells are washed in FACS buffer.
2. $3 \times 10^5$ cells are incubated in a 96-well rounded bottom microtiter plate with 3.43 nM of antibody–citrine fusion protein or isotype control antibodies to allow binding (see Note 2).
3. For detection of bound antibodies, secondary Cy5 labeled antibodies are added to the same final concentration of 3.43 nM for 30 min on ice.
4. The cells are washed in FACS buffer to remove unbound antibody and thereafter subjected to FACS analyses.
5. Cy5 which detects the antibody moiety is detected in the Cy5 channel, while citrine fluorescence is detected in the FITC channel.

## 4. Notes

1. The integrity and composition of antibody–citrine fusion proteins can be further determined by NanoElectrospray Q-TOF mass spectrometry.
2. Alternatively, $3 \times 10^5$ cells are incubated in a 96-well rounded bottom microtiter plate with 3.43 nM of antibody–citrine fusion protein or isotype control antibodies for 30 min on ice to allow binding, but prevent internalization.

### References


1. Casey JL, Coley AM, Tilley LM, Foley M (2000) Green fluorescent antibodies: novel in vitro tools. Protein Eng 13: 445–452
2. Griep RA, van TC, van der Wolf JM, Schots A (1999) Fluobodies green fluorescent single-chain Fv fusion proteins. J Immunol Methods 230:121–130
3. Morino K, Katsumi H, Akahori Y et al (2001) Antibody fusions with fluorescent proteins: a versatile reagent for profiling protein expression. J Immunol Methods 257: 175–184
4. Schwalbach G, Sibler AP, Choulier L et al (2000) Production of fluorescent single-chain antibody fragments in *Escherichia coli*. Protein Exp Purif 18:121–132
5. Ormo M, Cubitt AB, Kallio K, Gross LA, Tsien RY, Remington SJ (1996) Crystal structure of the *Aequorea victoria* green fluorescent protein. Science 273:1392–1395

6. Tsien RY (1998) The green fluorescent protein. Annu Rev Biochem 67:509–544
7. Griesbeck O, Baird GS, Campbell RE et al (2001) Reducing the environmental sensitivity of yellow fluorescent protein. Mechanism and applications. J Biol Chem 276:29188–29194
8. Haas AK, von SC, Matscheko D, Brinkmann U (2010) Fluorescent citrine-IgG fusion proteins produced in mammalian cells. MAb 2: 648–661
9. Merchant AM, Zhu Z, Yuan JQ, Goddard A, Adams CW, Presta LG, Carter P (1998) An efficient route to human bispecific IgG. Nat Biotechnol 16:677–681
10. Ridgway JB, Presta LG, Carter P (1996) 'Knobs-into-holes' engineering of antibody CH3 domains for heavy chain heterodimerization. Protein Eng 9:617–621
11. Nyfeler B, Michnick SW, Hauri HP (2005) Capturing protein interactions in the secretory pathway of living cells. Proc Natl Acad Sci U S A 102:6350–6355
12. Nyfeler B, Hauri HP (2007) Visualization of protein interactions inside the secretory pathway. Biochem Soc Trans 35:970–973
13. Burtrum D, Zhu Z, Lu D, Anderson DM, Prewett M, Pereira DS, Bassi R, Abdullah R, Hooper AT, Koo H, Jimenez X, Johnson D, Apblett R, Kussie P, Bohlen P, Witte L, Hicklin DJ, Ludwig DL (2003) A fully human monoclonal antibody to the insulin-like growth factor I receptor blocks ligand-dependent signaling and inhibits human tumor growth in vivo. Cancer Res 63:8912–8921
14. Gong Y, Yao E, Shen R, Goel A, Arcila M, Teruya-Feldstein J, Zakowski MF, Frankel S, Peifer M, Thomas RK, Ladanyi M, Pao W (2009) High expression levels of total IGF-1R and sensitivity of NSCLC cells in vitro to an anti-IGF-1R antibody (R1507). PLoS One 4:e7273

# Chapter 18

# Methods to Engineer and Identify $IgG_1$ Variants with Improved FcRn Binding or Effector Function


## Robert F. Kelley and Y. Gloria Meng



## Abstract

Antibodies as therapeutic agents have gained broad acceptance as shown by the number of antibodies in clinical use and many more in clinical development. This utility is an outcome of the high specificity and affinity of the antigen-binding site comprised of the heavy and light chain variable domains. In addition, the Fc portion of human or humanized $IgG_1$ antibodies promotes long half-life through interaction with the recycling FcRn receptor and effects killing functions through interaction with complement and Fcγ receptors. Engineering the Fc portion to increase half-life through stronger binding to FcRn, or to increase complement or cell-mediated killing may lead to improved therapeutic antibodies. These improvements may benefit the patients through convenience in dosing or increased efficacy. Here we describe protocols for generating Fc-engineered $IgG_1$ antibodies and assays to measure Fc receptor binding, antibody dependent cellular cytotoxicity activity, and complement dependent cytotoxicity activity to identify variants with improved FcRn binding or effector function.



**Key words:** Antibody engineering, FcRn binding, FcγR binding, ADCC, CDC


## 1. Introduction

Human IgG binds to neonatal Fc receptor (FcRn) at acidic pH to be protected from degradation and dissociates from FcRn at neutral pH to maintain a long circulating half-life (1). Broad expression of FcRn promotes recycling of IgG. Engineering the Fc portion to increase the binding affinity of therapeutic IgG to FcRn at acidic pH, but not at neutral pH, may improve the half-life and reduce the dosing frequency (2) (Fig. 1). In addition to the FcRn receptor, the Fc region of human IgG also interacts with Fcγ receptors (FcγRs) expressed on leukocytes to elicit effector function. $IgG_1$ is the major subclass of human IgG. It binds to FcγRI (CD64) with high affinity and to FcγRII (CD32) and FcγRIII (CD16) with low affinity (3). Both FcγRI and FcγRIIIa are signaling receptors but a


Gabriele Proetzel and Hilmar Ebersbach (eds.), *Antibody Methods and Protocols*, Methods in Molecular Biology, vol. 901, DOI 10.1007/978-1-61779-931-0_18, © Springer Science+Business Media, LLC 2012

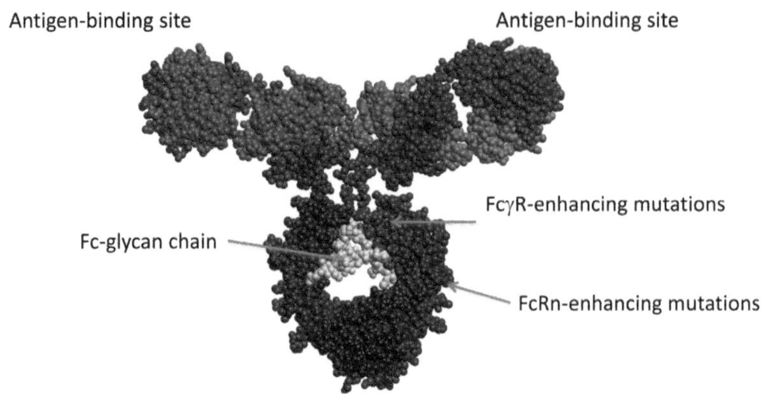


Fig. 1. Space filling model of IgG structure showing approximate location of Fc modifications resulting in altered effector function.

nonsignaling form of CD16 (FcγRIIIb) is found on neutrophils. FcγRII exists in activating (FcγRIIa, FcγRIIc) and inhibitory (FcγRIIb) forms. Human natural killer (NK) cells express FcγRIIIa and are the primary effectors for antibody-dependent cellular cytotoxicity (ADCC). NK cells isolated from some human donors also express FcγRIIc that may be capable of triggering cytotoxic events (4, 5). In addition, a subpopulation of NK cells displays surface expression of the inhibitory FcγRIIb receptor (6). Macrophages, γδ T cells and some monocytes also express FcγRIIIa.

A polymorphism (Val or Phe at 158) in human FcγRIIIa may affect the therapeutic response. Patients homozygous for the higher affinity Val158 allotype of FcγRIIIa show better response to Rituximab, suggesting that increasing the binding affinity of therapeutic $IgG_1$ to FcγRIIIa may improve the clinical outcome (7, 8). Improved binding to FcγRIIIa may be accomplished through amino acid substitutions in the Fc region (9, 10) (Fig. 1) or via glycosylation engineering by producing $IgG_1$ in *FUT8* knockout Chinese hamster ovary (CHO) cells (Biowa, Princeton, NJ) (11) or other glycosylation engineered CHO cells (12, 13). The Fc portion of human $IgG_1$ has a single N-linked glycosylation site at Asn297 that is required for FcγR and complement binding, but is dispensable for FcRn-binding. Modifications of the carbohydrate chain, in particular removal of the core fucose ("afucosylation"), can result in significant increased FcγRIIIa binding and antibody-dependent cellular cytotoxicity (ADCC). Human $IgG_1$ can also engage complement component C1q to initiate complement dependent cytotoxicity (CDC) for lysis of antibody-coated targets. Amino acid changes have been discovered that increase complement-mediated lysis (14).

To identify engineered $IgG_1$ variants with improved FcRn and effector function, we measure Fc receptor binding by Enzyme-Linked Immunosorbent Assay (ELISA) using soluble Fc receptors consisting of the extracellular domains. Previously, we compared binding of $IgG_1$ variants to Fc receptors in ELISAs using soluble Fc receptors or CHO cells expressing Fc receptors and obtained similar results (15). Since soluble receptor-based ELISA is easier to perform, we continue to use this format. We used these assays to identify $IgG_1$ variants with increased FcRn binding and unaltered FcγR binding or variants with increased FcγRIIIa binding and unaltered binding to FcRn or other FcγRs. The same assays can also be used to identify $IgG_1$ variants with decreased Fc receptor binding. In addition to ELISAs, we also measure binding of Fc receptors to immobilized $IgG_1$ variants by surface plasmon resonance using Biacore instruments. Moreover, we measure the ADCC and CDC activities to assess the effector functions of the $IgG_1$ variants. In this report, we describe protocols for generating $IgG_1$ variants with amino acid substitutions in the Fc regions and for the assays used to characterize the variants.

## 2. Materials

### *2.1. Plasmid Construction*

1. cDNA designed for mammalian expression of the target antibody heavy chain.
2. Oligonucleotide for mutagenesis.
3. *E. coli* strain CJ236 ($dut^-$ $ung^-$).
4. XL1-Blue Competent Cells (Stratagene, Santa Clara, CA, USA).
5. M13K07 helper phage (Stratagene).
6. Antibiotics: 5 mg/mL stock solutions of carbenicillin and kanamycin.
7. Luria-Bertani (LB) broth.
8. 2YT broth.
9. LB agar plates containing 50 μg/mL carbenicillin.
10. 5× KCM buffer: 0.5 M KCl, 0.15 M $CaCl_2$, 0.25 M $MgCl_2$.
11. LB/PEG/DMSO: LB broth adjusted to pH 6.1 with HCl, containing 100 g/L PEG 3350, 10 mM $MgSO_4$, 10 mM $MgCl_2$, 50 mL/L DMSO.
12. 20% PEG 8000/2.5 M NaCl.
13. Phosphate buffered saline (PBS): 8.0 mM $Na_2HPO_4$, 1.5 mM $KH_2PO_4$, 2.7 mM KCl, and 137 mM NaCl, pH 7.4.
14. M13 DNA Spin kit (Qiagen, Germantown, MD, USA).
15. 10× TM Buffer: 0.5 M Tris–HCl pH 7.5, 100 mM $MgCl_2$.
16. 10 mM rATP.

17. 100 mM dithiothreitol (DTT).
18. 25 mM dNTP mix (equal volumes of 100 mM each dATP, dCTP, dTTP, dGTP).
19. T4 polynucleotide kinase: 10 U/μL (New England BioLabs, Ipswich, MA, USA).
20. T4 DNA ligase: 400 U/μL (New England BioLabs).
21. T7 DNA polymerase, unmodified; 10 U/μL (New England BioLabs).

### 2.2. Reagents for IgG Production and Purification

1. Human embryonic kidney 293 T cells (catalog no. CRL-11268, American Type Culture Collection, Rockville, MD, USA).
2. 293 Cell growth media: 10% fetal bovine serum (catalog no. F2442, Sigma, St Louis, MO, USA), 2 mM L-glutamine, 10 mM Hepes, pH 7.2, 2.44 g/L $NaHCO_3$, F12:DMEM 50:50 (Invitrogen, Grand Island, NY, USA).
3. Heavy and light chain vectors.
4. FuGENE™ 6 transfection reagent (Roche Applied Science, Mannheim, Germany).
5. Transfection media: Gibco™ FreeStyle™ 293 Expression Medium (Invitrogen).
6. 10× Trypsin-EDTA (Gibco, Invitrogen): 0.5% trypsin, 5.3 mN EDTA.
7. T-150 sterile, filter-cap flasks (catalog no. 355001, BD Biosciences, Bedford, MA, USA).
8. Low protein binding filter flask (catalog no. 430767 or alike, Corning Life Sciences, Lowell, MA, USA).
9. Phenylmethanesulfonyl fluoride (PMSF) and bovine lung aprotinin (Sigma).
10. rProtein A agarose column (catalog no. IPA400HC, Repligen, Waltham, MA, USA).
11. 75 mM Tris–HCl, 1.5 M KCl, pH 8.
12. 100 mM acetic acid.
13. 1 M Tris–HCl, pH 8.
14. PD-10 desalting column (GE Healthcare, Piscataway, NJ, USA).
15. Centricon-10 (Millipore, Bedford, MA).

### 2.3. FcRn Binding ELISAs

1. 96-Well and 384-well MaxiSorp ELISA plates (Thermo Scientific, Nunc, Roskilde, Denmark).
2. Microwell plate washer and reader for 96-well and 384-well ELISA plates.
3. Shaker for ELISA plates.
4. Coat buffer: 0.05 M sodium carbonate, pH 9.6.

5. Wash buffer: 0.05% polysorbate 20 in PBS, pH 7.4.
6. Block buffer: 0.5% BSA, 15 part per million (ppm) ProClin in PBS, pH 7.4.
7. Assay buffer: 0.5% BSA, 0.05% polysorbate 20, 15 ppm ProClin in PBS, pH 7.4.
8. Horseradish peroxidase (HRP)-conjugated goat $F(ab')_2$ anti-human $F(ab')_2$ (catalog no. 109-036-097, 0.8 mg/mL) (Jackson ImmunoResearch, West Grove, PA, USA).
9. 1 M phosphoric acid.
10. Substrate: 3,3′,5,5′-tetramethyl benzidine (TMB) (Kirkegaard & Perry Laboratories, Gaithersburg, MD, USA).
11. Express soluble FcRn, a heterodimer consisting of FcRn ECD with a $His_6$ tag on the carboxy-terminus (FcRn-His) and β2-microglobulin, in CHO cells using the previously described plasmids and purify the soluble receptors using a nickel column (9).
12. Express non-His tagged FcRn in CHO cells similarly. Purify the FcRn from the cell culture media using a human IgG column (GE Healthcare) (see Note 1).
13. Acidify the cell culture media with 2-(*N*-morpholino) ethanesulfonic acid (MES) to final 100 mM MES pH 5.5 and load to the IgG column.
14. Wash the column and elute bound FcRn with 50 mM HEPES pH 8.0, 150 mM NaCl.
15. Biotinylate FcRn using biotin-X-NHS (Research Organics, Cleveland, OH) or other biotinylation reagents.
16. NeutrAvidin (Pierce, Rockford, IL).
17. pH 6.0 wash buffer: 0.05% polysorbate 20 in PBS, pH 6.0.
18. pH 6.0 assay buffer: 0.5% BSA, 0.05% polysorbate 20, 15 ppm ProClin in PBS, pH 6.0.
19. HRP-conjugated streptavidin (GE Healthcare).
20. Data analysis: four-parameter nonlinear regression curve-fitting program (XLfit, Guildford, Surrey, UK).

### 2.4. FcγR Binding ELISA

1. Equipment, reagents, and software as described in items 1–10 and 20 in Subheading 2.3.
2. Express soluble FcγRI, FcγRIIa(H131), FcγRIIa(R131), FcγRIIb, FcγRIIIa(F158), and FcγRIIIa(V158), consisting of the extracellular domain fused with Gly-$His_6$-glutathione-S-transferase at the carboxy-terminus (FcγR-His-GST), in CHO cells using the previously described plasmids and purify the soluble receptors using a nickel column (9).
3. Anti-GST. We used an in-house mouse anti-GST antibody.

4. F(ab′)$_2$ goat anti-human κ light chain antibody (catalog no. 0855059, MP Biochemicals, Burlingame, CA) or F(ab′)$_2$ goat anti-human λ light chain antibody (catalog no. AHI1901, BioSource, Camarillo, CA).

### 2.5. Surface Plasmon Resonance Methods to Measure FcRn Binding

1. Biacore 3000 or Biacore T-100 (GE Healthcare).
2. Prepare soluble non-His tagged FcRn.
3. CM5 or Series S sensor chips, amino coupling kit, normalization solution (70% glycerol) (GE Healthcare).
4. HBS-P running buffer: 10 mM HEPES, pH 7.4 containing 150 mM NaCl, 0.005% (v/v) Surfactant P20 (GE Healthcare).
5. 10 mM glycine-HCl pH 2.5 regeneration solution (GE Healthcare).
6. pH 5.8 running buffer for measuring FcRn binding: 25 mM MES, 25 mM HEPES, pH 5.8, 150 mM NaCl, 0.05% polysorbate 20.
7. pH 8.0 running buffer to dissociate IgG from FcRn immobilized on the chip: 25 mM MES, 25 mM HEPES, pH 8.0, 150 mM NaCl, 0.05% polysorbate 20.

### 2.6. Surface Plasmon Resonance Methods to Measure FcγR Binding

1. Biacore 3000 or Biacore T-100 (GE Healthcare).
2. Prepare soluble versions of the FcγRs lacking the GST fusion but with a His$_8$ tag.
3. CM5 or Series S sensor chips (GE Healthcare).
4. Amino coupling kit (GE Healthcare).
5. Normalization solution (70% glycerol) (GE Healthcare).
6. HBS-P running buffer: 10 mM HEPES, pH 7.4 containing 150 mM NaCl, 0.005% (v/v) Surfactant P20 (GE Healthcare).
7. 10 mM glycine-HCl pH 2.5 regeneration solution (GE Healthcare).
8. pH 5.8 running buffer for measuring FcRn binding: 25 mM MES, 25 mM HEPES, pH 5.8, 150 mM NaCl, 0.05% polysorbate 20.
9. pH 8.0 running buffer to dissociate IgG from FcRn immobilized on the chip: 25 mM MES, 25 mM HEPES, pH 8.0, 150 mM NaCl, 0.05% polysorbate 20.

### 2.7. ADCC Assay

1. 100 mL of heparinized normal human whole blood of the heterozygous FcγRIIIa(F158/V158) genotype (see Note 2).
2. RosetteSep (StemCell Technologies, Vancouver, BC Canada).
3. Target cells. For anti-CD20 IgG$_1$, we used WIL2-S B lymphoma cells (American Type Culture Collection).
4. Tabletop centrifuge. Allegra X-12R (Beckman Coulter, Brea, CA) or alike.

5. Cytotoxicity Detection Kit (Roche Applied Science, Indianapolis, IN).
6. Data analysis: four-parameter nonlinear regression curve-fitting program (KaleidaGraph, Synergy Software, Reading, PA).

### 2.8. CDC Assay

1. Whole blood.
2. RosetteSep B cell Enrichment Cocktail (StemCell Tech. Vancouver, BC, Canada).
3. PBS.
4. Fetal bovine serum (Biosource International, Invitrogen, Carlsbad, CA, USA).
5. Ficoll-Pague Plus (Amersham Biosciences, Piscataway, NJ, USA).
6. WIL2-S B lymphoma cells.
7. 96-Microwell plate (BD Biosciences, Santa Clara, CA, USA).
8. Normal human serum complement (Quidel, San Diego, CA, USA).
9. Alamar Blue (Invitrogen).
10. 37°C incubator.
11. Plate shaker.
12. Fluorescent plate reader (excitation wavelength: 530 nm, emission wavelength: 590 nm).
13. Data analysis: four-parameter nonlinear regression curve-fitting program (KaleidaGraph).

## 3. Methods

### 3.1. Plasmid Construction to Generate IgG Fc Variants

The protocol described here is for making amino acid substitutions in the Fc region of an antibody. Typically, two or more amino acid changes in a variant are required to make a significant change in effector function. Fc engineering can be applied to any antibody in recombinant form, irrespective of the discovery platform. A cDNA designed for mammalian expression of the target antibody heavy chain is required. We commonly use a protocol derived from the procedure of Kunkel et al. (16) that is based on oligonucleotide-directed mutagenesis of single-stranded DNA (ssDNA). This requires that the plasmid encoding the heavy chain DNA has an f1 origin of replication to drive replication in single-stranded form in *E. coli* (see Note 3). For mutagenesis of template ssDNA, an oligonucleotide specifying the amino acid change, but otherwise complementary to the template DNA, needs to be chemically synthesized. We typically use oligonucleotides that have 15 bp of complementarity on both the 5′ and 3′ side of the site of mutation. Examples of the kinds of mutations that can alter effector function or FcRn binding and the number of variants to characterize are provided by Shields (9), Lazar (10) and Yeung (2).

1. Prepare competent CJ236 cells in LB/PEG/DMSO (17) and DNA intended for mutagenesis in 1× KCM. Transform cells with DNA and plate on LB agar plate with 50 μg/mL carbenicillin following protocol described in Kunkel et al. (16).
2. Pick a single colony to inoculate 1 mL of 2YT broth containing 50 μg/mL carbenicillin, grow at 37°C for 6–8 h with continuous shaking.
3. Add 10 μL of $10^{12}$ pfu/mL M13K07 helper phage, continue shaking at 37°C for 15 min, then transfer 1 mL to 50 mL of 2YT broth containing 50 μg/mL carbenicillin and 50 μg/mL kanamycin in 250-mL shake flask and grow overnight at 37°C.
4. Centrifuge culture at 8,000 rpm (maximum 7,900 × *g* in a Sorvall SM-24 rotor) to remove cells, remove supernatant to new centrifuge tube, and add 1/5 volume of 20% PEG/2.5 M NaCl solution, invert to mix, and incubate for 10 min at room temperature to precipitate phage.
5. Centrifuge at 13,000 rpm (maximum 20,900 × *g*) for 15 min to collect phage pellet, wash pellet by resuspending in PBS, and recentrifuge.
6. Transfer supernatant to new tube and repeat PEG precipitation. Redissolve phage pellet in 1 mL PBS.
7. Prepare single-stranded (ss) DNA from phage pellet using Qiagen M13 spin kit following protocol included. Elute ssDNA from spin column with 100 μL elution buffer, measure absorbance at 260 nm to determine DNA concentration using A260 = 1 for 33 ng/μL ssDNA.
8. Phosphorylate mutagenic oligonucleotide (330 ng/μL stock concentration) by preparing in an Eppendorf tube a solution containing 2 μL oligonucleotide, 2 μL 10× TM buffer, 2 μL 10 mM rATP, 1 μL 100 mM DTT, and 12 μL $H_2O$.
9. Add 1 μL of T4 polynucleotide kinase to wall of tube, centrifuge briefly to mix, and incubate at 37°C for 30 min.
10. Anneal phosphorylated oligonucleotide with ssDNA prepared above. Mix 1 μg ssDNA, 2 μL of phosphorylated oligonucleotide solution, 2.5 μL 10× TM buffer and $H_2O$ to 25 μL in an Eppendorf tube.
11. Centrifuge to mix and incubate for 1 min at 90°C, then 5 min at 50°C, and then place on ice.
12. Initiate fill-in reaction by adding 1 μL 10 mM rATP, 1 μL 25 mM dNTPs, 1.5 μL 100 mM DTT, 0.6 μL T4 DNA ligase, 0.3 μL T7 DNA polymerase.

13. Centrifuge to mix and incubate at 37°C for 1.5 h.
14. Transform XL1-Blue Competent Cells and plate on LB agar plates containing 50 μg/mL carbenicillin.
15. Pick 4–6 single colonies, prepare dsDNA using Qiagen spin kit, and determine DNA sequence of Fc using dideoxynucleotide sequencing. DNAs from correct sequence clones are produced for transfection using the maxi protocol described by Qiagen.

### 3.2. IgG Production and Purification

Small scale transient transfections are performed in 293 T cells (see Note 4).

1. Grow 293 T cells in 293 cell growth media in T-150 flasks in a $CO_2$ incubator maintained at 37°C until confluency of 80% is reached.
2. Split cells 1:3 every 3 days.
3. To split, wash cells in 10 mL sterile PBS, then add 1.8 mL PBS and 0.2 mL 10× Trypsin. Place in incubator for 2 min then resuspend cells in 8 mL of growth media. Add 2 mL of resuspended cells to 23 mL of growth media in T-150 flask and return to incubator.
4. Split cells 1 day before transfection as described above. For each T-150 flask of 293 T cells, use 0.1 mL FuGENE™ 6 and 5 μg each of the heavy and light chain vectors (10 μg total endotoxin-free DNA) in a final volume of 1 mL transfection media (Freestyle™ 293 Expression Medium).
5. Transfect 2–5 T-150 flasks per antibody. For five flasks, add 4.5 mL 50:50 F12–DMEM media prewarmed to 37°C to a sterile 15-mL Falcon tube. Pipette 0.5 mL of FuGENE™ 6 reagent into media without allowing undiluted FuGENE™ 6 to touch sides of tube.
6. Mix by hand or vortex and let sit at room temperature for 5 min.
7. Add DNA and allow FuGENE™ 6-DNA complexes to form for a minimum of 20 min and maximum of 2 h, before adding to a T-150 flask containing 293 T cells in a final volume of 25 mL transfection media.
8. Add 1 mL of transfection mixture to each T-150 flask dropwise, swirl plates to evenly distribute DNA, and then return to incubator.
9. Conditioned media is collected 4–7 days post-transfection.
10. PMSF and bovine lung aprotinin are added to final concentrations of 1 mM and 1.2 μg/mL, respectively.
11. The media is filtered using a low protein binding polystyrene bottle with a 0.22 μm cellulose acetate filter to remove detached cells.

12. Purify IgG on a 0.5–1 mL of rProtein A agarose column. The column is washed in 25 mL of 75 mM Tris–HCl, 1.5 M KCl, pH 8 or PBS, pH7.4, before eluting with 2.5 mL 100 mM acetic acid, 150 mM NaCl.
13. Collect fractions in tubes containing a 1/10 volume of 1 M Tris–HCl, pH 8 to neutralize the solution. Buffer exchange into PBS using a PD-10 desalting column, followed by concentration using a Centricon-10.
14. Typically 2–5 T-150 flasks (50–125 mL supernatant) gave a yield of 0.2–1 mg antibody.

### 3.3. FcRn Binding ELISAs

We used two ELISA formats to measure FcRn binding (15). In the first format, plates are coated with NeutraAvidin followed by biotinylated soluble FcRn consisting of the extracellular domain α chain and β2 microglobulin. IgG is added to the plates and bound IgG is detected using anti-F(ab')$_2$-HRP. In the second format, plates are coated with antigen. IgG is added followed by biotinylated soluble FcRn. Bound FcRn is detected using Streptavidin-HRP. This format is less affected by the presence of IgG aggregate. Binding of IgG to FcRn is measured at pH 6.0 and dissociation of bound IgG at neutral pH is evaluated at pH 7.4.

1. For the NeutrAvidin coat format (see Note 5), coat 96-well ELISA plates with 100 μL/well of 2 μg/mL NeutrAvidin in coat buffer and incubated at 4°C overnight.
2. Wash the plates three times with 400 μL/well of wash buffer on the plate washer.
3. Block the plates with 150 μL/well of block buffer. Incubate at room temperature for 1 h with gentle shaking.
4. Wash the plates three times.
5. Add 100 μL/well of 2 μg/mL biotinylated FcRn in assay buffer and incubate for 1 h with gentle shaking.
6. Wash the plates three times.
7. Please note: pH 6.0 assay buffer and pH 6.0 wash buffer are used for the IgG binding and the detection antibody incubation steps below. Prepare seven serial twofold dilutions (3.1–200 ng/mL) of the IgG standard (see Note 6) and the samples as well as a 0 ng/mL buffer control in duplicate in pH 6.0 assay buffer. Add 100 μL/well to the plates and incubate at room temperature for 2 h with gentle shaking.
8. Wash each plate three times with pH 6.0 wash buffer and then rotate the plate on the washer and wash three times more.
9. Dilute F(ab')$_2$ anti-human IgG F(ab')$_2$-HRP 1:7,500 in pH 6.0 assay buffer (see Note 7). Add 100 μL/well to the plates and incubate at room temperature for 1 h with gentle shaking.
10. Wash the plates with pH 6.0 wash buffer as in step 8.

11. Add 100 μL/well of the substrate TMB to develop the plates. When the standards show a blue titration curve (see Note 8), add 100 μL/well of 1 M phosphoric acid to stop the reaction.
12. Read the absorbance at 450 nm using 630 nm for background subtraction.
13. For data analysis, determine the middle point absorbance (mid-OD) of the standard titration curve by averaging the absorbance readings of the lowest (3.1 ng/mL) and the highest (200 ng/mL) IgG standards. Calculate the corresponding concentrations of standard and samples using a four-parameter nonlinear regression curve-fitting program. Calculate the relative affinity by dividing the standard concentration by the sample concentration. The higher the ratio, the stronger the binding.
14. For assessing IgG-FcRn complex dissociation at pH 7.4, run two sets of standards and samples on the same ELISA plate. Carry out the assay steps 1–8 as described above and continue with a dissociation step. Add pH 6.0 assay buffer to one set of standards and samples and pH 7.4 assay buffer to the other set. Incubate for 45 min to allow dissociation. Wash the plates as in step 8 and continue the assay at step 9.
15. For the antigen coat format (see Note 5), coat the 96-well plates with 100 μL/well antigen (see Note 9). Wash and block the plates as described in steps 2 and 3 above. Prepare seven serial twofold dilutions (3.1–200 ng/mL) of the IgG standard (see Note 6) and the samples as well as a 0 ng/mL buffer control in duplicate in assay buffer.
16. Add 100 μL/well to the plates and incubate at room temperature for 2 h.
17. Wash the plates three times with wash buffer and rotate the plates and wash three times more. Please note: pH 6.0 assay buffer and pH 6.0 wash buffer are used for the following FcRn binding and streptavidin-HRP incubation steps. Add 100 μL/well of 0.125 μg/mL FcRn-bio in pH 6.0 assay buffer.
18. After a 1 h incubation, wash the plates with pH 6.0 wash buffer as in step 8. Add streptavidn-HRP (1:10,000 dilution in pH 6.0 assay buffer) and incubate for 30 min. Wash the plates with pH 6.0 wash buffer as in step 8.
19. Add the substrate to develop the plates and read the plates as described in steps 11 and 12 above.

### 3.4. Fcγ Receptor Binding ELISAs

To measure binding of IgG to FcγR by ELISA, plates are coated with anti-GST followed by soluble FcγR consisting of the extracellular domain with a His-GST tag (15). Noncomplexed IgG is added to the plates to measure high affinity FcγRI binding and complexed IgG is added to the plates to measure low affinity FcγRII and FcγRIII binding. Bound IgG is detected using anti-$F(ab')_2$-HRP.

1. Coat 384 well ELISA plates with 25 μL/well of 2 μg/mL anti-GST in coat buffer (see Note 10).
2. Wash the plates three times with 120 μL/well of wash buffer and block the plates with 80 μL/well of block buffer.
3. Wash the plates three times. Add 25 μL/well of 0.25 μg/mL FcγR-His-GST in assay buffer and incubate for 1 h.
4. Wash each plate three times with wash buffer and then rotate the plate on the washer and wash three times more.
5. For measuring high affinity FcγRI binding, prepare 11 serial threefold dilutions (0.0085–500 ng/mL) of the IgG standard (see Note 6) and the samples as well as a 0 ng/mL buffer control in duplicate in assay buffer. For measuring low affinity FcγRII and FcγRIII binding, crosslink IgG to increase binding avidity by preincubating 50 μg/mL IgG standard or samples with equal volumes of 100 μg/mL goat $F(ab')_2$ anti-human κ or anti-human λ antibody in assay buffer at room temperature for 1 h (see Note 11). Prepare 11 serial threefold dilutions (0.42–25,000 ng/mL) of the complexed IgG standard and the samples in assay buffer. Add 25 μL/well to the plates and incubate for 2 h.
6. Wash the plates as in step 4.
7. Dilute $F(ab')_2$ anti-human IgG $F(ab')_2$-HRP 1:10,000 in assay buffer (see Note 7). Add 25 μL/well to the plates and incubate at room temperature for 1 h with gentle shaking.
8. Wash the plates as in step 4.
9. Add 25 μL/well of the substrate TMB to develop the plates. When the standards show a blue titration curve (see Note 12), add 25 μL/well of 1 M phosphoric acid to stop the reaction. Read the plates and analyze the data as described above in steps 12–13 in the FcRn binding ELISA. For FcγRI binding data analysis, determine the mid-OD by averaging the absorbance readings of the 0.0085 and 500 ng/mL IgG standards. For FcγRII or FcγRIII binding data analysis, determine the mid-OD by averaging the absorbance readings of the 0.42 and 25,000 ng/mL IgG standards.

### 3.5. Surface Plasmon Resonance to Measure FcRn Binding

The following protocol is for steady-state measurements on the binding of FcRn to immobilized antibody using Biacore. Immobilization of the antibody avoids avidity affects that arise from 2:1 FcRn:IgG binding when the FcRn is immobilized. Given the weak affinity (500–1,000 nM $K_D$) of wild-type human $IgG_1$ for

FcRn, affinities are determined from steady-state rather than kinetic analysis.

1. Dock chip and normalize according to instrument manual.
2. Prime system with pH 5.8 running buffer. A separate immobilization is made for each IgG variant to be tested and up to three antibodies can be tested per sensor chip.
3. Immobilize IgGs (5–10 μg/mL) onto flow cells 2–4 of a Series S CM5 sensor chip for measurements on a Biacore T-100™ instrument, or a standard CM5 chip for measurements on a Biacore 3000 machine, using the amine coupling procedure according to the manufacturer's protocol. Immobilization levels should be not greater than 1,000 response units (RU) per flow cell, and ideally closer to 100 RU. Flow cell 1 is activated and blocked with ethanolamine and used as the reference cell.
4. Prepare eight serial threefold dilutions of FcRn (1.5 nM to 10 mM) in pH 5.8 running buffer.
5. Inject solutions of FcRn (low concentration to high) for 60 s at a flow rate of 50 μL/min followed by a dissociation phase of 30 s.
6. Regenerate surfaces between cycles by a single injection of pH 8.0 running buffer (30 s at 50 μL/min).
7. Analyze sensorgrams using evaluation software provided by manufacturer and fit to a simple 1:1 steady-state binding model.

### 3.6. FcγR Binding by Biacore

The following protocol is for steady-state measurements on the binding of FcγR to immobilized antibody. Given the weak affinity (100–1,000 nM $K_D$) of wild-type human $IgG_1$ for FcγR other than FcγRI, affinities are determined from steady-state rather than kinetic analysis.

1. Immobilize IgGs (5–10 μg/mL) onto flow cells 2–4 as described above. Immobilization levels should be not greater than 500 RU per flow cell, and ideally closer to 300 RU. Flow cell 1 is activated and blocked with ethanolamine and used as the reference cell.
2. Prepare eight serial threefold dilutions of FcγR (15.6 nM to 2 μM) in HBS-P running buffer as well as a zero FcγR concentration buffer control.
3. Inject solutions of FcγR (0 to high concentration) for 600 s at a flow rate of 10 μL/min followed by a dissociation phase of 30 s.
4. Regenerate surfaces between cycles by a single 60 s injection of 10 mM glycine-HCl, pH 2.5, at a flow rate of 10 μL/min.
5. Analyze sensorgrams using evaluation software provided by manufacturer and fit to a simple 1:1 steady-state binding model.

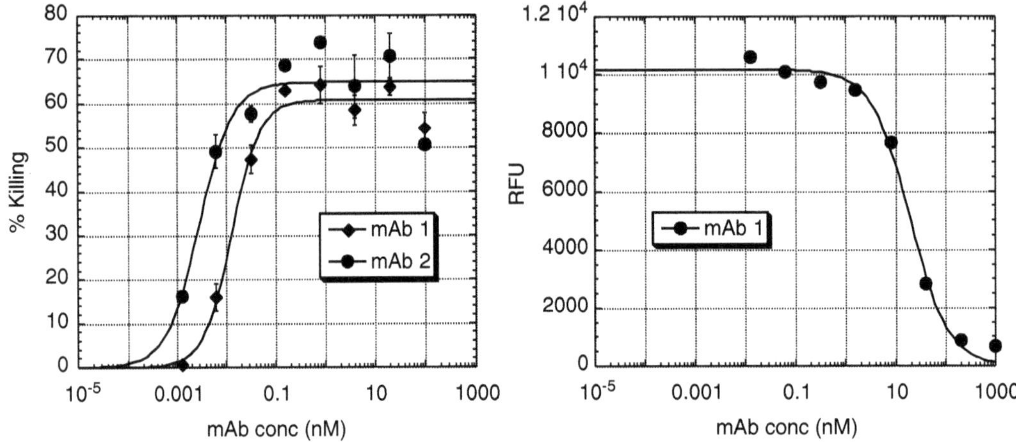


Fig. 2. Examples of antibody titration curves in the ADCC (*left*) and CDC (*right*) assays. *mAb*: monoclonal antibody.

### 3.7. ADCC Assay

1. Isolate NK cells from heparinized normal human whole blood of the heterozygous FcγRIIIa(F158/V158) genotype using RosetteSep following the manufacturer's protocol.
2. Add antibody (0.012 pM to 50 nM or 1.8 pg/mL to 7.5 μg/mL in fourfold serial dilution in duplicate in 50 μL) to 10,000 target cells in individual wells of a 96-well plate (see Note 6).
3. Incubate for 30 min at room temperature.
4. Add 50 μl of 30,000–50,000 effector NK cells and incubate for an additional 4 h at 37°C.
5. Centrifuge the plates at 1,000 rpm (230×*g* in a Beckman Coulter SX4750 rotor) for 5 min, transfer supernatant, and assay.
6. The level of cell lysis is determined by measuring the amount of lactate dehydrogenase released from cells using the Cytotoxicity Detection Kit.
7. Percent of cell lysis relative to antibody concentration is plotted and $EC_{50}$ values calculated using a four-parameter nonlinear regression curve-fitting program. Example cell lysis curves are shown in the left panel of Fig. 2.

### 3.8. CDC Assay

1. For antibodies directed to B cell surface antigens, suitable target cells are normal human B cells prepared by incubating whole blood in RosetteSep B cell Enrichment Cocktail.
2. Dilute whole blood with equal volume of PBS containing 2% fetal bovine serum.
3. Separate by gradient centrifugation over Ficoll-Pague Plus (see Note 13).
4. Target cells to be lysed, are washed in PBS and adjusted to a concentration of $1\times10^6$ cells/mL. Assays are performed in 96 microwell plate format.

5. Prepare 11 serial fourfold dilutions of antibody in PBS with a starting concentration of 1,000–3,000 nM.
6. Mix 50 μL of serially diluted antibody with 50 μL of target cells and 50 μL of a 1:4 dilution of normal human serum complement in individual wells of the microwell plate. Incubate for 2 h at 37°C.
7. Add 50 μL of Alamar Blue and incubate for an additional 18 h at 37°C.
8. Shake plates for 15 min and then read on a fluorescent plate reader (excitation wavelength 530 nm, emission wavelength 590 nm) to determine the relative fluorescent units (RFU).
9. Plot RFU value relative to concentration of antibodies in KaleidaGraph and analyze curves using a 4-parameter fit to calculate the $EC_{50}$ for lysis. An example CDC curve is shown in the right panel of Fig. 2.

## 4. Notes

1. For purification of non-His tagged FcRn on a human IgG column, it is important to prewash the IgG column with loading buffer and elution buffer to remove any loosely bound IgG. This reduces the amount of IgG contaminant in the purified FcRn. Since the IgG contaminant is biotinylated during the FcRn biotinylation step and can bind to the NeutrAvidin coated on the plate and be detected by the anti-human $F(ab')_2$-HRP detection antibody, the presence of IgG contaminant increases the assay background.
2. For measuring ADCC activity of antibodies, genotyping human donors for Val/Phe158 polymorphism was done using a PCR method similar to that described in Cartron (7).
3. Alternatively, PCR-based methods such as QuikChange® (site-directed mutagenesis kit from Stratagene) can be applied to double-stranded DNA.
4. CHO cells can also be used to express $IgG_1$. However, we recommend comparing $IgG_1$ variants produced using the same host cells.
5. For the FcRn binding ELISA using the NeutrAvidin coat format, it is important to compare wild type IgG preparations with similar amounts of aggregate since the presence of aggregated IgG increases the apparent binding affinity (15). However, we did not see obvious effect of the amount of aggregate on the binding affinity ranking of variants with non-detectable or increased binding affinity to FcRn (15). The antigen coat format is less sensitive to the presence of aggregate.

This format can be used to compare IgG variants with the same antigen binding sites if the antigen is available in a soluble form.

6. We include a designated lot of a wild type $IgG_1$ preparation as the standard in all our Fc receptor binding ELISAs. We calculate the relative binding affinities of the IgG variants to this standard. This allows for comparison of the relative binding affinities of variants that were assayed on different days. In addition, there can be lot-to-lot variation in the fucose level on an antibody resulting in slight differences in the FcγR binding affinity and ADCC activity. We recommend using a well-characterized lot of antibody with <5% afucosylation as the standard to calculate relative FcγR binding affinity and ADCC activity.
7. We used horseradish HRP-conjugated goat $F(ab')_2$ anti-human $F(ab')_2$ to detect IgG variants bound to the Fc receptors on the plates. $F(ab')_2$ does not have Fc and will not disturb the Fc receptor–IgG complex on the plate.
8. For the FcRn binding ELISAs, the substrate incubation time is about 10 min.
9. For the FcRn binding ELISA using the antigen coat format, we coated plates with 0.25–2 μg/mL antigen. For anti-Her2 variants, using 0.25 or 1 μg/mL of Her2 extracellular domain for coat gave similar relative FcRn binding results. However, the 1 μg/mL coat gave a slightly higher background. For anti-VEGF variants, we used 0.25 μg/mL of $VEGF_{165}$ for coat. We added anti-VEGF followed by biotinylated non-His-tagged FcRn. Biotinylated his-tagged FcRn was not used because it gave a high background. This background was not seen when $VEGF_{109}$ was used for coat (15).
10. For the FcγR binding ELISAs, the Fc portion of the anti-GST coat antibody may interact with the high affinity FcγRI. However, we compared using anti-GST IgG or anti-GST Fab for coat in the FcγRI binding ELISA and obtained similar relative affinities and continued to use anti-GST IgG for coat.
11. For the FcγRII and FcγRIII binding ELISAs, we used $F(ab')_2$ anti-light chain antibody to crosslink IgG variants to increase binding avidity. $F(ab')_2$ does not have Fc and will not compete with IgG variants for binding to Fcγ receptors on the plates.
12. For the FcγR binding ELISAs, the substrate incubation time is about 5 min. Use the same substrate incubation time for all IgG variants for FcγRI, FcγRII, or FcγRIII binding and keep the absorbance readings below 3.
13. For measuring CDC activity of anti-CD20 $IgG_1$ variants, we also used WIL2-S B lymphoma cells as target cells.

## Acknowledgments

We thank Devin Tesar for providing the protocol for surface plasmon resonance measurement of FcRn binding, Gerald Nakamura for advice on ADCC and CDC protocols, and Yanmei Lu for reviewing the Fc receptor binding ELISA protocols.

### References

1. Roopenian DC, Akilesh S (2007) FcRn: the neonatal Fc receptor comes of age. Nat Rev Immunol 7:715–725
2. Yeung YA, Leabman MK, Marvin JS et al (2009) Engineering human $IgG_1$ affinity to human neonatal Fc receptor: impact of affinity improvement on pharmacokinetics in primates. J Immunol 182:7663–7671
3. Gessner JE, Grussenmeyer T, Schmidt RE (1995) Differentially regulated expression of human IgG Fc receptor class III genes. Immunobiology 193:341–355
4. van der Poel CE, Spaapen RM, van de Winkel JG et al (2001) Functional characteristics of the high affinity IgG receptor, FcγRI. J Immunol 186:2699–2704
5. Metes D, Ernst LK, Chambers WH et al (1998) Expression of functional CD32 molecules on human NK cells is determined by an allelic polymorphism of the FcγRIIc gene. Blood 91:2369–2380
6. Dutertre C-A, Bonnin-Gelize E, Pulford K et al (2008) A novel subset of NK cells expressing high levels of inhibitory FcγRIIb modulating antibody-dependent function. J Leukoc Biol 84:1511–1520
7. Cartron G, Dacheux L, Salles G et al (2002) Therapeutic activity of humanized anti-CD20 monoclonal antibody and polymorphism in IgG Fc receptor FcγRIIIa gene. Blood 99:754–758
8. Weng WK, Levy R (2003) Two immunoglobulin G fragment C receptor polymorphisms independently predict response to rituximab in patients with follicular lymphoma. J Clin Oncol 21:3940–3947
9. Shields RL, Namenuk AK, Hong K et al (2001) High resolution mapping of the binding site on human $IgG_1$ for FcγRI, FcγRII, FcγRIII, and FcRn and design of $IgG_1$ variants with improved binding to the FcγR. J Biol Chem 276: 6591–6604
10. Lazar GA, Dang W, Karki S et al (2006) Engineered antibody Fc variants with enhanced effector function. Proc Natl Acad Sci USA 103:4005–4010
11. Yamane-Ohnuki N, Kinoshita S, Inoue-Urakubo M et al (2004) Establishment of FUT8 knockout Chinese hamster ovary cells: an ideal host cell line for producing completely defucosylated antibodies with enhanced antibody-dependent cellular cytotoxicity. Biotechnol Bioeng 87:614–622
12. Shields RL, Lai J, Keck R et al (2002) Lack of fucose on human $IgG_1$ N-linked oligosaccharide improves binding to human FcγRIII and antibody-dependent cellular toxicity. J Biol Chem 277:26733–26740
13. Mossner E, Brunker P, Moser S et al (2010) Increasing the efficacy of CD20 antibody therapy through the engineering of a new type II anti-CD20 antibody with enhanced direct and immune effector cell-mediated B-cell cytotoxicity. Blood 115:4393–4402
14. Idusogie EE, Wong PY, Presta LG et al (2001) Engineered antibodies with increased activity to recruit complement. J Immunol 166:2571–2575
15. Lu Y, Vernes JM, Chiang N, Ou Q et al (2011) Identification of $IgG_1$ variants with increased affinity to FcγRIIIa and unaltered affinity to FcγRI and FcRn: comparison of soluble receptor-based and cell-based binding assays. J Immunol Methods 365:132–141
16. Kunkel TA, Roberts JD, Zakour RA (1987) Rapid and efficient site-specific mutagenesis without phenotypic selection. Methods Enzymol 154:367–382
17. Chung CT, Miller RH (1988) A rapid and convenient method for the preparation and storage of competent bacterial cells. Nucleic Acids Res 16:3580

# Chapter 19

# Class-Specific Effector Functions of Therapeutic Antibodies

**Virginie Pascal, Brice Laffleur, and Michel Cogné**

## Abstract

Physiology usually combines polyclonal antibodies of multiple classes in a single humoral response. Beyond their common ability to bind antigens, these various classes of human immunoglobulins carry specific functions which can each serve specific goals. In many cases, the function of a monoclonal therapeutic antibody may thus be modulated according to the class of its constant domains. Depending on the immunoglobulin class, different functional assays will be used in order to evaluate the functional activity of a monoclonal antibody.

**Key words:** Antibody-dependent cell cytotoxicity, Antigen neutralization, Complement, Complement-dependent cytotoxicity, Human antibodies, Immunoglobulin

## 1. Introduction

Monoclonal antibodies (mAbs) constitute the fastest growing family of new therapeutic drugs, with hundreds of mAbs in preclinical development and clinical trials (1). Human antibodies or humanized antibodies may serve various goals through various effects. This can include neutralization of a circulating antigen or pathogen (e.g., by inhibition of receptor–ligand cognate interaction, inhibition of virus binding to the cell surface, inhibition of viral decapsidation (2)), modulation of a target cell fate (e.g., through inhibition of cell growth or induction of apoptosis (3)), and lysis of a target cell [either by complement-dependent cytotoxicity (CDC) or antibody-dependent cell cytotoxicity (ADCC)]. To yield such effects, antibodies need to bind the antigen with good affinity and specificity but also to exert adequate effector functions. In the case of cancer immunotherapy, most of the tumor-directed antibodies employed are chosen from the IgG1 isotype, due to its long plasma half-life (4) and their ability to trigger complement activation and ADCC. Nevertheless, given the functional

Gabriele Proetzel and Hilmar Ebersbach (eds.), *Antibody Methods and Protocols*, Methods in Molecular Biology, vol. 901,
DOI 10.1007/978-1-61779-931-0_19, © Springer Science+Business Media, LLC 2012

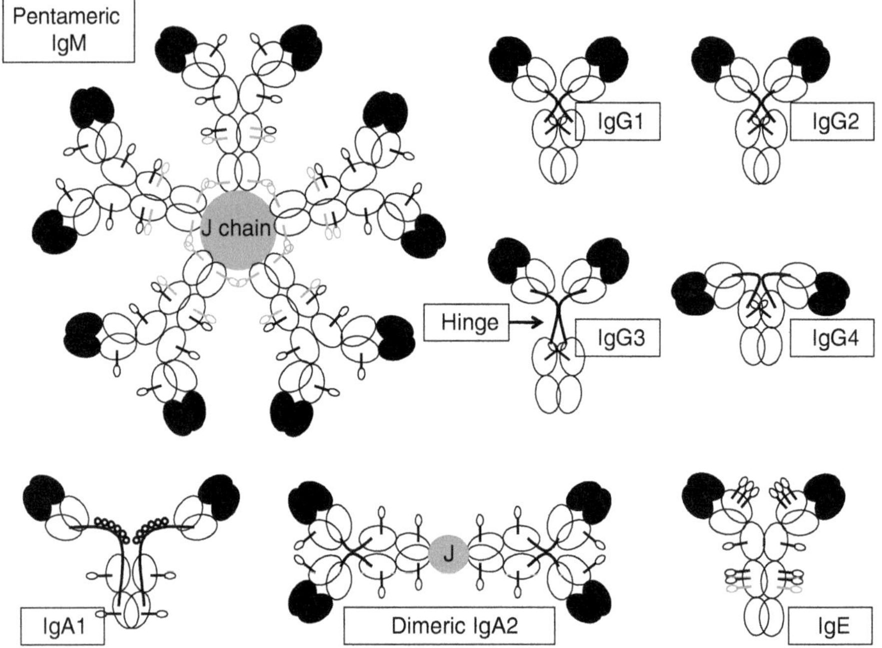


Fig. 1. Diagrammatic representation of human Ig showing variable (*black*) and constant (*white*) heavy and light chain domains. IgA and IgM interact with J chain (*gray*) to form polymers. Glycosylation is shown for complex (*black rackets*) or oligomannose (*gray rackets*) *N*-glycans and for clusters of *O*-glycans (*small black circles* of the IgA1 hinge region).

limitations of IgG regarding tissue accessibility or interactions with effector cells (5), many efforts have also recently been concentrated towards the development of novel molecules from other human immunoglobulin (Ig) classes, such as IgM, IgA, or IgE (6–8).

Human Igs belong to five classes based on the sequence of their heavy chain constant regions: IgM, IgD, IgG, IgE, and IgA. The IgG class is itself subdivided into four different subclasses (IgG1, IgG2, IgG3, and IgG4) and the IgA class into two isotypes (IgA1 and IgA2). The basic structure of each human Ig class and isotype is illustrated in Fig. 1. Although the Ig isotypes differ structurally, they are all built from the same basic units. All Igs have a four chain structure as their basic unit. They are composed of two identical light chains (23 kDa) and two identical heavy chains (50–70 kDa). Heavy chains include three or four constant domains, CH1, CH2, CH3, and CH4. The CH1 and CH2 domains are separated by a flexible region called the hinge region. IgM has four constant domains and can bind covalently via the CH4 domain another protein called the J chain, which promotes IgM polymerization into a pentamer or hexamer. In contrast, all IgG isotypes are monomers. The major singularities of the various IgG isotypes stand in their hinge regions. The IgG4 (as well as the IgG2) hinge is three amino acids shorter than the hinge of IgG1. Based on its shorter hinge, IgG4 was assumed to have a lower segmental flexibility (9). IgA is mainly monomeric in serum but IgA can also form polymers, bind to the J chain and be secreted as a dimer or a higher order polymer, and then be exported at mucosal surfaces (10). IgE is produced as a monomer.

Each class and isotype is specialized both regarding its localization in the body and regarding the functions it can assume (Table 1). IgM antibodies are found mainly in blood and are specialized in antigen neutralization and efficient complement activation upon binding antigen (11). As a consequence of its pentameric structure, IgM is also a strongly agglutinating Ig. IgG antibodies are usually of higher affinity and are found in blood and in extracellular fluids, where they can neutralize toxins, viruses, and bacteria, opsonize them for phagocytosis, and activate the complement system. IgA antibodies are synthesized as monomers, which enter blood and extracellular fluids, or as dimeric molecules in the lamina propria of various epithelia. IgA dimers are selectively transported across these epithelia into sites such as the gut lumen, where they neutralize toxins and viruses and block the entry of bacteria across the intestinal epithelium (12). IgA is the major Ig class in secretions (tears, saliva, colostrum, mucus). Most IgE antibodies are bound to the surface of mast cells that reside mainly just below body surfaces; antigen catching by mast cell-bound IgE triggers local defense reactions (13). Cell-bound IgE can also trigger efficient activation of basophils, eosinophils, and platelets, altogether yielding proinflammatory and ADCC reactions that are crucial for parasite immunology. Thereby, the heavy chain determines the intrinsic structural properties and immune effector functions of each Ig.

In conclusion, properties of therapeutic antibodies can generally be divided into two categories. The class I antibodies recognize cell-bound antigens and then lead to the target cell death. The Fc region effector functions usually play a major role in their action. The isotypes that can be used in this category are IgG1, IgG3, IgA, IgE, and IgM. Class II antibodies rather interact with cell-bound antigens in a way that rather blocks or enhances signaling pathways without recruiting effectors. In this second case, IgG2 and IgG4 isotypes are classically good candidates, although polymeric IgA also stands as an interesting challenger in this regard.

This chapter will focus on methods to characterize and measure these various effector functions of Igs in order to assess their capabilities as therapeutic antibody.

## 2. Materials

### *2.1. Antibody Purification*

1. G columns (GE Healthcare, UK).
2. 0.1 M Glycine (pH 2.5).

**Table 1**
**Effector functions of human immunoglobulins**

| | Main localization | Mean serum level (mg/mL) | Neutralization | Binding complement factor | CDC | Fc receptor | ADCC via NK cells | ADCC via neutrophils | Degranulation (mast cells, basophils) |
|---|---|---|---|---|---|---|---|---|---|
| IgM | Serum | 1.5 | ++ | C1q | +++ | pIgR; Fcα/μR<br>FcμR (TOSO) | – | – | – |
| IgG1 | Serum | 9 | + | C1q | ++ | FcγRI | ++ | – | + |
| IgG2 | Serum | 3 | + | C1q | + | FcγRII (CD32) | – | – | – |
| IgG3 | Serum | 1 | + | C1q | +++ | FcγRIII (CD16) | ++ | – | + |
| IgG4 | Serum | 0.5 | + | None | – | FcRn | – | – | – |
| IgA1 | Serum<br>Mucosa | 1.9 | +++ | Factor B; MBL | + | FcαRI (CD89)<br>pIgR | – | ++ | – |
| IgA2 | Mucosa | 0.2 | +++ | Factor B; MBL | + | Fcα/μR<br>ASGR | – | ++ | – |
| IgE | Tissus | $3.10^{-6}$ | + | None | – | FcεRI<br>FcεRII (CD23) | – | – | +++ |

3. 2 M Tris–HCl, pH 9.
4. Phosphate buffered saline (PBS).
5. Streptococcal IgA binding peptide (Sap).
6. 0.1 M Glycine, pH 3
7. 1 M Tris–HCl, pH 9.
8. Jacalin (Pierce, Rockford, IL, USA).
9. Soluble galactose.
10. Protein L (ThermoScientific, Rockford, IL USA).

#### 2.2. Antibody and Ligand Labeling

1. Labeling kit (Molecular Probes®, Invitrogen, Life Technologies, Carlsbad, CA, USA).
2. DyLight Antibody Labeling Kit (Pierce).
3. Lightning-Link™ kit (Innova Biosciences, Cambridge, UK).
4. 1 mCi $^{125}$I (Amersham, GE Healthcare).
5. PBS.
6. Chloramine-T in PBS.
7. Sodium metabisulfite.
8. Carrier protein: e.g., bovine serum albumin (BSA).
9. Sephadex G-75 (GE Healthcare).

#### 2.3. Target Cell Validation

1. Cell lines [American Type Culture Collection (ATCC) www.atcc.org/, Health Protection Agency Culture Collections (HPACC) www.hpacultures.org.uk/], the German Research Center for Biological Material (DSMZ) www.dsmz.de/, and the Riken BioResource Center Cell Bank (Riken) www.brc.riken.jp.
2. FITC BrdU Flow Kit (BD Pharmingen, San Diego, CA, USA).
3. Vybrant® MTT Cell Proliferation Assay Kit (Invitrogen).
4. AlamarBlue® Cell Viability Reagent (Invitrogen).
5. APO LOGIX™ Carboxyfluorescein Caspase Detection Kits (Cell Technology Inc, Mountain View, CA, USA).
6. Caspase-Glo® Assay (Promega, Madison, WI, USA).
7. Propidium iodide (PI) (Invitrogen).
8. Calcein-AM (R&D Systems, Minneapolis, MN, USA).
9. DELFIA Eu-Labeling kit (Perkin Elmer, Waltham, MA, USA).
10. Carboxyfluorescein diacetate, succinimidyl ester (CFSE) (Invitrogen).
11. CellTrace™ Far Red DDAO-SE (Invitrogen).

**2.4. Effector Cell Purification**

1. Human peripheral blood or peripheral blood mononuclear cells (PBMC).
2. NK cell isolation kit (Miltenyi Biotech, Bergisch Gladbach, Germany).
3. Ficoll-Hypaque™ (GE Healthcare).
4. MicroBeads.
5. Ficoll-Hypaque/Dextran sedimentation (Sigma Aldrich).
6. Mono-Poly™ Resolving Medium (MP Biomedicals, Solon, OH, USA).
7. Percoll gradient (Biochrom, Cambridge, UK).
8. RosetteSep® Human Monocyte Enrichment cocktail (StemCell Technology, Vancouver, BC, Canada).
9. Cytokines, such as granulocyte-macrophage colony-stimulating factor (GM-CSF) and macrophage colony-stimulating factor (M-CSF).

**2.5. Antibody-Mediated Inhibition of Receptor–Ligand Interaction**

1. Fluorescent labeled growth factors.
2. $^{125}$I-labeled growth factors.
3. Surface plasmon resonance system, e.g., Biacore (GE Healthcare).

**2.6. Apoptosis and Growth Inhibition Assays**

1. Propidium iodide (PI).
2. Fluorescein isothiocyanate (FITC)-labeled annexin V (BD Pharmingen).
3. PBS without $CaCl_2$ or $MgCl_2$, cold (4°C).
4. [$^3$H]thymidine.
5. MTS assay (Promega).
6. 96-Well plates for cell culture.
7. Test and control mAbs.
8. BrdU.
9. 2 N HCl.
10. FITC-conjugated anti-BrdU mouse mAb (BD Pharmingen).
11. PBS.

**2.7. Complement-Mediated Cytotoxicity Assays**

1. Target cells.
2. Unheated serum.
3. mAbs.
4. AlamarBlue® Cell Viability Reagent (Invitrogen).
5. CellTiter-Glo (Promega).

6. Lactate dehydrogenase (LDH) release assay (Promega).
7. Propidium iodide.
8. C1q protein depleted sera (Quidel, San Diego, CA, USA).
9. Factor B depleted sera (Quidel).
10. C1q protein (Quidel).
11. ImageStream system (Amnis, Seattle, WA, USA).
12. Amnis IDEAS software.
13. Paraformaldehyde.

#### 2.8. Antibody-Dependent Cell-Mediated Cytotoxicity Assays

1. PBMC.
2. Fluorescent dyes.
3. Lab-Tek II glass chamber slides.
4. Anti-CD14–R-phycoerythrin (RPE).
5. Fixative.
6. Carboxyfluorescein diacetate, succinimidyl ester (CFSE).
7. Phycoerythrin (PE)-Texas Red (ECD)-conjugated anti-human CD45 Ab.
8. PE-conjugated anti-human CD16 Ab.
9. Fluorescent DNA dye DRAQ5™ (Biostatus Limited).
10. ImageStream system (Amnis).
11. Amnis IDEAS software.
12. Target and negative control cells.
13. Purified PBMC or other preparations of killer cells.
14. 1% Triton X-100.
15. $^{51}Cr$-label.
16. Fluorescent dyes, such as calcein-AM, CFSE, or BCECF.
17. Saline.
18. 20 mM Eu(DH3C00)3+.
19. 100 mM Diethylenetriaminopentaacetate (DTPA).
20. 0.5 mg Dextran sulfate.
21. $CaCl_{2.}$
22. 96-Well round-bottomed microtiter plates.
23. Enhancement solution: a detergent causing the dissociation of europium ions to form a soluble and highly fluorescent component.
24. Time-resolved fluorometer (Arcus 1232 Delfia).
25. PBMC-derived cells or differentiated U937 (mononuclear).
26. Confocal microscopy.

27. Flow cytometry.
28. Fluorescence-activated cell sorting (FACS) tubes.
29. Anti-CD89-PE.
30. Propidium iodide.

#### 2.9. In Vivo Testing of Antibodies

1. Carboxyfluorescein diacetate succinimidyl ester (CFDA-SE) (Molecular Probes, Invitrogen).
2. CellTrace Far Red DDAO-SE (DDAO-SE) (Molecular Probes, Invitrogen).
3. Target cells.
4. Mice, e.g., NOD/SCID (e.g. NOD.CB17-*Prkdcscid*/J), NOD-scid IL2Rg$^{null}$ (NOD.Cg-*Prkdcscid Il2rgtm1Wjl*/SzJ), or NOD-Rag1$^{null}$ IL2Rg$^{null}$ (NOD.Cg-*Rag1tm1Mom Il2rgtm1Wjl*/SzJ) (The Jackson Laboratory, Bar Harbor, USA).
5. Cell culture medium.
6. Primary tumor cells.
7. Matrigel (BD Biosciences).
8. PMOD software (PMOD Technologies Ltd).

## 3. Methods

#### 3.1. Antibody Purification

Depending upon the Ig class, a variety of chromatography techniques can be employed for antibody (Ab) purification. All mouse and human IgG classes bind protein G columns. Once bound through their Fc region, IgG can be eluted with 0.1 M glycine, pH 2.5. The eluate then has to be neutralized immediately with 2 M Tris–HCl, pH 9 and dialyzed overnight to PBS (14).

Bovine and human IgA1 and IgA2 (but not mouse IgA) can be purified by chromatography using streptococcal IgA binding peptide (Sap) (15) coupled onto beads; IgA will be further eluted from column with 0.1 M glycine, pH 3 and neutralized with 1 M Tris–HCl, pH 9. Sap binds the CH2–CH3 interdomain region of the α H chain. IgA1 class antibodies are also classically purified through affinity for the lectin jacalin and then eluted with in the presence of soluble galactose. Whatever the H chain class, many antibodies can be purified by affinity onto protein L, which binds canonical motifs conserved in a majority of κ light chain V domains (16).

#### 3.2. Antibody and Ligand Labeling

Many assays require coupling of the antibody molecule itself (or of the antigen of interest) with a fluorescent or radioactive marker. Several commercial kits allow the labeling of protein or monoclonal antibodies with various dyes. Radiolabeling may be more difficult, since it requires materials for radioprotection and an authorization to manipulate radioelements. Two radioactive isotopes commonly used for conjugation with antibodies or ligands are iodine 125 ($^{125}I$) and tritium ($^{3}H$). Incorporation of iodine may be either by direct electrophilic substitution on the peptide or by intermediate fixation on a chemical reagent which is then grafted onto the peptide or the antibody of interest. In both cases, iodine in a reduced form (NaI) reacts with the phenol group of a tyrosine or with the side chain of a histidine residue. These groups are first oxidized with chloramine-T, lactoperoxidase, or iodogen. For example, a radiolabeled protein can be obtained by incubating 50 μg of the protein with 1 mCi $^{125}$l and 20 μg of chloramine-T in PBS, followed after 1 min by the addition of 48 μg of sodium metabisulfite and 6 mg of a carrier protein, e.g., BSA. The product is then gel-filtrated over Sephadex G-75 and the fractions corresponding to the main labeled macromolecular peaks are pooled (17).

### 3.3. Target Cell Validation

Established tumor cell lines and protocols exist for many different tissue systems, derived from human, mouse, or other mammalian tissues. Cell lines are available for example from the American Type Culture Collection (ATCC), the Health Protection Agency Culture Collections (HPACC), the German Research Center for Biological Material (DSMZ) and the Riken BioResource Center Cell Bank (Riken).

In some cases, antibody binding may cause measurable physiological changes within the targeted cell. One example is cell proliferation, which can be analyzed by measuring DNA synthesis by bromodeoxyuridine (BrdU) incorporation (e.g., FITC BrdU Flow Kit), evaluation of the mitochondria mass (MTT or MTS assay), or evaluation of some enzyme activity within the cytosol (alamarBlue® Cell Viability Reagent). In the same way, several methods are available to study cell death: caspase detection in apoptotic cells (Carboxyfluorescein Caspase Detection, Caspase-Glo® assays), or use of fluorescent molecules such as propidium iodide (PI) or the calcein-AM to discriminate dead cells from living cells.

Another important aspect of therapeutic antibody evaluation requires labeling of target cells in order to evaluate their fate either in vitro in a cytotoxicity assay or in vivo after injection into recipient animals. In the case of time-resolved fluorescent assays, target cells can be labeled with the DELFIA® Eu-Labeling kit. For in vivo studies, the dye carboxyfluorescein diacetate, succinimidyl ester (CFSE) is most commonly used. CFSE is colorless and passively diffuses into cells. After its acetate groups are cleaved by intracellular esterases, it becomes a highly fluorescent amine-reactive fluorophore, labeling covalently intracellular proteins and thus remaining strictly intracellular. The approximate excitation and emission peaks of CFSE after hydrolysis are 492 and 517 nm, respectively. This dye can be used in dual fluorescence with other cell tracers, such as the Far Red DDAO-SE ($\lambda$abs./$\lambda$em.: 647/657 nm).

### 3.4. Effector Cell Purification

Assays measuring ADCC usually require purification of a cytotoxic leukocyte population, most often from peripheral blood. CD16+ natural killer (NK) cells can easily be sorted from blood using magnetic beads (e.g., NK cell isolation kit). Human peripheral blood mononuclear cells (PBMC) from anticoagulated peripheral blood or buffy coat should be first isolated by density gradient centrifugation, e.g., using Ficoll-Hypaque. Non-NK cells are then indirectly magnetically labeled with a cocktail of biotin-conjugated antibodies against lineage-specific antigens and a cocktail of MicroBeads. Upon subsequent magnetic separation, the magnetically labeled non-NK cells are retained on the column, while the unlabeled NK cells pass through.

A variety of techniques and media for separating polymorphonuclear leukocytes (PMNs) from whole blood have been described, including Ficoll-Hypaque/Dextran sedimentation, Mono-Poly™ Resolving Medium, and Percoll gradient. In the first technique, the dextran sedimentation which removes most of the red blood cell (RBC) is followed by a hypotonic lysis eliminating any remaining RBC and platelets. Ficoll sedimentation allows the separation of mononuclear cells from neutrophils. The neutrophils sink to the bottom of the Ficoll, whereas mononuclear cells remain at the plasma–Ficoll interface. The Mono-Poly™ is a Ficoll-Hypaque medium which permits isolation of mononuclear and polymorphonuclear leucocytes from whole blood in one step without requirements of red blood cells lysis. To purify neutrophils, Percoll is usually used as a discontinuous gradient consisting of 70 and 63% Percoll. After centrifugation, neutrophils are collected from the interface between the two Percoll layers. Remaining erythrocytes are removed by ice-cold hypotonic lysis. All three separation techniques produce functionally active PMNs of high purity, but the use of Percoll gradients may be preferable when a quick method of separation minimizing PMN preactivation is required (18).

Monocytes can be prepared to 70–80% purity by The RosetteSep® Human Monocyte Enrichment cocktail. This product is designed to negatively select monocytes from whole blood. Unwanted cells are targeted for removal with tetrameric antibody complexes recognizing CD2, CD3, CD8, CD19, CD56, CD66b, and glycophorin A. When centrifuged over a buoyant density medium such as Ficoll-Hypaque, the unwanted cells pellet along with the RBCs. The purified monocytes are present as a highly enriched population at the interface between the plasma and the Ficoll. Cultivation of monocytes during 7 days in presence of the human cytokine GM-CSF or M-CSF promotes their differentiation into macrophages (19).

### 3.5. Antibody-Mediated Inhibition of Receptor–Ligand Interaction

Although the mechanisms by which therapeutic antibodies mediate their action in vivo are often a matter of controversy, this can be analyzed more easily using in vitro assays. Conceptually, therapeutic antibodies effects are classified into direct mechanisms, simply dependent from antigen (Ag)-binding V domains, and indirect mechanisms, needing molecular or cellular effectors recruited by Ig constant domains.

Some of the most commonly targeted tumor-associated structures are growth factor receptors, which are over-expressed in a number of malignancies. mAbs binding these receptors can normalize growth rates and sensitize cells to cytotoxic agents. MAb-based signaling inhibition can occur by blocking the oligomerization of the receptor or by interfering with ligand binding.

1. Fluorescent (7) or $^{125}$I-labeled (20) growth factors can be incubated with target cells in the presence of the inhibitory mAb. After washing, cells are analyzed by flow cytometry in the case of fluorescent ligand, e.g., EGF or with a scintillation counter after solubilization of cells incubated with the radiolabeled ligand, e.g., EGF. Inhibition of ligand binding is calculated by the formula:

$$\%\ \text{Inhibition of ligand} - \text{binding} = \frac{\begin{pmatrix}\text{relative fluorescence intensity (RFI) or} \\ \text{count without Ab} - \text{RFI or count with Ab}\end{pmatrix}}{\text{RFI or count without antibody}} \times 100.$$

2. The ability of mAbs to compete with an immobilized factor for binding to its solubilized receptor (extra cellular domain, ECD) can also be measured by surface plasmon resonance [(SPR) Biacore] (21). Here, the ligand is immobilized on a CM5 sensor chip using standard amine coupling. Binding is measured for a series of samples containing a fixed concentration of soluble receptor and increasing molar excesses of Ab. The equilibrium SPR response obtained is expressed as a fraction of the response with no added Ab in function of the amount of Ab (see also Chapters 11 and 12).
3. X-ray crystallography can determine the precise interaction between the Fab fragment and its ligand (21). However such studies are still challenging, time-consuming, and costly and may not be successful for all cases.

   Depending on the application, a specific Ig subtype may be chosen. Strong anti-inflammatory activities of IgG2 and IgG4 in comparison to IgG1 and IgG3 make them attractive for applications where recruitment of immune effectors is unnecessary or undesired (e.g., for receptor blocking without cell depletion). The IgA class could be preferred when only antigen binding but not proinflammatory signals are sought after. Especially polymeric IgA, which contains four potential antigen binding sites and therefore can more efficient compete with other ligands than IgGs (22).

### 3.6. Apoptosis and Growth Inhibition Assays

Various therapeutic antibodies have been developed to induce apoptosis after binding to surface receptors such as the "tumor necrosis factor-related apoptosis inducing ligand" TRAIL, or CD20

(23, 24). Proapoptotic activities are evaluated in vitro by flow cytometry after annexin-V and propidium iodide staining (25).

1. Briefly, relevant target cells are incubated with Ab at 37°C over 5 h, and then stained with fluorescein isothiocyanate (FITC)-labeled annexin V and propidium iodide (PI) in cold PBS–$CaCl_2$–$MgCl_2$. Flow cytometry discriminates living cells (Annexin $V^-/PI^-$), early apoptotic cells (Annexin $V^+/PI^-$), and late apoptotic/necrotic cells (Annexin $V^+/PI^+$). Percentage of apoptosis induced by the Ab is calculated with the following formula (see Note 1):

$$\text{\% of early apoptotic cells} = \frac{\%\ \text{Ann}^+\text{IP}^-_{\text{experimental}} - \%\ \text{Ann}^+\text{IP}^-_{\text{basal}}}{\%\ \text{Ann}^-\text{IP}^-_{\text{basal}}} \times 100;$$

$$\text{\% of late apoptotic cells} = \frac{\%\ \text{Ann}^+\text{IP}^+_{\text{experimental}} - \%\ \text{Ann}^+\text{IP}^+_{\text{basal}}}{\%\ \text{Ann}^-\text{IP}^-_{\text{basal}}} \times 100.$$

Beside inducing apoptosis, Ab binding to certain surface receptors and resulting signal transduction can cause growth inhibition by cell cycle arrest at the G1/S phase of the cell cycle, as observed for the chimeric anti-CD20 antibody rituximab (26). Ab-mediated inhibition of proliferation of a tumor cell line can be measured by quantifying DNA incorporation of $[-^3H]$thymidine (26) or by an MTS assay.

2. In the MTS assay, relevant target cells are cultured at 37°C in 96-well plates. Proliferation is assessed after 24, 48 or 72 h of exposure to various concentrations of the test or control mAbs. The amount of viable cells is determined by measuring the absorbance ($A_{490nm}$) of the dissolved formazan product after addition of MTS for 4 h. Cells incubated in medium without Ab are used as control. Growth inhibition is expressed as follows:

$$100 - \frac{\text{Mean DO}_{\text{exp group}} - \text{Mean DO}_{\text{medium}}}{\text{Mean DO}_{\text{control}} - \text{Mean DO}_{\text{medium}}} \times 100.$$

3. Cell cycle arrest can be evaluated by a BrdU pulse-labeling technique. Target cells are cultured at 37°C with or without relevant mAb. After 24 h, exponentially growing cells ($10^6$) are pulse-labeled with BrdU and fixed. Cells are then incubated with 2 N HCl to partially denature the DNA. Incorporated BrdU is stained with FITC-conjugated anti-BrdU mouse monoclonal antibody (mAb). Samples are washed and resuspended in PBS containing propidium iodide (PI). Bivariate distributions of BrdU amounts (FITC) versus DNA content (PI) are analyzed by flow cytometry and allow define the various regions corresponding to the $G_0/G_1$, S, and $G_2/M$ phases of the cell cycle.

In some instances, the direct in vitro effects of mAb have been shown to be increased by hyper-cross-linking using either anti-Ig antisera or mAb multimers or FcγR-bearing cells (27). By analogy to mAb multimers, polymeric IgA proved more effective for growth inhibition than IgG1 (28); the T-shape of the IgA molecule instead of the Y-shape of IgG might also limit steric hindrance and increase ability to cross-link targets expressed at the cell surface.

### 3.7. Complement-Mediated Cytotoxicity Assays

A major Fc-mediated cytotoxic effect of therapeutic antibodies is cell lysis resulting from complement activation. Complement-dependent cytotoxicity (CDC) assays can be performed by incubation of target cells at 37°C with relevant mAbs and unheated serum. CDC can be assessed by using cell viability reagents, such as Alamar Blue (29), CellTiter-Glo (30), lactate dehydrogenase (LDH) release (31), or propidium iodide staining.

1. In the case of PI staining, flow cytometry indicates the percentage of specific cytolysis, as calculated from cell counts by the following formula:

$$\%\text{ of specific lysis} = \frac{\%\ \text{IP}^+_{\text{experimental}} - \%\ \text{IP}^+_{\text{basal}}}{100 - \%\ \text{IP}^+_{\text{basal}}} \times 100.$$

   Complement activation follows three potential pathways initiated by different factors: C1q for the classical pathway, factor B for the alternative pathway and mannan-binding lectin (MBL) for the lectin pathway, respectively. To further explore which pathway is involved in CDC mediated tumor cell lysis, assays can be performed in the presence of sera depleted specifically for a single complement fraction (C1q, factor B or MBL).

2. C1q binding studies.
   Binding of C1q to the mAb Fc region initiates the classical complement cascade, ultimately leading to formation of the membrane attack complex and lysis of target cells. C1q binding assays have been developed for a number of platforms, including SPR (32) and enzyme-linked immunosorbent assays (ELISA) (33).

   By comparing the efficacy of C1q binding of several mAb isotypes with the same antigen specificity (11), it has been shown that radiolabeled C1q binds hapten-coated red cells in the presence of hapten-specific human IgM, IgG1, and IgG3mAbs (with IgG3 > IgG1 > IgM), but not IgG2, IgG4, or IgE. IgA is generally unable to bind C1q and activate the classical pathway (22, 34), but several reports have documented its activation of the alternative pathway by recruiting factor B, as also possibly the mannan-binding lectin initiating the lectin pathway (35–38).

3. The ImageStream multispectral imaging flow cytometer system has been used to study C1q binding on target cells opsonized by antibodies (39). This technique is based on high resolution digital imaging of thousands of cells in a flow cytometry environment, and allows quantitative determination of both the binding of different fluorescent probes as well as the degree of colocalization of the probes on individual cells. Target cells are incubated with varying amounts of recombinant C1q and Ab of interest. The mixture is incubated at 37°C for 60 min, washed three times, and fixed with paraformaldehyde. A total of 10,000 cells are analyzed and following data collection, images are analyzed using Amnis IDEAS software. Cells are gated based on light scattering to exclude small particles and cell aggregates. The degree of colocalization of C1q with bound mAbs is calculated by the bright detail similarity score feature (40).

### 3.8. Antibody-Dependent Cell-Mediated Cytotoxicity Assays

#### 3.8.1. Ability to Recruit Cytotoxic Effector Cells

ADCC results from the Ab ability to act as a flexible adaptor molecule, linking tumor-associated antigens and cytotoxic effector cells. This mechanism involves interaction of the constant domain of the antibody Fc region with specific Fc receptors (FcR) expressed on immune cells. Thus, in many studies, assessment of ADCC is preceded by the demonstration of an interaction between target and effector cells mediated by a specific antibody. To that goal, the recruitment of human monocytes on target cells can be imaged by immunofluorescence (41), using PBMC mixed with fluorescent dye prelabeled target cells (effector-to-target ratio 50:1) in the presence of the relevant mAb in a Lab-Tek II glass chamber slide. The cells are incubated at 37°C in a humidified atmosphere of 5% $CO_2$ for 30 min, washed, stained with the monocyte marker anti-CD14–R-phycoerythrin (RPE), washed, fixed, and observed using immunofluorescence microscopy.

Recruitment of effector cells can also be evaluated by the imaging flow cytometer system. We for example have used this technique to compare the ability of monomeric and dimeric forms of an IgA mAb to recruit PMN. Target cells are labeled with CFSE and incubated with the specific mAb at 4°C. After washes, opsonized and labeled target cells are mixed with purified leucocytes in a 1:1 ratio. After 30 min incubation at 4°C, the cells are stained with phycoerythrin (PE)-Texas Red (ECD)-conjugated anti-human CD45 Ab and PE-conjugated anti-human CD16, washed and fixed. All cell nuclei are labeled with a far-red fluorescent DNA dye DRAQ5™ just before acquisition in order to count all the cells and normalize. Following data collection with an ImageSream apparatus, images are analyzed using the Amnis IDEAS software. The percentage of target cells associated with at least one CD16+ effector corresponds to the formula:

$$\%\text{ of aggregated targets} = \frac{\begin{pmatrix}\text{Count of target CFSE + cells bound} \\ \text{with CD16 + effector cells}\end{pmatrix}}{\text{total count of target CFSE + cells}} \times 100.$$

*3.8.2. Antibody-Dependent Cell-Mediated Cytotoxicity Assays*

ADCC is probably the most studied activity of therapeutic mAbs, with a vast number of methods available. Antibody triggered target cell death can be assessed by measuring the release of cytosolic components, such as ATP or LDH (42). Target and negative control cells (50 μL of $10^6$ cells/mL) are mixed with purified PBMC or other preparations of killer cells to give an effector/target cell ratio of 14:1. Lysis is evaluated by lactate dehydrogenase activity in the media after 4 h of incubation at 37°C. Spontaneous lysis of target and effector cells without antibody, and maximal lysis with 1% Triton X-100 are used as controls.

ADCC can also be assessed by measuring the release of specific metabolites from prelabeled target cells, using $^{51}Cr$ or fluorescent dyes such as calcein-AM (43), CFSE (44) or BCECF (45). For example, Dechant et al. have recently used the chromium release assay to demonstrate the capability of a mAb to recruit effector cells on tumor target cells labeled with 200 μCi $^{51}Cr$ for 2 h and adjusted to $10^5$/mL (7). Purified effector cells and the specific mAb were distributed in round-bottom microtiter plates. The assay started by adding target cells (50 μL), resulting in a final volume of 200 μL/well and an effector-to-target cell ratio of 80:1. After 3 h at 37°C, plates were centrifuged and $^{51}Cr$ release from supernatants was measured from triplicates. Percentage of cellular cytotoxicity was calculated with the following formula:

$$\%\text{ of specific lysis} = \frac{(\text{experimental cpm} - \text{basal cpm})}{(\text{maximal cpm} - \text{basal cpm})} \times 100,$$

with maximal $^{51}Cr$ release determined by adding perchloric acid (3% final concentration) to target cells, and basal release measured in the absence of specific mAb and effector cells. The radioactive chromium release assay has a number of advantages: it is easy to perform, highly sensitive, gives low spontaneous release, and utilizes a label that is nontoxic to the cells (46). The limitations of the assay come from the use of a radioactive label, the short half-life of the label and strict regulations for handling and disposal of radioactive materials.

In comparison, simple fluorescence assays lack sensitivity (because of the high background fluorescence) until Blomberg et al. (47, 48) described a method based on the dissociation and release of a nonradioactive lanthanide, europium, from its chelate with diethylenetriaminopentaacetate (DTPA). Release of $Eu^{3+}$ into solution, where it forms a highly fluorescent chelate, can be measured rapidly and with a high level of sensitivity through the detection of time-resolved fluorescence (TRF) (49). This assay is sensitive, specific, nonradioactive, but measurements require a plate reader with a TRF option (50). Using this technique, Maley and Simon described a method for standardizing cytotoxicity assays by the use of cryopreserved fluorescently labeled target cells (9). The cells are labeled in batches with $Eu^{3+}$ and frozen in multiple aliquots. Replicate aliquots can be thawed on different days and used for cytotoxicity assays. More precisely, target cells are washed in saline to reduce extracellular $Ca^{2+}$ content. The cell pellet is resuspended in labeling buffer supplemented with 20 mM $Eu(DH3C00)^{3+}$, 100 mM DTPA, and 0.5 mg of dextran sulfate and incubated during 20 min at room temperature. Then, the labeling process is stopped by the addition of $CaCl_2$ and the cells are washed three times before being frozen. The day of the experiment, freshly thawed $Eu^{3+}$ target cells are dispensed into wells of 96-well round-bottomed microtiter plates ($5 \times 10^3$ cells/100 mL). An equal volume of effector cells is added to each well. Suspensions of effector cells are adjusted to give effector/target ratios ranging from 50:1 to 6:1, in the presence of various concentrations of the specific mAb to be assayed. The microplates are incubated for 4 h at 37°C. All assays are done in triplicate. After incubation, 20 μL of the supernatants are transferred to wells of a flat-bottom 96-well microplate, and 200 μL of enhancement solution (a detergent causing the dissociation of europium ions to form a soluble and highly fluorescent component) are added to each well. After mixing for 5 min, fluorescence is measured in a time-resolved fluorometer. The percentage of specific cytotoxicity is calculated as:

$$\frac{\text{experimental release} - \text{spontaneous release}}{\text{maximum release} - \text{spontaneous release}} \times 100.$$

Spontaneous release is determined by incubating the targets with 100 μL of culture medium instead of effector cells, and maximum release is determined by incubating the targets with 0.5% Triton-X.

#### 3.8.3. Antibody-Dependent Cellular Phagocytosis Assay

Antibody-dependent cellular phagocytosis (ADCP) measures the destruction of target cells via monocyte or macrophage-mediated phagocytosis. ADCP assays use PBMC-derived cells or U937 cells differentiated to the mononuclear type. Phagocytosis readout requires tracking fluorescently tagged target cells by either confocal microscopy (51) or flow cytometry (8). The latter three-color flow cytometric method allows assaying the contributions of cytotoxicity and phagocytosis in Ab-dependent cell-mediated target cell lysis. In this experiment, target cells are incubated with 20 μL of 5 mM CFSE for 10 min at 37°C and washed twice in culture medium at 4°C to stop the reaction. CFSE+ target cells are then incubated in triplicate in fluorescence-activated cell sorting (FACS) tubes with unstained monocytes and specific mAb at 37°C, 5% $CO_2$. The total number of cells in each tube is $2.6 \times 10^5$ in a 400 μL volume. Following an incubation of 2.5 h, cells and effector cells are labeled with anti-CD89-PE (10 μg/mL) at 4°C. Following a further wash, the cells are mixed thoroughly to interrupt cell–cell contact and labeled with propidium iodide to identify dead cells. The cells are then analyzed by flow cytometry. Calculations of

ADCC and ADCP are made using dot plots analyses where Region Rl includes events representing total CFSE+ targets cells. The CFSE+ cells may be present within PE-stained effector cells (after phagocytosis) and such events define Region R2 (CFSE+ PE+ events). Region R3 contains tumor targets killed externally by effector cells (cytotoxicity) and thus CFSE+/PI+. The basal Rl population is determined with a tube containing only effector and target cells without Ab and referred as the "Rl spontaneous loss (SL) control". The percentage of specific cytotoxicity (ADCC) is calculated as: $[(\text{R1 SL control} - \text{R1} + \text{R3})/\text{R1 SL control}] \times 100$.

The percentage of target cells phagocytosed (ADCP): $[\text{R2}/\text{R1 SL control}] \times 100$.

### 3.9. In Vivo Testing of Antibodies

Although in vitro assays are rapid, readily quantifiable, consistently reproducible and allow the assessment of various mechanisms, they do not mimic all interactions that occur in vivo. Furthermore, indirect effects of mAbs are difficult to reproduce. Therefore, whenever possible, in vitro assays should be carried out using appropriate target cells, preferably from more than one source, or more importantly, be followed and validated by in vivo assays. With this in mind, many efforts have been made for the development of in vivo cancer models, particularly in mice where tumor growth suppression can be evaluated and the mechanism(s) of tumor cell inhibition can be defined through the selective depletion of complement or of putative effector cell populations.

#### 3.9.1. In Vivo Target Cell Lysis

To allow an efficient assessment of candidate therapeutic antibodies, Guyre et al. have developed a flow cytometric-based method that rapidly and directly quantifies antibody-mediated killing in a short term in vivo assay (52). This in vivo antibody-mediated killing (IVAK) method uses two fluorescent dyes: carboxyfluorescein diacetate succinimidyl ester (CFDA-SE) and CellTrace Far Red DDAO-SE (DDAO-SE) to distinguish Ab target and internal reference populations. In this method, cells are labeled with 2 μM DDAO/0.1 μM CFDA-SE (dim reference cells) or 2 μM DDAO/2 μM CFDA-SE (bright target cells). Dim and bright cells are mixed ~1:1 and injected i.p. ($10^6$ in 200 μL) into mice (see Note 2) followed by i.p. injection of Ab (2, 20, or 150 μg in 200 μL). After 5 h, mice are euthanized and peritoneal washings are harvested individually. The cells are analyzed by flow cytometry. Regions drawn on cytograms define the target and reference cell populations and ratios are calculated as a percentage of target cells ($\text{CFDA}^{\text{hi}}$ $\text{DDAO}^{\text{hi}}$) divided by the percentage of reference cells ($\text{CFDA}^{\text{low}}$ $\text{DDAO}^{\text{hi}}$). Ratios from individual mice treated with specific mAb are then normalized to PBS-treated mice, and percent killing is calculated as follows:

$$1 - \frac{\text{ratio Ab treated mouse}}{\text{mean ratio of the PBS injected group}} \times 100.$$

*3.9.2. Tumor Grafts in Syngeneic Hosts or Immunodeficient Mice*

Tumor models can sometimes be easily established by grafting mouse tumors in hosts from the same genetic background that will not reject the tumor (see Note 2). For example, to study the mechanism of action of the anti-CD20 rituximab antibody in vivo, Gaetano et al. have set up a model of murine lymphoma that stably expresses the human CD20 molecule (53). Injection of $8 \times 10^3$ EL4-CD20$^+$ cells in the tail vein of C57BL/6 syngeneic animals produced tumors leading to death in 100% of animals within 30–40 days after tumor inoculation. In this study, 150 μg of specific mAbs were administered intraperitoneally (i.p.), 24 h after tumor graft and the authors evaluated the therapeutic efficacy by comparing the survival of treated to untreated animals.

Nevertheless, although syngeneic tumor grafts in mice allow to create simple models, they do not accurately depict the physiological histology and metastatic pattern of most human tumors. The development of immunodeficient mice able to allow human tumor growth was an important milestone for the development of in vivo antitumor strategies. *Nude* mice, characterized by thymic agenesis and deficiency of mature T lymphocytes, were the first immunodeficient mice used as recipients for human tumor cell engraftment (54). Severe combined immunodeficient (SCID) mice, lacking both mature T and B cells, have provided an alternative model for studying human tumors in vivo, which allows, unlike *nude* mice, engraftment of human hematopoietic cells (55). In 1992, RAG-1 and RAG-2-deficient mice were developed, characterized by the absence of functional B and T cells and at refs. 56, 57. The same year, the SCID mutation was backcrossed onto the nonobese diabetic (NOD) strain background characterized by reduced NK activity together with absence of macrophages and circulating complement (58). NOD-*scid* mice still present a residual innate immunity activity, and some remaining NK cell activity. This limitation was resolved by crossing RAG2−/− or RAG1−/− (NRG) (59) and NOD-scid mice with IL-2R γ knockout mice characterized by the absence of functional NK cells. The Rag2$^{-/-}$; γc$^{-/-}$ (60), the NOD-scid IL2Rg$^{null}$ (NOG or NSG) and NOD-Rag1$^{null}$ IL2Rg$^{null}$ (NRG) (61–63) murine models show no mature B and T lymphocytes and completely lack NK cells. These mouse strains and variants of these currently represent the most pertinent models for in vivo studies on tumor biology and therapy (64–66).

*3.9.3. Evaluation of the Therapeutic Efficacy of the Ab In Vivo*

A number of human cancer models have been created using immunodeficient mice. In these models, tumor transplantation can be achieved through different ways, including intradermal, subcutaneous (s.c.), intramuscular, intravenous (i.v.), or i.p.

For a breast cancer in model 100 μL of culture medium is mixed with 100 μL of matrigel containing $10^3$ primary tumor cells were transplanted into the mammary glands of 6-week-old female NOD/SCID mice by s.c. injection (67). Mice are treated with specific Abs administered i.p. twice a week at a dose of 8 mg/kg. Tumor growth is monitored weekly by palpation for 6 months or until the tumor size is $\leq$1,500 mm$^3$ (see Note 3).

In the case of hematopoietic malignancies, tumor implantations are generally done by i.v. injection into the lateral tail vein. For example, Nijmeijer et al. have described a model of acute lymphoblastic leukemia where female NOD/SCID mice were injected i.v. with 10$^7$ human leukemic cells (68). Antibodies were administered i.p. in 250 μL saline for 5 days per week over 3 weeks. Engraftment and progression of leukemia were monitored weekly by flow cytometric analysis of peripheral blood samples from individual animals, taken from the lateral tail vein. After red blood cell lysis, the percentage of human leukemic cells was determined by flow cytometry after staining with anti-mouse CD45 and anti-human CD45 mAbs.

The monitoring of tumor progression can be performed by noninvasive methods with assistance of luminescent, fluorescent or radioactive tracers. Positron emission tomography (PET) provides three-dimensional images and allows in vivo quantification of multiple functional processes. The system detects specific γ rays emitted by a tracer which is a positron-emitting radionuclide, after its introduction into the body within a biologically active molecule. Tumors generally differ from healthy tissue with regard to metabolism, hypoxia, cell proliferation, bone remodeling, or tumor-receptor density. For example, PET analysis after injection of $^{18}$F-FDG (fluorodeoxyglucose) reveals the increased glycolytic rate of malignant cells in tumors, compared with surrounding normal tissues (69, 70). Although FDG in the most common tracer for PET scan, other molecules can help to differentiate tumor from healthy tissue. A recent study used fluorine-18-fluoromisonidazole ($^{18}$FMISO) retained in hypoxic tumor tissues to evaluate Ab efficacy against a graft of tumoral endothelial cells ($0.5 \times 10^6$ cells injected in 100 μL PBS s.c. in the flank) (71). To follow the development of the tumor, mice are injected with $^{18}$F-FMISO ($14.9 \pm 4.9$ MBq in 100 μL) in the tail vein. After 4 h, an image is acquired using a small animal dedicated tomography. For the assessment of tumor $^{18}$F-FMISO uptake, all studies are exported and analyzed using the PMOD software. Maximum standardized uptake value (SUV) was calculated for each tumor using the formula:

$$\text{SUV} = \frac{\text{tissue activity concentration (Bq/cm}^3\text{)}}{\text{injected dose (Bq)}} \times \text{body weight (g)}.$$

Another major obstacle to predicting the clinical effectiveness of engineered antibodies with animal models and especially with mice is the difference of their immune systems from that of humans particularly in terms of FcR function and distribution (72). Murine models integrating human-derived effector elements are thus valuable, either by grafting human effector cells into mice (73) or by establishing transgenic mice expressing human FcγRIIIa (74), FcεRIα (75) or FcRn (76).

## 4. Notes

1. Apoptosis can be also assessed by a caspase 3 or caspase 7 assays (77).
2. Either the mice need to be syngeneic to the target cells to avoid rejections or immunodeficient mice need to be used.
3. The tumor size limit in mice is usually defined by the Institutional Animal Care and Use Committee.

### References


1. Carter PJ (2006) Potent antibody therapeutics by design. Nat Rev Immunol 6:343–357
2. Law M, Hangartner L (2008) Antibodies against viruses: passive and active immunization. Curr Opin Immunol 20:486–492
3. Wiezorek J, Holland P, Graves J (2010) Death receptor agonists as a targeted therapy for cancer. Clin Cancer Res 16:1701–1708
4. Ghetie V, Ward ES (2000) Multiple roles for the major histocompatibility complex class I-related receptor FcRn. Annu Rev Immunol 18:739–766
5. Cartron G, Dacheux L, Salles G et al (2002) Therapeutic activity of humanized anti-CD20 monoclonal antibody and polymorphism in IgG Fc receptor FcgammaRIIIa gene. Blood 99:754–758
6. Azuma Y, Ishikawa Y, Kawai S et al (2007) Recombinant human hexamer-dominant IgM monoclonal antibody to ganglioside GM3 for treatment of melanoma. Clin Cancer Res 13:2745–2750
7. Dechant M, Beyer T, Schneider-Merck T et al (2007) Effector mechanisms of recombinant IgA antibodies against epidermal growth factor receptor. J Immunol 179:2936–2943
8. Bracher M, Gould HJ, Sutton BJ et al (2007) Three-colour flow cytometric method to measure antibody-dependent tumour cell killing by cytotoxicity and phagocytosis. J Immunol Methods 323:160–171
9. Maley DT, Simon P (1990) Cytotoxicity assays using cryopreserved target cells pre-labeled with the fluorescent marker europium. J Immunol Methods 134:61–70
10. Mostov KE (1994) Transepithelial transport of immunoglobulins. Annu Rev Immunol 12: 63–84
11. Bruggemann M, Williams GT, Bindon CI et al (1987) Comparison of the effector functions of human immunoglobulins using a matched set of chimeric antibodies. J Exp Med 166: 1351–1361
12. Mestecky J, Russell MW, Elson CO (1999) Intestinal IgA: novel views on its function in the defence of the largest mucosal surface. Gut 44:2–5
13. Kawakami T, Galli SJ (2002) Regulation of mast-cell and basophil function and survival by IgE. Nat Rev Immunol 2:773–786
14. Eliasson M, Olsson A, Palmcrantz E et al (1988) Chimeric IgG-binding receptors engineered from staphylococcal protein A and streptococcal protein G. J Biol Chem 263: 4323–4327
15. Sandin C, Linse S, Areschoug T et al (2002) Isolation and detection of human IgA using a streptococcal IgA-binding peptide. J Immunol 169:1357–1364
16. Nilson BH, Solomon A, Bjorck L et al (1992) Protein L from *Peptostreptococcus magnus* binds to the kappa light chain variable domain. J Biol Chem 267:2234–2239
17. Aalberse RC, van der Gaag R, van Leeuwen J (1983) Serologic aspects of IgG4 antibodies. I. Prolonged immunization results in an IgG4-restricted response. J Immunol 130:722–726
18. Venaille TJ, Misso NL, Phillips MJ et al (1994) Effects of different density gradient separation techniques on neutrophil function. Scand J Clin Lab Invest 54:385–391
19. Bender AT, Ostenson CL, Giordano D et al (2004) Differentiation of human monocytes in vitro with granulocyte-macrophage colony-stimulating factor and macrophage colony-stimulating factor produces distinct changes in cGMP phosphodiesterase expression. Cell Signal 16:365–374
20. Sunada H, Magun BE, Mendelsohn J et al (1986) Monoclonal antibody against epidermal growth factor receptor is internalized without stimulating receptor phosphorylation. Proc Natl Acad Sci USA 83:3825–3829

21. Li S, Schmitz KR, Jeffrey PD et al (2005) Structural basis for inhibition of the epidermal growth factor receptor by cetuximab. Cancer Cell 7:301–311
22. Lohse S, Derer S, Beyer T et al (2011) Recombinant dimeric IgA antibodies against the epidermal growth factor receptor mediate effective tumor cell killing. J Immunol 186: 3770–3778
23. Falschlehner C, Ganten TM, Koschny R et al (2009) TRAIL and other TRAIL receptor agonists as novel cancer therapeutics. Adv Exp Med Biol 647:195–206
24. Shan D, Ledbetter JA, Press OW (1998) Apoptosis of malignant human B cells by ligation of CD20 with monoclonal antibodies. Blood 91:1644–1652
25. Guo Y, Chen C, Zheng Y et al (2005) A novel anti-human DR5 monoclonal antibody with tumoricidal activity induces caspase-dependent and caspase-independent cell death. J Biol Chem 280:41940–41952
26. Rose AL, Smith BE, Maloney DG (2002) Glucocorticoids and rituximab in vitro: synergistic direct antiproliferative and apoptotic effects. Blood 100:1765–1773
27. Shan D, Ledbetter JA, Press OW (2000) Signaling events involved in anti-CD20-induced apoptosis of malignant human B cells. Cancer Immunol Immunother 48:673–683
28. Ghetie MA, Bright H, Vitetta ES (2001) Homodimers but not monomers of Rituxan (chimeric anti-CD20) induce apoptosis in human B-lymphoma cells and synergize with a chemotherapeutic agent and an immunotoxin. Blood 97:1392–1398
29. Lazar GA, Dang W, Karki S et al (2006) Engineered antibody Fc variants with enhanced effector function. Proc Natl Acad Sci USA 103:4005–4010
30. Zhao X, Singh S, Pardoux C et al (2009) Targeting C-type lectin-like molecule-1 for antibody-mediated immunotherapy in acute myeloid leukemia. Haematologica 95:71–78
31. Sepp A, Binns RM, Lechler RI (1996) Improved protocol for colorimetric detection of complement-mediated cytotoxicity based on the measurement of cytoplasmic lactate dehydrogenase activity. J Immunol Methods 196: 175–180
32. Blanquet-Grossard F, Thielens NM, Vendrely C et al (2005) Complement protein C1q recognizes a conformationally modified form of the prion protein. Biochemistry 44:4349–4356
33. Idusogie EE, Wong PY, Presta LG et al (2001) Engineered antibodies with increased activity to recruit complement. J Immunol 166: 2571–2575
34. Daha MR, Gorter A, Rits M et al (1989) Interaction of immunoglobulin A with complement and phagocytic cells. Prog Clin Biol Res 297:247–260, discussion 260–261
35. Chuang PD, Morrison SL (1997) Elimination of N-linked glycosylation sites from the human IgA1 constant region: effects on structure and function. J Immunol 158:724–732
36. Roos A, Bouwman LH, van Gijlswijk-Janssen DJ et al (2001) Human IgA activates the complement system via the mannan-binding lectin pathway. J Immunol 167:2861–2868
37. Hiemstra PS, Gorter A, Stuurman ME et al (1987) Activation of the alternative pathway of complement by human serum IgA. Eur J Immunol 17:321–326
38. Pfaffenbach G, Lamm ME, Gigli I (1982) Activation of the guinea pig alternative complement pathway by mouse IgA immune complexes. J Exp Med 155:231–247
39. Pawluczkowycz AW, Beurskens FJ, Beum PV et al (2009) Binding of submaximal C1q promotes complement-dependent cytotoxicity (CDC) of B cells opsonized with anti-CD20 mAbs ofatumumab (OFA) or rituximab (RTX): considerably higher levels of CDC are induced by OFA than by RTX. J Immunol 183: 749–758
40. Beum PV, Lindorfer MA, Hall BE et al (2006) Quantitative analysis of protein co-localization on B cells opsonized with rituximab and complement using the ImageStream multispectral imaging flow cytometer. J Immunol Methods 317:90–99
41. Karagiannis SN, Wang Q, East N et al (2003) Activity of human monocytes in IgE antibody-dependent surveillance and killing of ovarian tumor cells. Eur J Immunol 33:1030–1040
42. Wang Y, Fei D, Vanderlaan M et al (2004) Biological activity of bevacizumab, a humanized anti-VEGF antibody in vitro. Angiogenesis 7:335–345
43. Tai YT, Li X, Tong X et al (2005) Human anti-CD40 antagonist antibody triggers significant antitumor activity against human multiple myeloma. Cancer Res 65:5898–5906
44. Gomez-Roman VR, Florese RH, Patterson LJ et al (2006) A simplified method for the rapid fluorometric assessment of antibody-dependent cell-mediated cytotoxicity. J Immunol Methods 308:53–67
45. Kolber MA, Quinones RR, Gress RE et al (1988) Measurement of cytotoxicity by target cell release and retention of the fluorescent dye bis-carboxyethyl-carboxyfluorescein (BCECF). J Immunol Methods 108:255–264
46. Whiteside TL, Bryant J, Day R et al (1990) Natural killer cytotoxicity in the diagnosis of

immune dysfunction: criteria for a reproducible assay. J Clin Lab Anal 4:102–114

47. Blomberg K, Granberg C, Hemmila I et al (1986) Europium-labelled target cells in an assay of natural killer cell activity. I. A novel non-radioactive method based on time-resolved fluorescence. J Immunol Methods 86:225–229
48. Blomberg K, Granberg C, Hemmila I et al (1986) Europium-labelled target cells in an assay of natural killer cell activity. II. A novel non-radioactive method based on time-resolved fluorescence. Significance and specificity of the method. J Immunol Methods 92:117–123
49. Hemmila I, Dakubu S, Mukkala VM et al (1984) Europium as a label in time-resolved immunofluorometric assays. Anal Biochem 137:335–343
50. von Zons P, Crowley-Nowick P, Friberg D et al (1997) Comparison of europium and chromium release assays: cytotoxicity in healthy individuals and patients with cervical carcinoma. Clin Diagn Lab Immunol 4:202–207
51. Wallace PK, Kaufman PA, Lewis LD et al (2001) Bispecific antibody-targeted phagocytosis of HER-2/neu expressing tumor cells by myeloid cells activated in vivo. J Immunol Methods 248:167–182
52. Guyre CA, Gomes D, Smith KA et al (2008) Development of an in vivo antibody-mediated killing (IVAK) model, a flow cytometric method to rapidly evaluate therapeutic antibodies. J Immunol Methods 333:51–60
53. Di Gaetano N, Cittera E, Nota R et al (2003) Complement activation determines the therapeutic activity of rituximab in vivo. J Immunol 171:1581–1587
54. Rygaard J, Povlsen CO (1969) Heterotransplantation of a human malignant tumour to "Nude" mice. Acta Pathol Microbiol Scand 77:758–760
55. Reddy S, Piccione D, Takita H et al (1987) Human lung tumor growth established in the lung and subcutaneous tissue of mice with severe combined immunodeficiency. Cancer Res 47:2456–2460
56. Shinkai Y, Rathbun G, Lam KP et al (1992) RAG-2-deficient mice lack mature lymphocytes owing to inability to initiate V(D)J rearrangement. Cell 68:855–867
57. Mombaerts P, Iacomini J, Johnson RS et al (1992) RAG-1-deficient mice have no mature B and T lymphocytes. Cell 68:869–877
58. Prochazka M, Gaskins HR, Shultz LD et al (1992) The nonobese diabetic scid mouse: model for spontaneous thymomagenesis associated with immunodeficiency. Proc Natl Acad Sci USA 89:3290–3294
59. Brehm MA, Bortell R, Diiorio P et al (2010) Human immune system development and rejection of human islet allografts in spontaneously diabetic NOD-Rag1null IL2rgammanull Ins2Akita mice. Diabetes 59:2265–2270
60. Colucci F, Soudais C, Rosmaraki E et al (1999) Dissecting NK cell development using a novel alymphoid mouse model: investigating the role of the c-abl proto-oncogene in murine NK cell differentiation. J Immunol 162:2761–2765
61. Ito M, Hiramatsu H, Kobayashi K et al (2002) NOD/SCID/gamma(c)(null) mouse: an excellent recipient mouse model for engraftment of human cells. Blood 100:3175–3182
62. Shultz LD, Lyons BL, Burzenski LM et al (2005) Human lymphoid and myeloid cell development in NOD/LtSz-scid IL2R gamma null mice engrafted with mobilized human hemopoietic stem cells. J Immunol 174: 6477–6489
63. Pearson T, Shultz LD, Miller D et al (2008) Non-obese diabetic-recombination activating gene-1 (NOD-Rag1 null) interleukin (IL)-2 receptor common gamma chain (IL2r gamma null) null mice: a radioresistant model for human lymphohaematopoietic engraftment. Clin Exp Immunol 154:270–284
64. Suemizu H, Monnai M, Ohnishi Y et al (2007) Identification of a key molecular regulator of liver metastasis in human pancreatic carcinoma using a novel quantitative model of metastasis in NOD/SCID/gammacnull (NOG) mice. Int J Oncol 31:741–751
65. Le Devedec SE, van Roosmalen W, Maria N et al (2009) An improved model to study tumor cell autonomous metastasis programs using MTLn3 cells and the Rag2(−/−) gammac (−/−) mouse. Clin Exp Metastasis 26: 673–684
66. Bertilaccio MT, Scielzo C, Simonetti G et al (2010) A novel Rag2-/-gammac-/−xenograft model of human CLL. Blood 115:1605–1609
67. Nakanishi T, Chumsri S, Khakpour N et al (2010) Side-population cells in luminal-type breast cancer have tumour-initiating cell properties, and are regulated by HER2 expression and signalling. Br J Cancer 102:815–826
68. Nijmeijer BA, van Schie ML, Halkes CJ et al (2010) A mechanistic rationale for combining alemtuzumab and rituximab in the treatment of ALL. Blood 116:5930–5940
69. Gambhir SS (2002) Molecular imaging of cancer with positron emission tomography. Nat Rev Cancer 2:683–693
70. McLarty K, Fasih A, Scollard DA et al (2009) 18F-FDG small-animal PET/CT differentiates trastuzumab-responsive from unresponsive

human breast cancer xenografts in athymic mice. J Nucl Med 50:1848–1856

71. Palazon A, Teijeira A, Martinez-Forero I et al (2011) Agonist anti-CD137 mAb act on tumor endothelial cells to enhance recruitment of activated T lymphocytes. Cancer Res 71: 801–811
72. Bergman I, Basse PH, Barmada MA et al (2000) Comparison of in vitro antibody-targeted cytotoxicity using mouse, rat and human effectors. Cancer Immunol Immunother 49:259–266
73. Niwa R, Shoji-Hosaka E, Sakurada M et al (2004) Defucosylated chimeric anti-CC chemokine receptor 4 IgG1 with enhanced antibody-dependent cellular cytotoxicity shows potent therapeutic activity to T-cell leukemia and lymphoma. Cancer Res 64:2127–2133
74. Stavenhagen JB, Gorlatov S, Tuaillon N et al (2007) Fc optimization of therapeutic antibodies enhances their ability to kill tumor cells in vitro and controls tumor expansion in vivo via low-affinity activating Fcgamma receptors. Cancer Res 67:8882–8890
75. Nigro EA, Brini AT, Soprana E et al (2009) Antitumor IgE adjuvanticity: key role of Fc epsilon RI. J Immunol 183:4530–4536
76. Zalevsky J, Chamberlain AK, Horton HM et al (2010) Enhanced antibody half-life improves in vivo activity. Nat Biotechnol 28:157–159
77. Pathan NI, Chu P, Hariharan K et al (2008) Mediation of apoptosis by and antitumor activity of lumiliximab in chronic lymphocytic leukemia cells and CD23+ lymphoma cell lines. Blood 111:1594–1602

# Index

## A



## B




Gabriele Proetzel and Hilmar Ebersbach (eds.), *Antibody Methods and Protocols*, Methods in Molecular Biology, vol. 901, DOI 10.1007/978-1-61779-931-0, © Springer Science+Business Media, LLC 2012

## C



## D



## E

## M



## N



## O



## P



## Q

## R



## S



## T

## U



## V



## W



## Y



## Z

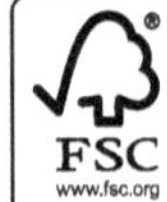


MIX
Papier aus verantwortungsvollen Quellen
Paper from responsible sources
FSC® C105338

If you have any concerns about our products,
you can contact us on
**ProductSafety@springernature.com**

In case Publisher is established outside the EU,
the EU authorized representative is:
**Springer Nature Customer Service Center GmbH**
**Europaplatz 3, 69115 Heidelberg, Germany**

Printed by Libri Plureos GmbH
in Hamburg, Germany